Families in the Intensive Care Unit

AF694407

Ashlee J. Vance • Deena Kelly Costa
Giora Netzer
Editors

Families in the Intensive Care Unit

A Guide to Understanding, Engaging, and Supporting at the Bedside

Second Edition

Springer

Editors
Ashlee J. Vance
Health Policy and Health Services
Henry Ford Health System
Detroit, MI, USA

Deena Kelly Costa
School of Nursing
Yale University
New Haven, CT, USA

Giora Netzer
University of Maryland Medical System
Baltimore, MD, USA

ISBN 978-3-031-83788-3 ISBN 978-3-031-83786-9 (eBook)
https://doi.org/10.1007/978-3-031-83786-9

© The Editor(s) (if applicable) and The Author(s), under exclusive license to Springer Nature Switzerland AG 2018, 2025

This work is subject to copyright. All rights are solely and exclusively licensed by the Publisher, whether the whole or part of the material is concerned, specifically the rights of translation, reprinting, reuse of illustrations, recitation, broadcasting, reproduction on microfilms or in any other physical way, and transmission or information storage and retrieval, electronic adaptation, computer software, or by similar or dissimilar methodology now known or hereafter developed.
The use of general descriptive names, registered names, trademarks, service marks, etc. in this publication does not imply, even in the absence of a specific statement, that such names are exempt from the relevant protective laws and regulations and therefore free for general use.
The publisher, the authors and the editors are safe to assume that the advice and information in this book are believed to be true and accurate at the date of publication. Neither the publisher nor the authors or the editors give a warranty, expressed or implied, with respect to the material contained herein or for any errors or omissions that may have been made. The publisher remains neutral with regard to jurisdictional claims in published maps and institutional affiliations.

This Springer imprint is published by the registered company Springer Nature Switzerland AG
The registered company address is: Gewerbestrasse 11, 6330 Cham, Switzerland

If disposing of this product, please recycle the paper.

To our families, the very essence of it all.

Foreword

Excellent, individualized care of the contemporary critically ill patient is impossible without active involvement of their families, who advocate and assist in directing care. We simply face too many decisions that are preference sensitive, too many high-tech test results that require the context of detailed history, and too often therapeutic choices about how invasive to be—or when to stop—that must be guided by a nuanced understanding of individual values which the patients are often too sick to provide themselves. And all of this is before considering the instrumental role of these family members, who are also highly effective at reducing delirium, relieving anxiety, and encouraging physical therapy.

And yet, in the contemporary ICU, care partners find themselves in foreign environs, bombarded by unfamiliar terminology and asked to make high-stakes decisions that they may face only once or twice in a lifetime [1]. The problem is pervasive with over 60% of care partners experiencing symptoms of burnout [2]. Families are often unable to participate emotionally and cognitively because of unmet basic needs [3]. A high percentage of these care partners experience learned helplessness [4].

Supporting such overwhelmed and distracted family members is a source of burnout and overwork for clinicians who are extraordinarily skilled at saving lives in the ICU but may have no expertise in helping care partners find a place to sleep. Even worse, providing care by default or from clinical inertia to patients, when those clinicians fear that the patient may not actually want, is a tremendous driver of burnout.

Frontline critical care teams, patients, and families around the world are slowly admitting this reality. Even in 2024, what we heard were recurrent stories of clinicians working to make sure that families' logistical and emotional needs were met. Care partners vocalized that the little emotional and intellectual reserve they have in these moments cannot be wasted. Yet, every day, lack of forethought and design brought distractions and frustrations like parking or difficulties to acquire food, because they cannot leave their loved one's side to feed the parking meter or wait in a 15-min line for sustenance.

We, like you, dear reader, are trying to fix that.

Fundamentally, we have come to believe that hospitals should invest in innovative and sustainable solutions to close these gaps, both the strains of supporting critical care for loved ones and trying to care for selves. As we work to build the model that will work for our particular institutions, we have found the wisdom in this book invaluable. Here are leaders from around the world, grappling with theory and data and practice and operational constraints. There are no easy answers, particularly in a world that imagines ICUs primarily as a cost- rather than a lifesaving service. But some things are clear.

We can do better. We can learn from each other. And it is the right thing to do. We look forward to trying and learning and sharing and trying other things and learning more and working—together, always together—to do better for our patients, their loved ones, and our care teams. This is the way.

References

1. Azoulay E, Pochard F, Kentish-Barnes N, et al. FAMIREA Study Group Risk of post-traumatic stress symptoms in family members of intensive care unit patients. Am J Respir Crit Care Med. 2005;171(9):987-994.
2. Ybema, Jan F., et al. Caregiver burnout among intimate partners of patients with a severe illness: an equity perspective. Pers Relatsh. 2002;9(1):73–88.
3. Verceles AC, Corwin DS, Afshar M, Friedman EB, McCurdy MT, Shanholtz C, Oakjones K, Zubrow MT, Titus J, Netzer G. Half of the family members of critically ill patients experience excessive daytime sleepiness. Intensive Care Med. 2014;40(8):1124–31. https://doi.org/10.1007/s00134-014-3347-z. Epub 2014 Jun 5. PMID: 24898893; PMCID: PMC4500523.
4. https://www.ncbi.nlm.nih.gov/pmc/articles/PMC3515025/.

Department of Health Policy and Management
Johns Hopkins Bloomberg School of Public Health
Johns Hopkins University
Baltimore, MD, USA

Jack Iwashyna

Preface

Being at the bedside as a family member—not as a clinician—was the transforming experience that led to this book's first edition. In healthcare, we use terms like "patient centered" but often overlook that family is integral to personhood. A recent study found that Americans view time with their family as the most important thing in their lives [1], and yet, we often overlook families or, worse, limit their presence and roles at their loved ones' sides. More so, the key role families play in our patients' long-term trajectories is disregarded, as is their suffering as human beings.

This second edition seeks to help us better understand how best to partner with families to provide better care and how we can support fellow human beings watching the suffering of those they love. Emerging from the maelstrom of the COVID pandemic, this is more urgent than ever.

Furthermore, this second edition incorporates lessons learned from the COVID pandemic that can help us be more equipped to navigate future public health crises that do not sideline the most important people in a patient's life: so that no pregnant person ever labors and delivers a baby alone, no parent is restricted from being with their infant or child while hospitalized, or no one ever dies alone.

Reference

1. Cerda A. Family time is far more important than other aspects of life for most Americans. Pew Research Center. Accessed August 22, 2024. https://www.pewresearch.org/short-reads/2023/05/26/family-time-is-far-more-important-than-other-aspects-of-life-for-most-americans/.

Detroit, MI, USA — Ashlee J. Vance
New Haven, CT, USA — Deena Kelly Costa
Baltimore, MD, USA — Giora Netzer

Acknowledgments

Families are at the heart of everything I do both personally and professionally. The desire to be involved in this work comes from a deep appreciation and gratitude to my own family who has supported me throughout my life and career journey. To my parents, who gave me space to blossom and showed up every time I needed help moving! To my siblings, who continually amaze and surprise me with their own paths and adventures. To my spouse, Travis, thank you for a beautiful life and believing in my dreams as much as I do.

Many thanks to the excellent mentors who have supported me throughout my professional journey, notably, Jackie McGrath, Debra Brandon, Kathleen Knafl, Deena Costa, Jack Iwashyna, and Nicole McDonald. Thank you for investing in my growth and your generosity of wisdom. I would not be where I am today without your immense guidance and valuable advice. I also extend my thanks to my work colleagues and Director, Brian Ahmedani, of the Center for Health Policy and Health Services Research at Henry Ford Health. I am grateful for your leadership and independence to pursue meaningful projects, such as this. I am so fortunate to work in a system where our ideas are valued and supported. With Grace—Ashlee Vance.

The work that I do has always been about people—the teams that care for patients, the families that support those patients, and the colleagues that I have the privilege to work alongside. Many thanks to all of you—mentors, friends, colleagues, patients, teams, and co-editors, Ashlee Vance and Giora Netzer—who make the work easy and so very fulfilling. And particular thanks to Guy, his family, and the SICU nurses—my interest in supporting families and teams is a direct result of our time together. To my parents: thank you for nurturing my endless curiosity with compassion and kindness. To my sisters: thank you for inspiring me to be a good person, good mom, and good sister. To my husband, Anthony: thank you for supporting me, loving me, and encouraging me, *always*. To our boys, Douglas and August: always know that we love you, adore you, and cannot wait to see how you will make this world a better place.—Deena Costa.

This book, and my life, reflects the gifts given by the family that raised me, the family that sustains and grows me, my teachers and mentors, and my patients who have taught me some of my most profound lessons. My mentors, thank you: Thomas

Shaffer, Marla Wolfson, Gregory Tino, John Hansen-Flaschen, Jason Christie (whose teaching and guidance were and are pivotal), Jack Iwashyna (who always makes me better), John Hess, Dale Needham, Anthony Harris, Michael Terrin, Chuck Callahan, Ken Wood, and Judy Davidson. A special thank you to Lisa Rowen, for taking me under her wing, bestowing her wisdom, and teaching about leadership and organizational change. I am grateful to colleagues and leaders at the University of Maryland Medical System, which has supported the family-centric mission. The Society of Critical Care Medicine and the American College of Chest Physicians have helped advance the awareness and support of families through guidelines, scholarship, and education. We appreciate Springer Press for their publication of the first edition of Families in the ICU and thank them for the opportunity to update and expand this body of work with the second edition. I am indebted to my co-editors, Ashlee and Deena, for their vision and brilliance for creating a work that provides so many insights and tools to advance our work with families.

Thank you, Ima and Abba, for imprinting on me the sanctity of family and to my sister and her family for lessons learned. My family is the center of everything. Alison, you made it all possible, all of it. Hannah, David, and Jacob, you are the greatest gift of all.—Giora Netzer

Contents

Chapter 1
Introduction to the Second Edition

Ashlee J. Vance, Deena Kelly Costa, and Giora Netzer

Defining Family

Throughout this book, the term "family" is defined and used. The definition for family is that used by the Society of Critical Care Medicine's original guidelines on family-centered care [1]:

> Family is defined by the patient or, in the case of minors or those without decision-making capacity, by their surrogates. In this context, the family may be related or unrelated to the patient. They are individuals who provide support and with whom the patient has a significant relationship.

Families' Lived Experience in the ICU

Broadly, families living the nightmare of their loved one being close to death are barraged with high intensity emotions. They are stressed, anxious, and depressed [2, 3]. Many have post-traumatic stress disorder (PTSD) before even leaving the intensive care unit (ICU) [4]. Sleep deprivation further torments them [5]. Unable to process these insults, they may turn to maladaptive coping, further exacerbating their suffering [6]. Thinking about the possible death of their loved one further deteriorates their social problem-solving skills [7]. Presented with data, they suffer the

A. J. Vance (✉)
Henry Ford Health, Detroit, MI, USA
e-mail: avance2@hfhs.org

D. K. Costa
Yale School of Nursing, New Haven, CT, USA

G. Netzer
University of Maryland Medical System, Baltimore, MD, USA

© The Author(s), under exclusive license to Springer Nature Switzerland AG 2025

A. J. Vance et al. (eds.), *Families in the Intensive Care Unit*,
https://doi.org/10.1007/978-3-031-83786-9_1

same biases we all do in daily life but now with greater consequences [8, 9]. As they gather, families grapple with the agonizing process of having to speak for their loved one in a unified voice, despite often being wracked by disagreement [10].

Notwithstanding the description above, intuitively, it is easy to imagine why sick patients, particularly those critically ill, might want loved ones at their bedside. Such face validity is even better appreciated in patients without autonomy or the ability to convey needs (as described in Chaps. 16 and 17 on pediatric and neonatal patients) or for those with impaired decision-making capacity caused by brain injury, impaired consciousness or some other neurologic condition (Chap. 13). Perhaps unsurprisingly then, a plethora of data demonstrates that the presence of families, loved ones and/or caregivers offers patients substantial benefit. Patients without families or loved ones at the bedside have been shown to have increased delirium, increased safety events (falls, healthcare-acquired infections and healthcare-acquired pressure injury) and more difficulties with discharge planning. Family members at the bedside can participate in delirium monitoring, aid with activities of daily living and engage more fully in care, especially for neonatal and pediatric patients. Importantly, family members also play a vital emotional support role for critically ill patients.

Creating Partnership with Families

It's said that more than the calf wants to suckle, the cow wants to nurse [11]. A parent's instinct is to give. Families have a natural instinct to protect those they love [12]. They ask us what they can do to help [13]. By communicating with and caring for families, valuing their presence, and engaging them in bedside activities, we help them to make sense of the situation and their new role [14].

Family Engagement Improves Patient Outcomes

In short, putting families to work helps our patients while simultaneously bringing meaning and coping to the families themselves. Numerous studies have documented the increased stress, presence of post-traumatic stress disorder and post-intensive care syndrome (PICS-F) for family members of a patient that is cared for in the ICU. Understanding how best to support families and patients together is integral to high-quality ICU care. For example:

- Families can increase rates of early mobilization, reducing the length of mechanical ventilation and ICU length of stay [15, 16]
- Liberalizing family presence at the bedside reduces ICU delirium [17]
- With families joining bedside rounds, ICU throughput improves [18]

- When parents participate in care in the neonatal ICU, their infants gain more weight and are more likely to breastfeed at discharge [19]
- Families participating in care have reduced anxiety levels [20]
- Families can keep an ICU diary, reducing their loved one's PTSD symptoms [21]
- Families are far more effective at detecting errors and adverse events than hospital safety systems [22]

We Need Families for the Health of ICU Survivors and of Our Community as a Whole

Survivorship is one of the defining challenges of critical care in the twenty-first century [23]. A large proportion of ICU survivors require family caregiving for the activities of daily living [24, 25]. Moreover, families are key determinants in whether the physical limitations incurred during critical illness result in disability [26]. In one example, the support provided by families, both instrumental and emotional, is significantly associated with the degree of recovery after stroke [27]. In the United States (conservatively), 200,000 older survivors are our neighbors [28], not even counting younger survivors. Given the role that families play in caring for our ICU patients after discharge, and modifying their post-ICU trajectories; as ICU clinicians, we must recognize that caring for families in the ICU is caring for the community itself [29].

Family Engagement Is Good for Us as a Healthcare Team

Families also provide benefits to ICU clinicians. Data suggests that one crucial role families serve for clinicians is the sharing of information about the patient [30]. Such information for noncommunicative patients would be unavailable to ICU clinicians and as described in Chap. 2 (Family Voices), families and clinicians recognize the importance of such information to patient care. Clinicians are also suffering—high rates of burnout and moral distress abound—and connecting with a loving family can support clinician's well-being. While we embrace the ICU for its energy and excitement, burnout is a significant problem among ICU providers [31]. When families are unsupported, conflict is more likely; that conflict, in turn, further increases burnout risk [32, 33]. As Joe Bienvenu points out [34], an intervention of targeted communication with families reduces staffing burnout as well [35]. In this sense, engaging families may benefit us as much as it does our patients and their loved ones. However, family presence in the ICU can have important implications. As described in Chap. 5 (Conflicts and the Family), conflict between the family and the patient or the family and the ICU team is not rare. Understanding how to navigate such conflict to ensure each and every patient receives the best care possible, with the most support from loved ones, can be a difficult needle to thread for many ICUs that are working with less staff, more and sicker patients than ever before.

Lessons Learned from the COVID-19 Pandemic

The COVID-19 pandemic reshaped how we think about public health; it exposed flaws in healthcare systems, particularly in the U.S.A. It also transformed the dynamic between healthcare providers, patients, and families in ways few anticipated. For years, healthcare providers made great strides in welcoming and valuing family involvement, recognizing the importance of their presence and perspective. Yet, almost overnight, pandemic-driven policies sidelined that progress. Restrictive visitor polices left families disconnected from loved ones, intensifying emotional strain and depriving patients of vital support [36–39]. One of the pandemic's lasting challenges is balancing public health safety with the undeniable value of family presence. For ICU patients, whose care often involves family members, this balance is crucial. It is essential that we restore the pre-pandemic focus on caregiver involvement as a key element of hospital care. Evidence consistently shows the benefits of family involvement, from improving patient outcomes to enhancing family or parental well-being and confidence.

To reshape family engagement in the ICU, we must integrate lessons learned from the pandemic into everyday practice. This starts with creating flexible, yet resilient, visitor policies that prioritize family involvement while adapting to varying public health conditions. Technology, which played a crucial role during the pandemic, should remain central to this effort. Virtual visits, for instance, allowed families to connect with patients when physical presence wasn't possible, and this can be expanded to supplement in-person visits, especially in restricted settings. Additionally, healthcare teams must actively include family members in decision-making processes, ensuring their voices are heard in the care plan. Training staff to facilitate better communication with families—both in person and through virtual means—will create a more inclusive, supportive ICU environment. See Chaps. 4, 7, and 9 to guide these efforts.

Looking forward, these strategies can also help us prepare for the next public health crisis. A key takeaway from the COVID-19 pandemic is that emergency protocols should not undermine patient care or the emotional well-being of families. As we develop future pandemic response plans, we must build systems that preserve family presence and engagement without compromising safety. Clear, adaptable policies can prevent the chaotic shifts seen during COVID-19 and ensure that families remain part of the care team, even in times of crisis. By embedding family-centered care into emergency preparedness, we can create a more compassionate, flexible healthcare system ready to navigate future challenges.

In sum, as you explore the following chapters, you will see a recurring theme: the need to realign healthcare policies with family-centered and family-affirming care. Use the information provided to assist you and your teams' efforts to transform and improve the quality of critical care. By acknowledging the vital role families play in critical care—whether for neonatal, pediatric, or adult patients—as the foundation of any effort to provide high-quality, compassionate care, we can enhance patient outcomes and caregiver well-being and strengthen our preparedness for future public health crisis.

References

1. Davidson JE, Aslakson RA, Long AC, et al. Guidelines for family-centered care in the neonatal, pediatric, and adult ICU. Crit Care Med. 2017;45(1):103.
2. Choi J, Sherwood PR, Schulz R, et al. Patterns of depressive symptoms in caregivers of mechanically ventilated critically ill adults from intensive care unit admission to 2 months postintensive care unit discharge: a pilot study. Crit Care Med. 2012;40(5):1546–53. https://doi.org/10.1097/CCM.0b013e3182451c58.
3. Pochard F, Darmon M, Fassier T, et al. Symptoms of anxiety and depression in family members of intensive care unit patients before discharge or death. A prospective multicenter study. J Crit Care. 2005;20(1):90–6.
4. Paparrigopoulos T, Melissaki A, Efthymiou A, et al. Short-term psychological impact on family members of intensive care unit patients. J Psychosom Res. 2006;61(5):719–22. https://doi.org/10.1016/j.jpsychores.2006.05.013.
5. Verceles AC, Corwin DS, Afshar M, et al. Half of the family members of critically ill patients experience excessive daytime sleepiness. Intensive Care Med. 2014;40(8):1124–31. https://doi.org/10.1007/s00134-014-3347-z.
6. Sullivan DR, Liu X, Corwin DS, et al. Learned helplessness among families and surrogate decision-makers of patients admitted to medical, surgical, and trauma ICUs. Chest. 2012;142(6):1440–6. https://doi.org/10.1378/chest.12-0112.
7. Glick DR, Motta M, Wiegand DL, Range P, Reed RM, Verceles AC, Shah NG, Netzer G. Exploratory study of anticipatory grief among surrogate decision makers of patients admitted to medical, surgical, and trauma intensive care units. Am J Respir Crit Care Med. 2017;195:A7101.
8. Leiter N, Motta M, Reed RM, et al. Numeracy and interpretation of prognostic estimates in intracerebral hemorrhage among surrogate decision makers in the neurologic ICU. Crit Care Med. 2018;46(2):264–71. https://doi.org/10.1097/CCM.0000000000002887.
9. Zier LS, Sottile PD, Hong SY, Weissfield LA, White DB. Surrogate decision makers' interpretation of prognostic information: a mixed-methods study. Ann Intern Med. 2012;156(5):360–6. https://doi.org/10.7326/0003-4819-156-5-201203060-00008.
10. Schenker Y, Crowley-Matoka M, Dohan D, Tiver GA, Arnold RM, White DB. I don't want to be the one saying 'we should just let him die': intrapersonal tensions experienced by surrogate decision makers in the ICU. J Gen Intern Med. 2012;27(12):1657–65. https://doi.org/10.1007/s11606-012-2129-y.
11. Bavli T. Schottenstein Edition. 1st ed Pesachim Volume 3. ArtScroll Mesorah Publications; 1998.
12. McAdam JL, Arai S, Puntillo KA. Unrecognized contributions of families in the intensive care unit. Intensive Care Med. 2008;34(6):1097–101. https://doi.org/10.1007/s00134-008-1066-z.
13. Zimmerman BA. A piece of my mind. Patient's sister, seeking job. JAMA. 2013;309(19):2003–4. https://doi.org/10.1001/jama.2013.2864.
14. Davidson JE, Zisook S. Implementing family-centered care through facilitated sensemaking. AACN Adv Crit Care. 2017;28(2):200–9. https://doi.org/10.4037/aacnacc2017102.

15. Rukstele CD, Gagnon MM. Making strides in preventing ICU-acquired weakness: involving family in early progressive mobility. Crit Care Nurs Q. 2013;36(1):141–7. https://doi.org/10.1097/CNQ.0b013e31827539cc.
16. Lai CC, Chou W, Chan KS, et al. Early mobilization reduces duration of mechanical ventilation and intensive care unit stay in patients with acute respiratory failure. Arch Phys Med Rehabil. 2017;98(5):931–9. https://doi.org/10.1016/j.apmr.2016.11.007.
17. Rosa RG, Tonietto TF, da Silva DB, et al. Effectiveness and safety of an extended ICU visitation model for delirium prevention: a before and after study. Crit Care Med. 2017;45:1660. https://doi.org/10.1097/CCM.0000000000002588.
18. Muething SE, Kotagal UR, Schoettker PJ, Gonzalez del Rey J, DeWitt TG. Family-centered bedside rounds: a new approach to patient care and teaching. Pediatrics. 2007;119(4):829–32. https://doi.org/10.1542/peds.2006-2528.
19. O'Brien K, Robson K, Bracht M, Cruz M, Lui K, Alvaro R, da Silva O, Monterrosa L, Narvey M, Ng E, Soraisham A, Ye XY, Mirea L, Tarnow-Mordi W, Lee SK, FICare Study Group, FICare Parent Advisory Board. Effectiveness of Family Integrated Care in neonatal intensive care units on infant and parent outcomes: a multicentre, multinational, cluster-randomised controllled trial. Lancet Child Adolesc Health. 2018;2(4):245–54.
20. Skoog M, Milner KA, Gatti-Petito J, Dintyala K. The impact of family engagement on anxiety levels in a cardiothoracic intensive care unit. Crit Care Nurse. 2016;36(2):84–9. https://doi.org/10.4037/ccn2016246.
21. Parker AM, Sricharoenchai T, Raparla S, Schneck KW, Bienvenu OJ, Needham DM. Posttraumatic stress disorder in critical illness survivors: a metaanalysis. Crit Care Med. 2015;43(5):1121–9. https://doi.org/10.1097/CCM.0000000000000882.
22. Khan A, Coffey M, Litterer KP, et al. Families as partners in hospital error and adverse event surveillance. JAMA Pediatr. 2017;171(4):372–81. https://doi.org/10.1001/jamapediatrics.2016.4812.
23. Iwashyna TJ. Survivorship will be the defining challenge of critical care in the 21st century. Ann Intern Med. 2010;153(3):204–5. https://doi.org/10.7326/0003-4819-153-3-201008030-00013.
24. Im K, Belle SH, Schulz R, Mendelsohn AB, Chelluri L, Investigators Q-M. Prevalence and outcomes of caregiving after prolonged (> or =48 hours) mechanical ventilation in the ICU. Chest. 2004;125(2):597–606.
25. Griffiths J, Hatch RA, Bishop J, et al. An exploration of social and economic outcome and associated health-related quality of life after critical illness in general intensive care unit survivors: a 12-month follow-up study. Crit Care. 2013;17(3):R100. https://doi.org/10.1186/cc12745.
26. Iwashyna TJ, Netzer G. The burdens of survivorship: an approach to thinking about long-term outcomes after critical illness. Semin Respir Crit Care Med. 2012;33(4):327–38. https://doi.org/10.1055/s-0032-1321982.
27. Tsouna-Hadjis E, Vemmos KN, Zakopoulos N, Stamatelopoulos S. First-stroke recovery process: the role of family social support. Arch Phys Med Rehabil. 2000;81(7):881–7. https://doi.org/10.1053/apmr.2000.4435.
28. Iwashyna TJ, Cooke CR, Wunsch H, Kahn JM. Population burden of long-term survivorship after severe sepsis in older Americans. J Am Geriatr Soc. 2012;60(6):1070–7. https://doi.org/10.1111/j.1532-5415.2012.03989.x.
29. Netzer G, Davidson JE. Creating patient- and family-focused care in the intensive care unit. In: Zimmerman DO-H, Osborn-Harrison DG, editors. Person-focused health care management. Springer; 2017.
30. Boltey EM, Wright N, Mosley EA, et al. Exploring the process of information sharing in an adult intensive care unit: an ethnographic study. J Interprof Care. 2022;36(2):168–76. https://doi.org/10.1080/13561820.2021.1899147.
31. Moss M, Good VS, Gozal D, Kleinpell R, Sessler CN. An official critical care societies collaborative statement: burnout syndrome in critical care health care professionals: a call for action. Am J Crit Care. 2016;25(4):368–76. https://doi.org/10.4037/ajcc2016133.

32. Embriaco N, Azoulay E, Barrau K, et al. High level of burnout in intensivists: prevalence and associated factors. Am J Respir Crit Care Med. 2007;175(7):686–92. https://doi.org/10.1164/rccm.200608-1184OC.
33. Burghi G, Lambert J, Chaize M, et al. Prevalence, risk factors and consequences of severe burnout syndrome in ICU. Intensive Care Med. 2014;40(11):1785–6. https://doi.org/10.1007/s00134-014-3454-x.
34. Bienvenu OJ. Is this critical care clinician burned out? Intensive Care Med. 2016;42(11):1794–6. https://doi.org/10.1007/s00134-016-4497-y.
35. Quenot JP, Rigaud JP, Prin S, et al. Suffering among carers working in critical care can be reduced by an intensive communication strategy on end-of-life practices. Intensive Care Med. 2012;38(1):55–61. https://doi.org/10.1007/s00134-011-2413-z.
36. Vance AJ, Malin KJ, Benjamin A, Shuman CJ, Moore TA, Costa DK. Pandemic visitor policies: parent reactions and policy implications. Acta Paediatr. 2022;111(3):604–6. https://doi.org/10.1111/apa.16208.
37. Vance AJ, Malin KJ, Miller J, Shuman CJ, Moore TA, Benjamin A. Parents' pandemic NICU experience in the United States: a qualitative study. BMC Pediatr. 2021;21(1):558. https://doi.org/10.1186/s12887-021-03028-w.
38. Andrist E, Clarke RG, Harding M. Paved with good intentions: hospital visitation restrictions in the age of coronavirus disease 2019. Pediatr Crit Care Med. 2020;21:e924. https://doi.org/10.1097/PCC.0000000000002506.
39. Baumbusch J, Lloyd JEV, Lamden-Bennett SR, Ou C. The unintended consequences of COVID-19 public health measures on healthcare for children with medical complexity. Child Care Health Dev. 2022;48:970. https://doi.org/10.1111/cch.12968.

Chapter 2
Voices from the Intensive Care Unit: Family and Clinician Perspectives

Nathan C. Wright, Ella Christoph, and Deena Kelly Costa

Introduction

Patients and their families are increasingly recognized as an integral part of the intensive care unit (ICU) team, particularly in adult ICUs [1]. From a patient-centered perspective, high-quality ICU patient care is supported through leveraging a patient's and/or family's knowledge of the patient's health, personality, and behaviors; keeping the family/patient informed about the patient's care via open communication; and including the patient and/or family in the decision-making process [2]. Oftentimes, many patients in the ICU are mechanically ventilated and therefore unable to speak and interact with clinicians on their own behalf [3]. In this context, family members' involvement and voices take on extra significance as part of the care team and as an advocate for the patient. However, not all family involvement supports a healing care environment for the patient, and not all clinicians take the same approach to including families in the care team [4]. In focused discussions, ICU patients and ICU clinicians illuminate how family members can best be involved to support their loved one, prefer to be involved in care, and impact both the patient's care directly and the clinicians delivering care.

N. C. Wright
Yale School of Nursing, West Haven, CT, USA

E. Christoph
Section of Pulmonary, Critical Care and Sleep Medicine, Yale School of Medicine, New Haven, CT, USA

D. K. Costa (✉)
Yale School of Nursing, West Haven, CT, USA

Section of Pulmonary, Critical Care and Sleep Medicine, Yale School of Medicine, New Haven, CT, USA
e-mail: deena.costa@yale.edu

© The Author(s), under exclusive license to Springer Nature Switzerland AG 2025
A. J. Vance et al. (eds.), *Families in the Intensive Care Unit*,
https://doi.org/10.1007/978-3-031-83786-9_2

In this chapter, families speak to their experiences in the ICU and the ways in which they interacted with and were included in patient care. Clinicians also share their perspectives about including family members in ICU care and how this affects the care they deliver in the ICU. The experiences and stories presented below are part of a larger, multi-ICU qualitative research study examining team dynamics as well as the patient/family member's role as part of the ICU team. Data were collected over May 2016–March 2021 in four ICUs in three health care systems (one academic health care system and two community hospitals); two medical ICUs, one mixed-medical surgical ICU, and a surgical ICU. From these ICUs, we conducted 63 h of observation, 23 shadowing experiences of ICU clinicians, and 30 semi-structured interviews (7 with family members of ICU patients and 23 with ICU clinicians) across the four ICUs.

In the following chapter, our goal was to use primary interview data from the above-described study to highlight family members' unique perspectives as much in their own words as we can. Family members of ICU patients are faced with the difficult and emotional task of navigating their loved one's care, a process that is influenced by many factors (e.g., health literacy, clinical/health professional experience, medical history, past experiences in the ICU) [5]. A better picture of family members as part of the ICU team emerged from these interviews. These interviews also offer insight into the unique benefits and challenges of family engagement in the ICU.

Family and Clinician Views on Family Engagement in the ICU

Positive Perspectives of Families Feeling Included, Supported, and Engaged Through Guidance and Communication

For family members, feeling included by clinicians in the patient's care was integral to feeling engaged and supported while in the ICU. Different families sought different levels of engagement and appreciated a variety of ways to be included. Families appreciated clinicians who provided clear and effective communication, offered information and guidance around decision-making, and attended to their family member's needs and well-being with care and support.

A daughter whose father was in the ICU discussed how she and her family were impacted by information about their loved one:

> *When he was in the [ICU], I was actually extremely impressed with how much I was included in just even the most basic things that they were doing. The nurse just would come in to change a bag out on the dialysis machine, and they'd be like, "Okay, well this is what we're going to do," and I'm like, "Okay, great." Everyone from the nurses to the respiratory therapist to all of the doctors…they got really used to seeing me, but every time I would see them, or even if I was in the hallway outside of the unit, they'd be like, "Okay, here's an update on your dad. This is what's going on." So they were really inclusive, which kind of surprised me…I kind of expected, you know, when they come in and do their checkups or*

whatever, that they would, you know, tell me what's going on or rounds…I'd be able to hear what's going on, but every time they saw me…I actually saw one of his doctors down in the cafeteria, and they [were] like, "Okay. Here's an update. This is what is going on," and I was like, "Okay, great." I can't say anything bad what those people were able to do during the time he was in that unit. (Site 1, family member 1)

…there were times that we'd sit down and we'd have… "Okay, this is…We need to discuss this." They were very willing to give the time. It wasn't like, "Okay, I have to…Let's run through this really quick." They were really good about giving the time and letting me ask all the questions that I needed to ask or if…you know, as it came towards the end…my brother wasn't there…he was at home dealing with our animals, and we had initially discussed, you know, that we were probably going to have to withdraw care for my father. I said, "Okay, great. I understand where you guys are coming from. I agree with this, but I'm not going to make any decisions until I talk to my brother, and he can't get here for another hour or so." They're like, "That's fine. When he gets here, let the nurse know so that we can all come back and have another meeting about it so that he feels completely included." So it wasn't just me. They were really willing to work with what we could make available. So even if we weren't there right then…it was okay, too. "Alright, we can do it all again, start from the complete beginning in an hour." So they were really inclusive. I guess 'inclusive' isn't the word I'm looking for, but willing to do everything multiple times just so that we felt like we had all the information, and everyone who would be included in the decision-making process had all the information. We never felt rushed to be like you have to do this right now, or you have to make a decision right now on this or whatever. So they were really good about it. (Site 1, family member 1)

I really don't think there were any times that I felt like I needed more information than they were giving me, or that they weren't telling me things, or I wasn't being included or whatever. They were always really good about letting me know or seeking me out for making decisions or anything…And I don't know if that's because I was there so often that it was just convenient for them to include me in things, or if that's just how they work, but for me I never felt like I needed more from them than what they were giving me. (Site 1, family member 1)

For other family members, inclusion required honesty from the clinicians about the state of the patient's health:

They always talk to me and let me know exactly what's going on and stuff, and they was always honest about the situation. So I appreciated that, even though I didn't like what they was saying, but I'd rather for them to tell me the truth than, you know…you know, getting hopes up for nothing, you know,…so that I could prepare for the worst if I had to. I ain't want the worst, but tell me the worst, but, you know, I'm trying to be strong and be realistic about things. (Site 1, family member 2)

Well, they haven't really talked to me much. But they do include me in all the, you know, what's going on or whatever. It's like I asked the doctor yesterday. "So give me just the straight facts. What do you think?" (LAUGHTER) "Is she dying? You know, just give it to me because I can handle it." You know, the truth for me, since I'm already trying to accept things…I just want to know the truth. That's it. So she did talk to me about that and stuff. So I'm like, "Alright. I've got that part, you know?" (LAUGHTER) But like they've always talked about what they want to do and what, and I just kind of say like, "Okay. As long as you guys think that this is the best thing for her, then I'm okay with that…but, again, it's going to be different family members too. So it's kind of a borderline like…Like I wouldn't want them to tell my mom or dad, you know what I mean? (LAUGHTER) But it's like I can handle the truth. (Site 2, family member 1)

> *Yeah, I understand. Like they can't do it all the time, I get it, but it would be like a life and death situation. "Do you really think she's going to be okay? Do you really think that she is going to pull through? What do you really think honestly as a doctor? If you've seen this stuff multiple times, what's the chances?" And I think that is important to me because like so I could have something positive to look forward to, you know, or negative and to get me prepared to whatever is…pulls ahead of me. It's that accepting and trying to have that grief to yourself that you can start to have that process, you know? And if it's something positive, you know, give me something for me to look forward to, you know? (Site 2, family member 1)*

Clinicians who communicated openly and shared information instilled confidence in families, helping them feel supported by the ICU team and capable of making difficult decisions, especially when it came to end-of-life and withdrawing care:

> *The team initiated the conversation because…he had this setback because he had gotten this other infection. So we had the conversation that this is now what's going on and that he has not made any real improvement in the time that he had been in the [ICU]. He had made like…He would make a small step forward, but then he'd, you know, have another setback. So he never made any significant improvement to getting better. He was basically the same, and as one of the attendings told me, staying the same isn't getting better; it's actually getting worse…and that kind of made sense to me as in, you know, if you're not gonna improve, staying in this situation isn't good for you either. So that made sense to me. So when he had this last setback, they had the conversation with me…and they were like, "This is what happens, this is what's going on, and he's already on the treatment for this situation."…Because they never actually found the source of the initial infection…So he was being treated with really broad-spectrum antibiotics and everything to try and cover everything. And they said, "Well, he's already being treated for this, and he's not responding to it, and he's getting worse. So it's time to think about what he would want going forward." And my brother and I's first question was, "is there another treatment for it?" So they brought in the Infectious Disease team to consult and see if there was a different medication that he should be on…Unfortunately, there wasn't. Then our next question was, "Okay. There is no other treatment he should be on…And he's not responding to the one that he should possibly be responding to. Is there a possibility that he could get better, and if he does get better, what is his quality of life going to be like at that point?" And they were very honest with us and said, "you know, honestly we don't think that he'll be able to get through this hurdle to get over this infection." Then they said, "But there's this small chance that he could, but if he does, he's most likely going to be in a bed for the rest of his life, on a ventilator for the rest of his life," and they were very honest about what his life would look like, and that was the decision…(tearful) the deciding factor for my brother and I to make the decision to withdraw care because our father wouldn't want to live like that…(Tearful) Even if he had got past it, but he wouldn't have wanted to live in a bed for the rest of his life on a ventilator. It had been hard enough on him when he was waiting for a transplant because he couldn't do everything that he normally would have done. It slowed him down a bit. So, not being able to do really anything would have been the worst, and he would never have wanted to stay on a ventilator and stay on care if he wasn't going to get better…So they said, "Well, we can leave him, you know, continue to treat him and see if, you know, he responds, but most likely he won't," and he wouldn't have wanted that. If there was such a little chance of him getting better, he wouldn't have wanted to continue being hooked up to so much…So my brother and I were able to make the decision that, yes, we wanted to withdraw care for him. We made that decision, but we had a couple of family members that couldn't get there to say goodbye until the next day…So, you know, we asked the doctors, "Is that going to be okay? Can we hold on until we can get everybody here?" And they said, "Absolutely, no big deal. We'll just continue care as is until, you know, you get everybody that you want to be there," and they were really good about it. They said, "You can change your mind at any point"…(Tearful) Even right up until the second that we were literally taking him off the*

ventilator and everything, they said, "You can change your mind at any point. So don't feel like making this decision now, you can't change your mind," which was comforting knowing that if we needed that extra 10 minutes, that we didn't have to be like set in stone to be like, well, we made that decision. It has to happen right this second. (Site 1, family member 1).

Providing Information as a Key Benefit of Patient and Family Engagement in the ICU

Both family members and clinicians often cite the ability of family members to provide useful information about the patient as a benefit of patient and family engagement in the ICU. Indeed, our prior work in these ICUs demonstrated the aspects and benefits of information sharing [6]. Family members can contribute to patient care by offering insight to clinicians regarding the patient's "normal" behaviors and other personal preferences or idiosyncrasies.

Yeah. And they did…They liked any information we had about her and her personality and stuff like that, because like I told them, that's why they said they don't bother her because she always throwing her arm up like this and I said, "That's how she sleep." (LAUGHTER)…And they don't bother her arm no more…Well, when they was saying about her arm and stuff, I said, "Well, she sleep like that," and they said, "Oh, okay." (LAUGHTER)…Because that's just how she sleep all the time. You look at her, she be like this. (LAUGHTER) (Site 1, family member 2)

Oh, yes. And just with the daily care, you know. Now they…They don't…They always want to make sure I know I don't have to do this. But when I say, "Well, I'll help. You know, I do this all the time at home anyway." And they'll say, "Well, we want you to know you can… You don't have…" They always stress that I don't have to assist, but I like doing it, you know? It gives me something to do, and in that way I can kind of calm her and see what her reaction is, allow them to do the mechanical things that they need to do, you know? It works out pretty well. I can't even…I can't even think of the last time I felt like any of the staff, from RT to Nursing to the physicians, ever made me feel like I shouldn't be involved or that I shouldn't say something or that I had no, you know, and then didn't want to hear what I had to say. They do want to hear it because, you know, especially with people like Penny or anyone who is semi-conscious. The family can pick up these little cues and subtle behaviors that the staff doesn't know what that is, you know? So when you say, you know, "Well, this is what she does when it hurts," or this is…They're like, "Oh, okay. Thank you for telling me that because we didn't know that. We didn't know that she doesn't like being on this side or that she doesn't want a pillow under her head." Because with Penny, you know, sometimes they have a pillow under her head, and I'm like, "No. She's not going to like that." And then she just pulls her head up further…That's just how she reacts to it. And they're like, "Well, she doesn't look comfortable." I'm like, "Nope. No pillow." And then they remember…You know, it's amazing. I don't know how they…Yes. I don't know how they keep it all in their heads. (Site 1, family member 4)

We've actually gotten it from the doctors, too, because when…Before she started having her problems, they were like, "Can you think of another time when she acted like this?" I had to think about it because it was years ago, but she had a lung collapse once and she was acting…That kind of just general thrashing in discomfort and obviously there was something going on, and he came back later and said, "Wow. That was close. It was like a mucous plug, but that is, you know, helpful because you…" He asked me direct because he said, "We don't know what's going on. We can tell something is going on…something's wrong, but what it is, I don't know." So they asked me, "Can you think of any other time when she acted like this or something similar happened," because, you know, they can't go through her entire, extremely extensive medical history, you know, just looking randomly for things that might explain it. So really I get…I feel that way from pretty much everybody. You know, even the RTs. When they come in, they're like, "Is there any particular way you do this at home?" "Do you do this at home?" "Is there something that comforts her, something you want us to do to make it?" Because being nasally suctioned is a miserable experience no matter what. And they realize and acknowledge it and say, "If there is anything that we're doing or you want us to do to make it as comfortable as possible," you know? So I think they're really, really good about that. (Site 1, family member 4)

So someone went, and I kind of think it might have been the infection doctor who visited Jody for quite a while yesterday, and it was kind of cute because Jody needed suctioning. I'm on the opposite side. And I realize she doesn't need suctioning through the trachea; she needs it in her mouth. So I jumped up and finally the infection doctor said, "You know more about this than I do. Just go ahead." And that was good. She didn't try to cover up. You know, she was honest about it. I think sometimes medical tries to stay way up here, and not realize that there are things that you have some common sense about or that you've been doing for a number of years. I'm sure they get patients back here that the family's been doing more than what they think they have, and there's got to be a trust. (Site 2, family member 3)

Clinicians echoed the utility of family input but also highlighted some instances in which family input was challenging to handle.

I think engagement makes everything human. So, you know, we get very technical, and we focus on the numbers and things in the chart, but sometimes it's good to have that engagement where the family member can speak to, "Oh, this isn't how they normally are," or tell us, you know, what is different. So they know the patient best and they know if something is off, or even…they're the ones there every day. So when they provide us insight, it kind of adds to what we're trying to accomplish. And then also sometimes, you know, there is that engagement where we have the moment where the family kind of is upset or starts crying. So then it kind of takes a step back too to remind us why we're there and what…what the goal is, and sometimes…You know, I definitely think it's humbling to us because sometimes it's clear that the team is rushing or maybe not being as empathetic, and then the family kind of like pull us back and make us talk about things that we were trying to maybe breeze past. So I think it's just kind of having them always there and like able to answer questions and help address concerns too is helpful. (Site 4, registered dietician)

Sometimes it's not helpful. I mean sometimes you have that kind of toxic family member that is making everything worse instead of better, but for the most part, when the family is involved, I think it just provides more in-depth information for the patient that we just don't know, and they know their family member better than we know them. So sometimes they can be like, "Yeah." Like I think the patient looks comfortable, and they're like, "Ya. I can tell by the way he's furrowing his eyebrows that he's not happy." You know and it's like, "Oh, I wouldn't have caught that." So I for the most part find the family very helpful and, you know, like I have witnessed rounds where the family has like provided key information that really was helpful or beneficial. (Site 2, nurse 3)

Additionally, family members chose a level of involvement that suited their medical knowledge and their personal desire to receive as much information as possible—or as little information as necessary.

...I like so much information, and I'm really good at taking the information I need to make a decision, and the information I don't need I can just kind of push aside or just let go. So I never felt like I was getting too much information. It was always...Because I like to get lots of information, I never had that information overload moment. (Site 1, family member 1)

I mean it made it easier to know that...I mean, my brother did kind of default back to me, and he'd be like, "Well, what do you think?" ...I have some medical knowledge. So everything wasn't way above my head like it is with him...So he'd kind of default back to me. He'd be like, "Okay," and he'd listen, and then he'd look at me and he'd say, "Well, what do you think? Is there something else that I need to know?" So I could then take all that information. Even though the doctors and the nurses were really good about not using jargon and talking above his head and explaining things...They were really good at explaining things...He would look to me to be like, "Okay, what are you doing?" So, yeah, even though I was basically the primary decision maker, they never insisted that it was just me making the decision. They were really good about making sure that everybody that I wanted included was included. (Site 1, family member 1)

I mean I didn't go to medical school. I didn't go to nursing school. So I don't know what's the best option for him. I can listen, and if they present me options, I can ask questions, but, you know, I don't know what this medication does versus a different medication. That's not what I know. But they were all very good at...Whenever they would come in to do something, they would let me know what they were doing or, "we're just giving him this medication," or whatever, which was nice...It kind of made...I guess it kind of makes you feel included so that you know what's going on all of the time...I do remember one time I told the nurses...They were like, "Oh, this is what we're doing," and I was like, "Great. I trust you"...They were like, "Well, we just want to make sure you know what's going on, and that we're not doing anything that we really shouldn't be doing." I was like, "I trust you, and I'm here all the time. I know what's going on. If I think you're doing something that's weird or maybe not appropriate, I would be like, hey, what's going on? Why are we doing that?" But that was never the case. Everything...always seemed normal to me or what they should be doing. (Site 1, family member 1)

But the fact that the doctors here and the nurses...Everyone that's attending to him is willing to say to us, "This is why we're here and this is what we're doing." And for someone like my husband and myself, we appreciate that. Perhaps there are people who don't. Perhaps they don't even understand it, but for us personally, that is extremely helpful, and it makes us feel as if they care because they're willing to spend the time it takes to sit down and talk to you. The doctors will come in and sit on the end of the bed and talk and explain what they were thinking, what they would like, where they were going. They even had me go home on Sunday night so that I could go to the imaging place to get the disc from the last report from the previous Thursday report because they had the paper report, but they really wanted the disc. So I went home on Sunday night and then went to the imaging place on Monday morning and grabbed the disc, and then came here so they could have it before they took him into surgery...But just the fact that...I think it was Dr. Pastore that came in and explained how much that would be helpful... It's just that they... They all came in and explained within their specialty what they were going to do or why they thought, "this is what we should do." It could be this or this, but they felt this was the option to take. (Site 1, family member 3)

Direct Participation in Care by Family Members

Family members contributed to patient care through direct and active participation, typically through more routine care procedures like grooming and positioning.

> *Oh, yeah. We was helping them lift her up in her bed and stuff and, you know...And I try to help keep her comfor when I'm here...Like that one arm. So, I try to move it around a little bit for her. You know, try to keep it active since she cannot move it herself and stuff in her fingers and try to make sure her legs get moved around and propped up... You know, stuff like that, just trying to, you know, do whatever I can and stuff. I wish I could comb her hair, but I can't. (LAUGHTER)...She decided to go all natural, but she didn't know this was going to happen. (Site 1, family member 2)*

> *No, I haven't, but I'd be perfectly willing to do it, but I'm looking at his situation and he's... You know, he's been in bed for so long that he's quite weak now, and I think that perhaps until he gets just a little bit stronger, I'd hate to... I wouldn't be able to support him if he were to slip or something in the shower, and I wouldn't want to jeopardize him. It's not that I wouldn't want to do it for him, but I have to look at that bigger picture. But, he loves to be tucked in. I tuck him in. He likes... They put the sheets, and they kind of put them over the back of the bed, but he likes to have his toes wrapped up...So I tuck them back in. And he likes to be cocooned almost, and that's fine. And then they come in. "Oh, can we look at this? Can we look?" And they're very nice, and then they go away, and now we have to cocoon him again. And that's okay... no problem. Yesterday, for the first time... He hasn't eaten anything since Sunday. So yesterday for the first time, he'll go on clear liquids. So we had... I was helping him to... He had a little chicken broth. He had a little Hawaiian punch. He had... I got a lemon ice and then let it melt, and then he had a little Ensure. I'm, you know, holding the straw while he can get it because, you know, that's what you do. You know? We've been married 40 years, you know, and it's (LAUGHTER) So, whatever it would take, I would have no problem with that at all...But I'm just thinking at this moment in time because Julia, who is his nurse right now, told me when he comes back from this procedure, they're going to wash him and clean him and change everything, and I think with how he is, somewhat incapacitated, you know,...I'm only 4...about 4′10″ right now. So this is where it becomes a disadvantage. I'm thankful he's not 6 foot tall. It would be impossible...But even...Even now, moving him physically for me when he can only give me a limited amount of assistance, I would rather that they do it. When he gets...When he's starting to get it together, shall I say, and we can do it together and no problem with that, but feeding him, you know, and anything like that, it would not be a problem. (Site 1, family member 3)*

Clinicians described an appreciation for helpful family members but also expressed caution when it comes to exactly how families contribute, highlighting a difference between "participation" and "involvement" in care.

> *I would say participating and involvement...I don't think family can participate in care. I don't think it's possible. I think they can be involved in care, but I don't think they can participate in care...I think family can be involved in rounds in terms of listening to where we're going. They can ask questions. They can raise concerns, but I think participating in care is actually doing care...There are very few families that I feel can participate in care...Yesterday, I had a patient who was...We extubated him. He wanted something to eat, and so I tested him with food and he was okay, but I could tell that he was drinking super fast... When I was leaving for the day, I looked into the room. His wife and his family were there, and the family goes, "Can he have something to drink?" And I told the nurse who took over for him...I go, "Listen." I go, "I would make sure that he is up because he doesn't know when to stop. He can go, go, go." I was about to turn around and tell them. You know,*

I was going to let her tell them that, the nurse, and the next thing I know I turn around, and I see the wife...The patient is now in the bed, scrunched down, head forward, and his wife is giving him something to drink. I go, "This man is going to aspirate." You know what I mean? She gave him a sip, and then she took it away... Then I turned to the nurse. I go, "Listen. He really needs to be up." And I feel that sometimes families will do anything to make their family feel better...food or something like that, but doing...You know, I don't think they know those details. (Site 1, nurse 1)

Patient Rounds as a Space for Engaging Families

Daily rounds were a common setting for family involvement. Many family members highlighted how morning rounds helped them feel included by providing a space for clinicians to include them in discussions of a patient's care. Family members were able to choose their degree of involvement on rounds based on their comfort level. Some family members just listened at rounds to stay up to date on new information, while others were more active in their participation.

It initially started after morning rounds...They were doing morning rounds, and it was the day that he got the new attending. They were doing morning rounds, and they had gotten a new lab report that had showed that my dad had declined. He ended up having yeast in his blood, and the attending stepped away from rounds and went in personally to look at my dad. Then we had a brief conversation about what this new information meant and what his likely outcomes were. He said, "Okay. Sit with this information. After rounds, we'll come back and we'll have a more in-depth conversation." And that's what they did, and then we were able to...Then I had...Then I brought my brother in, and we had another conversation about it...The doctors were really good about initiating it in my situation. (Site 1, family member 1)

...but as far as the staff...They go as far as...I mean, they're wonderful as far as making sure you're included in rounds...And asking you, "Is there anything you want to say? Is there anything we need?" Not just the nurses, the physicians, too. Everybody here has been just wonderful about doing that...Now part of that is, I've just been doing this for a long time. Because they include you...Or they didn't initially in the old days when they didn't want you to sleep in the room, but they started that a while back in Peds too, in making sure to include the family in the rounds and the discussion and the plan for the day and, you know, all of that type of thing. So I have been doing this for a while. So I think I'm probably...Where like we were talking about...Some of these people are here as a result of a traumatic injury or accident, and they've never been in a medical setting before. I have a grasp of the terminology, too, that sometimes...You know, if you're a newbie, you're like, "What the heck are they talking about?" You don't chime in because you have no idea what they're talking about...And they can't, I mean... "Dumb it down" is the wrong way to say it, but I mean it's a teaching hospital, and the residents and fellows and, you know...That's part of what they're rounding is school for them, you know. So they are going to be speaking in a way that you may not, and I don't always get everything they're saying, but I have a pretty good grasp, and especially of her particular medical problems because we've been down this road so many times...And I've never been made to feel like I shouldn't, you know what I mean? Or like, "What the heck is she talking for," you know? (LAUGHTER) They've really, really been wonderful in that regard. I have no complaints there. (Site 1, family member 4)

I don't go out in the hall with them. I guess I have enough trust that I don't have to...With the other group that they used to have here, it was never even a...even an offer. I...I don't know what the agreement is. (LAUGHTER) I think the first morning...I never...I've never really thought that I'd be invited, although I know if they have any conversation about Jody, I want her to be able to be in on it. I didn't like some of the...The one time when we were here, I got this...the thought that the medical team thought that we weren't being aware of the prognosis or that we weren't being...we weren't facing up to reality...I'm grateful that Rosalie [the nurse] was here and she knew better. I knew some of the tests that they were ordering, the medical team was ordering, was to prove to themselves that Jody's MS had exacerbated and was...everything was from that. I could tell by the fact that they had a new neurologist come up and I thought, "Okay. They're just trying to discount," and we know what's behind this. We know that Jody has medical problems. We know that her...some of her...the majority of her medical problems, we know, weren't caused by her MS, but because of other issues and treating and saying it's the MS isn't going to get her past the other thing, and then they can blame everything on the MS. (LAUGHTER) (Site 2, family member 3)

Many clinicians discussed how families are encouraged to listen in to rounds and be present to ask questions of the clinical team.

So I think, you know, patient and family engagement is to make certain that the...you know, the patients and families know where they are in the scope of their acute critical illness and know what the steps are...the big broad goals are for their care for that day or where things are generally going. So I think that means including them as a part of rounds and...I'm sorry...I didn't include the patient on my list of people who are a part of rounds, but I think that they are certainly...if they are able to be awake and participate...Many people, of course, who are critically ill are not, but I think it's important to have a family member present so that they can be a part of the conversation that's happening about their loved one. So I think to the best of their ability to be a part of that conversation, and typically before the end of rounds, I'll ask the patient...I'll say "hi" to the family member before we start. I'll say, "Hey, we're going to be talking about your loved one. Feel free to come and join us." So that's something that I will commonly say to make them feel welcome. And then at the end of it, I'll see if they have any questions, or I'll just give a brief summary to them to make certain that they...if there's a procedure that's happening that day, if we're going to do dialysis that day or what we're trying to do, because many times, even though we spend 15 minutes rounding on a person, the distillation of their plan is a couple of things. So I just try and make certain that they understand what those things are. (Site 4, physician 2)

However, some clinicians recognized challenges to including families in rounds and did not unilaterally agree on the benefits of including families. These clinicians also discussed strategies they used to navigate such challenges during rounds.

So family-centered rounds are nonsense. They're complete nonsense. And I have had this opinion since I was rounding in Children's Hospital, and here's the reason why. There are 3 reasons why they're nonsense. Reason #1. It isn't...The purpose of rounds...The purpose of communication on the physician team is to talk about the patient in the most concise, but yet most information-dense way possible... That is directly opposed in family-centered rounds, because family-centered rounds says that you should only talk in ways that families can understand, and the problem is that you can't function as physicians doing that. And so I think that there are times when you need to talk doctor-to-doctor, again in "doctor talk" as I like to say, and then there need to be times when you need to basically transform that and address it to families.... So I believe very strongly that, you know, rounds should be rounds and that discussions with the family should be discussions with the family, and I think that you need to have both. If a family member wants to join us on rounds and wants to overhear what we're talking about, I actually have no problem with them doing that, but then I think at the end of rounds, what at least I like to do when I'm the fellow on the unit, is I like to address the family member and say, "So let me just summarize that for you." And then kind of bring it down into a small...Not a small, but like more manageable terms... Issue #2 with family-centered rounds is that I think there are...When you're a resident and you're in front of a family member, you act differently. It's the observation effect, right? So you will act differently and you will say things differently in front of a family member than you would otherwise, and sometimes that's not really a good thing. You know, I think in rounds you need to be truthful and you need to talk about things, and you need to brings things up and sort of be in your own way. I think as soon as you add a family member in there, it changes the way that people say things because they're concerned or they're worried or what have you. Again, I think that that is not really ideal. The third thing is a practical thing. Sometimes people on the team don't fully understand what's going on, and so every once in a while you have an intern who doesn't understand what's going on, and they say something which is either wrong or not completely cognizant, and then the family hears that and then there's like, "Oh." Well, then we take it back. I think that there's just a lot of miscommunication there. I don't know, maybe those are all variations on the theme, but I think that, you know, having people not being able to communicate effectively is one thing. Number 2, censoring what you say and what information you release or not is different. (Site 1, physician 1)

Clinicians Caring for Family Needs as Separate from Patient Needs

Aside from caring for the patient, family members described ways in which clinicians would make sure to care for family members as well, whether by explicitly providing opportunities to share their own feelings about their experience and emotions or by offering small gestures to make them feel as comfortable as possible as they dealt with the impact of the ICU.

I remember the morning that we...this whole thing started. I had to call my brother into the hospital, and I was sitting in his room just, I guess, digesting the information, and I didn't really cry a lot when I was at the hospital while he was being treated, but I was...It was a hard...It was a hard conversation to have with my brother saying "you have to come to the hospital because we have to discuss this," and really knowing kind of what the outcome of the discussion was going to be. It was really hard, and I was sitting in the room just kind of crying to myself, and I wasn't asking for anybody or anybody to talk to, but Heidi [the nurse]...She went and she called Dale, the reverend, to come and just chat with me...(Tearful) And even though we're not a religious family, it was...It was really kind of a nice gesture for her to see that I was not doing so well...(Tearful) She brought him in, and I had met him before, and we discussed the fact that we're not really religious, but he came in and he was really good about just being a person to talk to...(Tearful) And Heidi [the nurse] stayed, and we all kind of just had a nice conversation. It kind of made me feel a little better that, you know, we were making the right decisions, and, yeah, it sucked, but this is what he would want and it was...It felt...Even though I wasn't the patient, I felt very cared for there. (Site 1, family member 1)

I think everyone that I kind of came across was really helpful. I remember the respiratory therapists were always really great. They would come in and be like, "Alright, I'm so and so from Respiratory, and I'm gonna do this," and they were really good about explaining things, too. At the end when we had made that decision, I left the room to go to the bathroom, and I was waiting in the hallway to get into the bathroom, and one of the respiratory therapists that he had had multiple times walked by and she saw me and she was like, "Are you okay?" And I said, "Well, no, not really," and I kind of told her what was going on, and she just gave me like a big hug. She's like, "I'm so sorry," (tearful) and it was kind of nice to have that. Even though she wasn't the one taking care of him that day, it was nice to have that little bit of support…(Tearful) And then…I don't remember her name, but the unit host. She was really good about…She'd stop in every day and say, "You need anything?" I said, "No." I tried to be pretty low key. Everyone has so many important jobs to do there that I didn't really want people having to do extra stuff. But she was like, "If you need anything, you just let me know." Everyone was really good about making sure not only (tearful) my dad was taken care of, but if my brother and I or anybody who happened to be there that day to see him was taken care of as well, whether it was just, "Do you want me to go get you a glass of water from the nutrition room," or calling Dale or whatever. They were all really good about making sure that whatever we needed was taken care of as well. (Site 1, family member 1)

Yeah. They always offer me something to drink or something, but I…I don't eat too much…Anyhow, they offer me something to drink or something like that. Even one nurse went and bought me a cup of coffee because their machine was down. (LAUGHTER)…Oh, yeah. That was real nice of her. Yeah, they've been real nice. I couldn't ask for no different. (Site 1, family member 2)

Well, I guess there's two different point of views on that, I guess, because I'm sitting back and I watch them, not to be nosy, not…You know, because I'm not concerned about her care. I'm the type of person who wants to know things and I learn from it. Okay? So I'm learning all this new stuff. So I've asked a couple of times like, "You want me to help?" (LAUGHTER) It's just that I'm not used to sitting around. They're like, "oh, that's okay." But I never interfered because I don't want to interfere into the treatment or anything that they're doing because they know what they're doing. And I really don't unless they…And I don't want to mess anything up. You know, but I offer, you know? But the staff… The nurses have been, you know, pretty decent with me. I…Oh, that one girl said…My sister was messing with…Trying to get out of the bed or something, and I'm like, "No, sis. Just relax. You've got tubes in your mouth. You're still at the hospital. I'm here," kind of thing, and I'm like…I looked at the nurse like…because I don't know if I'm doing this right or wrong, and she's like, "Oh, no. You're fine." I was like, "I just don't want to get, you know, all messed up or anything. (LAUGHTER)" She's like, "No, that's fine. You're actually helping." So she's the only one that had told me that I was actually doing good because I've been kind of afraid to talk to her or whatever. (LAUGHTER) But yeah, that was…That was nice. (Site 2, family member 1)

Bias and Burden as Contributing to Negative Views on Family Engagement

Not all family member experiences were positive, however. Family members had both positive and negative interactions with clinicians, often over the course of one ICU stay. The ICU setting itself, and the acuity of ICU patient needs, often contributed to their negative experiences. Family members may be overwhelmed, clinicians have many patients to care for, and the clinician team changes constantly, especially from the perspective of family members of a patient with a prolonged ICU stay.

One family member described how she felt the clinicians were only treating her sister as an addict and that those impressions affected the way that they planned and delivered care:

> *Well, there's a couple of them that I notice…The doctors don't know who they are. They come in, they check her, listen to her, and then they kind of just go on their little way. And I'm like (LAUGHTER), you know, "talk to me. Just tell me what you think and be real and truthful, you know? It's what I want to know." But yeah, that little part I don't care too much for. There's another doctor [that] was not very nice either. So for a minute there, I was thinking, you know, I don't want her to be treated as an addict. That's one thing. She's always afraid of going to the doctors, going to the hospital, you know, going anywheres just because everybody treated her as an addict. So that's what her fear was, and so I never took her. And, you know, then she was embarrassed because of, you know, her tracks and stuff. So that's kind of how I was feeling with that doctor. Like he's not going to fix her because she's an addict. Well, she's here. She's recovering. She's past that withdrawal. She's gonna be here long-term for at least 6–8 weeks. Maybe that's not enough for recovery for her for her drugs, but it's a start. And what I want is for her…I'm hoping this is going to be the end, but a beginning of a new life for her. So maybe if we can just, you know, push her into getting…giving her something to look forward to, you know, give her a fresh start. But he just don't want to do it because she's gonna go out here and relapse, and then it's not gonna be no good and stuff. I get that but I kind of…I'm not a professional like that. So, whatever they think is best for her. I just felt like he was treating her like an addict. (Site 2, family member 1)*

> *Since our last visit here, the person…The doctor that was in charge is no longer here, and that is a blessing. We had had some very edgy words with him over her treatment here before, and we're totally, totally astounded at the difference in treatment this time. They have addressed, without us giving them a whole lot of flak, each one of our concerns, and the first one was the CAT scan downstairs that showed…She got a better diagnosis than what she's had previously. Anyone walking around could have that diagnosis. It had nothing to do with her MS. Where in years past that she's been here, that was their big thing. "Well, you know she has MS," "you know this and everything else." So we've lost a lot of time over the years. Just the change in the medical staff. Nursing has always been favorable here. Every once in a while you'll get someone that doesn't realize that yes, she does have a little problem because she has MS, and that's in her temperature control. If it gets too warm, she loses it all. So occasionally a nurse, but we now hear nurses saying, "Don't you let Jody's temperature get above this certain thing." So just like I told the nurses when we left…"Her temperature is stable. I even have a little blanket on her, and we'll watch it the rest of the day." So that way she doesn't have to take any medication, which we don't like her to…And she doesn't like to take a lot of medication too. (Site 2, family member 3)*

Family members were negatively impacted when they felt as though they were being dismissed by clinicians, or that their presence in the ICU was more of a burden to the clinicians than a support to the patient.

> *So one of the nurses last week…And I don't talk to her. I just say, "Hey, sis, I'm here," or "Bye, sis, I'll be back," or whatever…You know, just little conversations kind of thing. So we came back from eating…Me, my mom and my dad came back from eating…I don't know what day it was. I told Rosalie [the nurse]…I think, is that her name? Last week, I thought it was Thursday or something. Well, me and my dad have been trying to like make one day…You know, he'll be here during the day, and then I'll be here, and then we'll be like switching on and off, you know? But that day, it was just me and my mom…Yeah, my mom,*

my dad and me, and one of the nurses was like...I come in and I said, "Hey, sis I'm back," and I was putting on...We were putting our gowns and stuff on at the same I was talking to her, and she come in all rude like, "Limit your talking to her. There's not supposed to be 3 of you guys in here. The rules are...There are only allowed 2 people in here, and you're lucky that I'm letting all 3 of you in here. The next nurse might not be so nice." I was like...I didn't say nothing. You know I got...I just kind of walked by Brooke and I just went and sat down. I'm like...My mom and dad (LAUGHTER) is like "uh oh." They could tell I was thinking in my head, you know. I just was dwelling on it, like "wow," you know? So I went and told the doctor like, "Look, you know, I don't appreciate it. We have been here from Day 1 for one. I understand the rules. I get it, you know. Not making exceptions but, you know, if we were rude to you guys, I would expect something back. It's unethical. You know, we're family." So I talked to him about it and stuff. So he's like, "I'm so sorry that had to happen." I'm like, "It's one thing just to tell me and let me know something," but it's another thing to be treating me disrespectful. ***INTERVIEWER****: Yeah. Did you feel comfortable enough to be able to like talk to the doctor and address that?* ***PARTICIPANT****: I did. I did with the doctor because he's really nice, and I didn't know which one was her doctor. (LAUGHTER) So I'm like...Because it's on the board. I'm like, "I don't even know who Mr. Garnett is or Dr. Garnett is." So I found out who it was. Because I've talked to so many doctors. I'm like...I don't even know. (LAUGHTER) So you know? So I'm like...So I did talk to him, and I told him, you know, about it and stuff, and it was just like kind of an unappreciated kind of thing. You know, I wasn't being rude to her or being disrespectful. I didn't even say anything to her. It just like...It threw me back, like "what?" (Site 2, family member 1)*

Most of the time, it's been, "This is what we're doing." And I understand some of the things...You know, you have to go ahead and just do them. They've understood early on that Jody does not have a Do Not Resuscitate clause. So they would have to come to us with some...And I remember one time when her temperature was going up and I had...This was in the early, early stages of being here, and I said, "We're going to be in trouble if that temperatures goes much higher." Nobody seemed to pay any attention. So maybe they could listen too, but then I know that at some point, they can't listen to everything. I mean I understand that too, and sometimes my husband even says to me, "Just shut up for a while." But anyway, in this instance when her temperature had gone up, and her mother-in-law was there too, and I said, "I've had it." So I wasn't getting anywhere with them. So I just started pulling gloves down and filling them with ice and packing her with ice. Then it got to be even more uncontrollable. So they wanted to code her, and I said, "no." I mean the first word was "no," and they took that as, "you don't want her coded?" I said, "yes, but not now. I want an ice machine." I said, "I want..." I had worked pediatrics for a number of years, and so we had an ice mattress that we could get. Well, they didn't know what it was up here, and I said, "Go to Pediatrics and get one. They'll know. Just tell them what you want, and they'll get it." Well, they sent somebody down. That was the first time they ever listened to me up here. Anyway they sent somebody down, and they brought back the ice mattress which is much more significant than what we used to have. I mean, we had to fill it with ice. But I mean this was all electronic. If the condition hadn't been so serious, they put it on top of her (LAUGHTER) instead of underneath her, and I said, "No, no. It has to be underneath her." So they did that, and we were fine. She never had to be coded or...No vent that time, but what would have happened if I hadn't been there. They still would have never attributed it. They would have never taken our word what cooling her off was going to do. (Site 2, family member 3)

The doctor kind of picked and choose. I wasn't too happy about that, because see my mother don't understand. I always had to explain everything to her, and my dad...He likes me to know. Like for them to tell me, and then he just kind of watches what I do, you know? And then afterwards we kind of talk about it and be like, "Okay, this is what he has said or whatever," for that situation. And it was nice the other day when her mother-in-law was here yesterday, and the doctor had came in…One of the doctors…I don't know which one it was…had came in and said, "Are you…" He looked at her mother-in-law and said, "Are you mom?" She's like, "No." And then she had asked me if it was okay to speak freely, which was nice. I'm like, "Yeah," even though I didn't want to, but I'm like, "Yeah, it's okay." So it was nice that she even asked. I probably wouldn't have said "no," (LAUGHTER) but it was the fact that they…(Site 2, family member 1)

Poor Communication Between Family and Clinicians

Family members found it difficult and concerning when they could not speak to a clinician and receive updates on a patient's care or progress, or if they were told information in a way they could not understand.

Like I said, they just been real good about everything, you know. When I call, like, you know…Except for one night, but they apologized…Because I called…Because I don't get off work until…Sometimes I don't get off work till 12:00, you know, and I always call when I get home to check on her, and I called, and the first line kept being busy, and so I called through the hospital operator until I got hooked to the floor, and then they told me…They was going to call me back. And I sat up until 2:30 in the morning. I had to end up calling them back and stuff. So I wasn't too happy about that, but I told them about it, and they was, "Oh, we're so sorry." It probably wasn't the ones that was talking to me's fault. It was the people before, but, again, I know they get busy up here. They doing things, you know, because I never know…Any patient could have…You know, they could have been really busy, so…I didn't get too mad because I finally got through to somebody…I wasn't gonna stop until I did. (LAUGHTER)…Because I get scared when I can't talk to somebody…Yeah. I be worrying that they working on her, something wrong, you know? That's why, you know, just to hear that she okay and stuff…That's all I want to hear, you know? Oh, yeah. She told that. They talked to me and told me she was okay. They apologized, you know, but…Like I said, me sitting at home and trying to call and sitting there waiting and waiting…I got a little frustrated…I was like, "Oh, somebody gonna talk to me." (LAUGHTER) (Site 1, family member 2)

I just had one experience last Saturday, I guess, when the PA came in. I didn't understand how he was trying to explain everything. It kind of bothered me. So I spoke with the nurse after he left, and he's been…He's been a lot better in communicating now. Sometimes you have to speak up…And not something intentionally to be mean towards someone, but you've got to be careful when you go to try to relay stuff to the family members because if they don't understand what you're saying, it'd be like, "What are you talking about?" (Site 2, family member 2)

Clinicians Described a Tension Between Caring for Patients and Engaging Families

Clinicians hold varying opinions about the optimal level of family involvement in the ICU as well as the benefits and challenges of family presence during ICU-level patient care. Speaking with clinicians highlighted the importance that individual clinicians place on family engagement but also demonstrated the necessity of defining family engagement in ways that are conducive to patient care. Medical providers deliver intensive, oftentimes complex care to ICU patients, and this care may be affected by family engagement. Some clinicians asked for more clarity around what leadership or administration means when they encourage increased family engagement. They noted that their primary responsibility is to the patient, and described how in some cases they felt a tension between their responsibility to the patient and engaging the family in care.

> *I still don't know what "patient/family-centered care" means. I don't know what that means…We're including the family in their care. Well, what does that mean? Give me an example of that…I'm here to do my job and that's to take care of this patient, you know what I mean? And once the patient is taken care of, then I will move on to the family. But if I'm trying to keep this patient alive and mom is having a hard time, I can't…I'm gonna keep the patient alive, and mom is just gonna have to kind of tough it out until hopefully somebody…Or I can flag a nurse down or flag somebody who is good with that type of communication who can assist her, you know, a social worker or other nurse or the chaplain….I can never get a true definition of what does that mean[s]…you know, "[patient/family] centered care." (Site 1, nurse 1)*

Additionally, one physician felt that sometimes patient and family engagement was used as a way of discussing ICU care without offering clinicians any tangible ways to engage them.

> *And I think even sometimes the physicians…They're like, "Oh, yeah, well empowering…That's a nursing thing. Have the nurses talk to them about, you know, doing the swabs or feeding the patient or doing things like…" They try to make it a nursing thing because they don't want to be involved in the hard thing, and I think daily communication with families is actually very difficult, and I think that that…is very difficult, has a large time burden, a large soul burden in doing it and talking to them, and so I think that, you know, a lot of people are looking for a lot of quick fixes, and I don't think there are any, and I think our critical care societies just by saying "empower patients," is a way to like…be like, "Ah hhhh. Look. Don't we look good and feel good about ourselves," but don't actually give us any real tools or solutions in how to do that. (Site 1, physician 1)*

Other clinicians described compartmentalizing and approaching the patient and the family as two separate entities, balancing their separate needs as the situation required.

> *I see them as two different things maybe because I, as I previously said, believe that a third of the time the family doesn't actually have the patient's own well-being at heart. So I tend to kind of divorce them in my mind. Now, I think as a physician you have to certainly include the family and, you know, talk with them regardless of whether they're an intubated patient who can't answer for themselves or anyone. I mean I do think you have to utilize and empower the family to do certain things. However, I tend not to ever, at least in my practice…I tend to put the family over here and the patient there and kind of look at them, you know, slightly differently and not lump them together as one unit. (Site 1, physician 1)*

> *That being said, many of our patients in the ICU aren't able to communicate for one reason or another because they're intubated, because they're sedated, because they're confused or agitated or comatose. There are a number of reasons why they can't communicate, and then it becomes the job of the team to engage the family as the surrogate decision makers for the patient. You know, it's always important as much as possible to ask the family to advocate,*

you know, what the specific patient would want him- or herself under the circumstances based on what he/she has written or said in the past or his style of living or his priorities or his religious beliefs or whatever it may be. That's what it comes down to is respecting the wishes of the patient or what you think the wishes of the patient are. There are times where you get a sense that either families or doctors are sort of doing what they want, which is not necessarily coming from what they think the patient wants, but from what their own biases or priorities are. Though I think it's essential to engage families as surrogates for the patient, but I often find myself making the point, "you know, what we really need to focus on is what the patient, you know, would want under the circumstances, rather than what I want or what you want or what anybody else says they want." And I have had situations...You know, this is not a big problem, but there's been a big push for patient- and family-centered care, and I've had patients in the past who have been upset that their family members were involved in their care when they were perfectly able to take care of themselves and wanted to maintain their own privacy and autonomy to make their own decisions. So it's not automatic to me that every family needs to be involved for every patient, and if they are involved it has to be as surrogates for the patient as opposed to an independent group that needs to be taken care of themselves. (Site 4, physician 1)

However, clinicians did express hesitation around some forms of family involvement and share cautionary examples of families who they perceived as having a negative impact on a patient's care. Engaging families in the ICU needs to be done intentionally and with care, given how families can affect the patient and the ICU care team's ability to deliver high-quality, timely care.

You can see, if you walk into any ICU and there's a difficult family, you can see and feel the tension around that room and how it results in poor morale and how it results in bad patient care. I had a patient over here at the Teaching Hospital. I was on for a Saturday, and I had a very demanding family who was causing a lot of problems for the nurses, and it interrupted patient care. I had to call the house manager and have them escorted out of the hospital, but you could just see every single time you walked past that room just how upset and demoralized the physician team taking care of them was and the nurses taking care of them were. (Site 1, physician 1)

Many clinicians did offer positive reflections on their experiences engaging families in the ICU setting, with a heavy focus on how families can provide unique insight into the patient, particularly when a patient may be ventilated and unable to speak for themselves.

Well, I think it's integral to have them involved because, like I said at the beginning, without the family involvement...If the patient is not able to speak for himself, we depend greatly on the family to fill in the blanks for us, and even if they can speak, sometimes they don't always say what...the truth like, you know, if the patient has a high pain tolerance and doesn't want to complain, the patient might tell me that they're not in pain, but the wife might pull me aside and say, "You know what? He has a tendency not to complain about pain. I can tell he's in pain for these reasons," and then that allows me to go back and reassess the patient in a different way. So without my families' involvement, I can't do my job. Now sometimes a family can be on the other side of the coin and it's a little too involved... you know, and then you can't do your job either because families are getting in the way. But, in general, without them, their care is not specialized or individualized to the patient themselves. So you need to...They have to be involved. They have to have...As I said at the very beginning, they are part of the team, and without their involvement, we can't give the best care to the patient. (Site 4, nurse 1)

Conclusion

Family members are an integral part of ICU patient care through their presence as advocates and as support for patients. ICU clinicians have a responsibility to ensuring that families have the necessary information to make informed decisions and to raise concerns about the care patients receive. These processes involve information sharing, open communication, and creating spaces for family members to ask questions or express their views. As many of the family members included here discussed, when clinicians included families in these ways, it improved the ICU experience for families and offered a positive space for patients to receive care. However, as many clinicians expressed, successful family engagement in the ICU is not clearly defined, and increasing family engagement in the ICU also poses new challenges. By highlighting family voices in parallel with clinicians, this chapter demonstrates the importance of family engagement in the ICU. Family engagement in the ICU is a dynamic, multifaceted process that requires attention to the unique needs of the patient, the family, and the clinicians as individuals who must work together in a high-pressure setting to ensure quality care for the patient.

Acknowledgments We thank the ICU clinicians and family members for their participation and willingness to participate in our study. All names of people and places in the quotations provided have been changed and replaced with pseudonyms to protect the participants' confidentiality.

Funding This study was funded by the University of Michigan Center for Complexity and Self-Management of Chronic Disease pilot project (P20NR015331) and Agency for Healthcare Quality and Safety (K08HS024552, PI Costa). Funders had no role in the design, interpretation or reporting of results.

References

1. McAdam J, Araj S, Puntillo K. Unrecognized contributions of families in the intensive care unit. Intensive Care Med. 2008;34:1097.
2. Davidson J, Aslakson R, Long A, Puntillo K, Kross E, Hart J, et al. Guidelines for family-centered care in the neonatal, pediatric, and adult ICU. Crit Care Med. 2017;45:103–28.
3. Smedira NG, Evans BH, Grais LS, Cohen NH, Lo B, Cooke M, et al. Withholding and withdrawal of life support from the critically ill. N Engl J Med. 1990;322:309–15.
4. McConnell B, Moroney T. Involving relatives in ICU patient care: critical nursing challenges. J Clin Nurs. 2015;24:991–8.
5. Burns K, Misak C, Herridge M, Meade M, Oczkowski S, Patient and Family Partnership Committee of the Canadian Critical Care Trials Group. Patient and family engagement in the ICU. Untapped opportunities and underrecognized challenges. Am J Respir Crit Care Med. 2018;198:310–9.
6. Boltey E, Wright N, Mosley E, White M, Iwashyna T, Manojlovich M, Costa D. Exploring the process of information sharing in an adult intensive care unit: an ethnographic study. J Interprof Care. 2022;36:168–76.

Chapter 3
Family-Centered Communication in the ICU During the SARS-CoV-2 Pandemic

Ji Won Shin, Emika S. Miller, Judith A. Tate, JiYeon Choi, and Mary Beth Happ

Introduction

Family-centered care is an "approach to health care that is respectful of and responsive to individual families' needs and values" [1]. Critical illness represents a major life-altering event for both patients and their families. Often, admission to an intensive care unit (ICU) is unplanned and associated with a life-threatening illness. Families experience high levels of stress as their family member's condition changes unpredictably, and the outcomes are uncertain. Family-centered care in the ICU supports the recognition of the essential role of families to serve as the patient's voice and advocate while they are critically ill. Communication is an important component of family-centered care in the ICU [1].

In this chapter, we will describe the unique effects of SARS-CoV-2 on communication between patients and families and ICU staff and families as the need to eliminate viral transmission overshadowed the needs of patients and families to have contact and communicate. We will address lessons learned about communication, family-centered care, and critical illness that were gleaned from our clinical experiences with the pandemic.

J. W. Shin (✉) · E. S. Miller · J. A. Tate · M. B. Happ
The Ohio State University College of Nursing, Columbus, OH, USA
e-mail: shin.527@osu.edu

J. Choi
Yonsei University College of Nursing, Seoul, South Korea

© The Author(s), under exclusive license to Springer Nature Switzerland AG 2025

A. J. Vance et al. (eds.), *Families in the Intensive Care Unit*,
https://doi.org/10.1007/978-3-031-83786-9_3

Communication Among Patients, Families, and Clinicians

For critically ill patients, the inability to communicate is one of the most distressing experiences of their ICU stay [2–4]. Many patients have difficulty communicating because of the seriousness of their illness, sedating medications or mechanical ventilation with an endotracheal tube, a physical barrier to communicating with their voice. Patients who have difficulty communicating experience fear, anxiety, and frustration as they are unable to make their needs understood by those around them [5–11].

Often, communicating with voiceless ICU patients is not a high priority for ICU staff [12–14]. Many staff feel underprepared to communicate with patients who cannot vocalize their needs as this content is not included in educational preparation for many health care clinicians. Because nurses lack both training and confidence in their ability to communicate with voiceless ICU patients, nurses often resort to strategies like trial and error to make sense of patients' communication attempts [12, 15]. Such trials are mostly ineffective and can lead to inaccurate or abandoned communication, which can impact safety and quality of patient care.

Communication impairment during critical illness is troubling for families as many of them are not familiar with patients' attempts to make nonvocal communication. Families have difficulty interpreting accurate messages related to patients' basic needs, while more complex messages are often abandoned. Missed or unsuccessful communication attempts provoke a range of negative emotions, such as distress, loss, and frustration, in families [16–18]. Families feel unprepared to communicate with nonvocal patients, which is a challenging concern, especially when the patient is most vulnerable [16]. Given the lack of communication training for ICU staff, staff support is missing for families as they also struggle to communicate with the patient. Moreover, ICU staff tend to rely on families' interpretation to understand what the patient is trying to communicate [19–21]. Families' discomfort with communication impairments may worsen frustration and distress in patients.

A crucial component of family-centered care in the ICU includes communication between families and the ICU staff. In a review, families of the critically ill identify reassurance and information sharing as the highest priorities [22]. Proximity to the patient, comfort, and support are additional priorities for families [23, 24]. Poor family-clinician communication can result in misunderstanding of the patient's condition and treatments. For this reason, families identify good communication from clinicians as the one key determinant of family satisfaction that needs improvement [25].

Pandemic Impact on Families of ICU Patients

The SARS-CoV-2 outbreak is a critical event that further challenged and demanded the adoption of alternate approaches to family communication in critical care settings. Due to the highly contagious nature of the disease, hospitals initiated policies to protect patients and health care workers and to contain the spread of SARS-CoV-2 [26]. Family visitation was restricted at the height of the pandemic with the intent to protect patients, families, and health care workers by minimizing exposures [27, 28] and to ration personal protective equipment (PPE), which was in short supply early in the pandemic. These restrictions resulted in dramatic decreases in family engagement in the ICU [29]. Contact with families was reported as one of the most important strategies to lower risk of delirium [30]. While more evidence is on the way, studies have consistently reported that restriction of visitation and separation resulted in increased feelings of uncertainty, guilt, helplessness, and negative impact on physical and mental health for family members of critically ill patients [31, 32].

These restrictions resulted in three major challenges to patient communication in the ICU. First, PPE obscures important verbal and nonverbal cues that patients rely on to interpret and comprehend messages. Next, restrictions were instituted on non-disposable equipment entering patient rooms. This would exclude many communication aids that could enhance patient communication. Finally, visitor restrictions resulted in fewer communication opportunities for patients. These included both communication exchanges with clinicians and with families.

Technology Adoption During the SARS-CoV-2 Pandemic

As technology has become more central in our lives, health care settings have also adopted technology in many ways. During the SARS-CoV-2 pandemic, we saw rapid expansion and use of communication technologies as alternatives for oral communication among patients, providers, and family members or family communication with providers in the ICU.

Communication technologies (e.g., electronic devices) and tools (e.g., picture-word communication boards, alphabet boards, writing tools) are forms of aided augmentative and alternative communication (AAC). AAC refers to all the ways we share ideas and feelings without talking [33].

In an integrative literature review on the use of communication technologies in adult acute-critical care settings across a 5-year period (2017–2022), we identified 71 relevant articles consisting primarily of qualitative accounts and descriptions of providing AAC. Patient-family video visits were mentioned or the focus of 32 articles and 33 articles reported on testing ICU patient communication devices or device reviews [34]. Overall, our literature review showed new focal areas in patient communication technologies in acute-critical care settings relevant to the

SARS-CoV-2 pandemic: video calls and electronic tablet applications. Published case studies portray the usage of a range of AAC technologies and techniques in complex cases of adult and older adult ICU patients with SARS-CoV-2 infection [35, 36]. Even with individualized speech and physical therapy interventions, time points for achieving communication goals were prolonged for SARS-CoV-2 patients [35, 36].

Box 3.1 Case Exemplar of a Communication Strategy [36]
A 70-year-old Spanish-speaking patient with acute respiratory distress syndrome and microhemorrhages (stroke) was so seriously ill that communication assessment and intervention did not begin until the patient's 57th day in the ICU. Answering simple yes/no questions was complicated by the need for an interpreter, the use of PPE on the part of providers, and the patient's extreme weakness and problems with cognition. The communication intervention for this patient included the use of a video interpreter and yes/no questions from a prepared Spanish-English question list, repeating questions, and reducing environmental distractions. The intervention decreased the patient's frustration and helped nurses feel more comfortable communicating with him.

According to a recent integrative review on the use of technology to engage family members in the ICU, a few studies used technology-based strategies to improve family communication in the ICU during the SARS-CoV-2 pandemic [37]. These studies aimed to enhance family members' participation and provide daily clinical updates via remote family conferences [38] or enable virtual ICU visitation via smartphones, tablets, or computers [39]. These studies provide examples of the recent science of technology use for family communication during the SARS-CoV-2 pandemic. The review findings suggest that future studies need to consider the inclusion of patient and family clinical outcomes to test the effectiveness of technology and involve more active family engagement in developing and implementing technology-based communication strategies [37].

Video Calls

Videoconferencing was (and continues to be) used worldwide during the pandemic as a method to enable virtual family presence at the bedside in intensive care, in communication about treatment decision-making, during end-of-life care, and throughout recovery [38–41]. Video visits during critical illness are delivered on special secure platforms or via Zoom or FaceTime. While these video visits provide many benefits, including a means to include remote family members in family meetings and decision-making and patient visits, videoconferencing should not replace in-person meetings [42]. Video visits may help reassure family members by seeing the patient's level of comfort and care [43, 44]. Conversely, some family members reported that visualizing the patient presented a distressing picture and was emotionally difficult [43–46]. Clinician time in facilitating the video visits and patient visual and/or hearing impairments were identified as barriers to using video visits [46]. Other concerns about video visits include equitable access to videoconferencing technology and the authenticity of technology-assisted interactions [46].

Negro and colleagues (2020) created a useful check list to guide planning and implementation of video visits (see Figs. 3.1 and 3.2) [47]. This guidance emphasizes the importance of preparing patients and family for what to expect, advising families on the technological requirements, and having a designated staff member to assist patients and families with the call. In some cases, this may include interpreting a nonvocal patient's messages using available AAC tools.

In addition to web-based remote family conferences and video calls with conscious patients, diaries, drawings, text messages, media groups, and virtual ICU visits were all instituted and utilized during the pandemic [48].

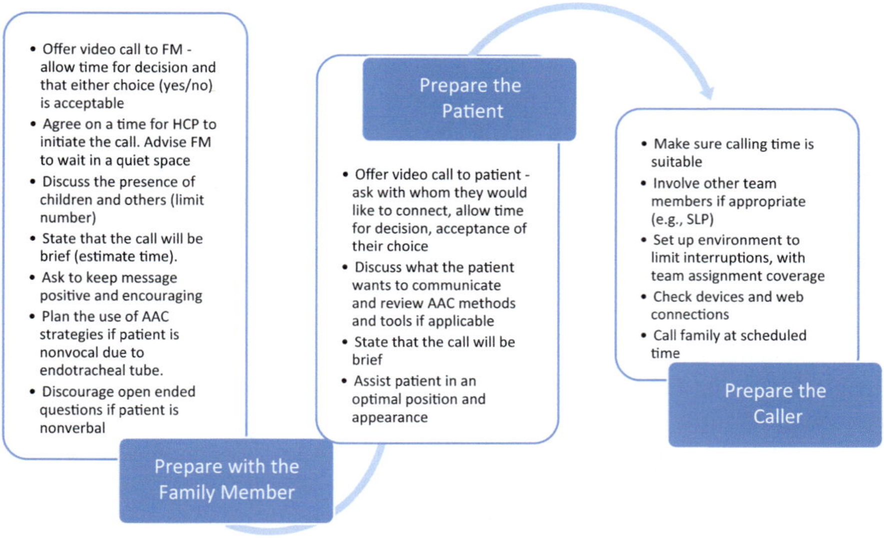

Fig. 3.1 Preparing for the video call in the ICU [47]. *FM* family member, *HCP* health care provider, *AAC* augmentative and alternative communication, *SLP* speech language pathologist. (Adapted from Negro A, Mucci M, Beccaria P, et al. Introducing the video call to facilitate the communication between health care providers and families of patients in the intensive care unit during COVID-19 pandemia. *Intensive & critical care nursing*. 2020;60:102893)

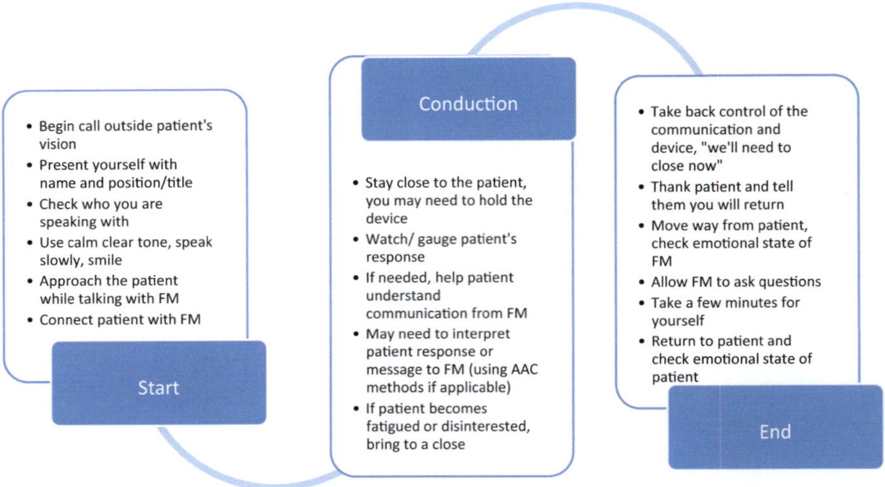

Fig. 3.2 Conducting the video call in the ICU [47]. (Adapted from Negro A, Mucci M, Beccaria P, et al. Introducing the video call to facilitate the communication between health care providers and families of patients in the intensive care unit during COVID-19 pandemia. *Intensive & critical care nursing*. 2020;60:102893)

Electronic Tablet Applications

With the influx of iPads and android tablets to the ICU to facilitate video visits, patient communication applications became more available for use in the ICU. For example, the VidaTalk™ patient communication application was offered free of charge for a limited period.

Research conducted prior to the pandemic provided evidence of the impact of communication via the patient communication application on family members' experience of communication interactions with their critically ill patient [49].

Dr. Ji Won Shin conducted a series of qualitative interviews with seven family visitors of mechanically ventilated ICU patients who received an electronic tablet with the VidaTalk™ patient communication application [18]. This study was nested within a randomized controlled trial testing the efficacy of the application. The study found that family members perceived the use of an electronic communication application to be helpful in "opening up" communication with their nonvocal patients by allowing clearer communication and expanding communication content. Family members reported feeling happy, thankful, and relieved to be able to communicate with the patient [18]. Family members described feeling less frustrated and less stressed when using the application in communication with patients. Patients were able to express their feelings using the application and patients and families often said "I love you" to each other.

Resources

Given the changing landscape related to communication with ICU patients and their families post-SARS-CoV-2, there are a variety of resources available to assist clinicians and family members. For example, a national group of interprofessional experts formed a SARS-CoV-2 task force to inform clinicians about best communication practices in these circumstances and to create a suite of free communication tools, language translations, and tips which are available on the Patient-Provider Communication website (https://www.patientprovidercommunication.org). Our research team also made video examples of communication techniques available as quick communication support demonstrations on the SPEACS-2 website (https://nucleus.con.ohio-state.edu/media/speacs2/speacs.htm). In addition, we collaborated with the American Thoracic Society Nursing Assembly to produce a podcast on "Tips for Communicating with your COVID-19 Patients on Mechanical Ventilation" [50].

Summary

The SARS-CoV-2 pandemic placed an urgency on the dissemination of communication materials and education and support for bedside providers [51]. Clinicians in the ICU need access to simple communication tools to quickly and reliably interpret patient messages and to help patients understand instructions and messages from care providers who are wearing PPE. Speech-language pathologists are experts in the assessment and provision of AAC and are essential to the provision of communication support for communication-impaired patients. However, basic communication assessment skills and the appropriate selection and use of simple AAC tools to facilitate communication should be standard competencies for all critical care clinicians.

Critical illness represents a significant source of stress and psychological crisis for families of patients in the ICU. Families have been recognized as crucial members of the care team with their physical presence at the bedside to facilitate trust, communication, and shared decision-making. Since the SARS-CoV-2 pandemic, restrictions to family visitation were imperative to protect all stakeholders from viral transmission despite many known adverse consequences to patients, families, and health care workers. This historical crisis has expedited adoption of technological interventions as viable opportunities for contact and communication between the patient and their family members. Many of these strategies should be continued in the post-pandemic era for selected situations when the family is unable to be present at the ICU bedside.

References

1. Davidson JE, Aslakson RA, Long AC, et al. Guidelines for family-centered care in the neonatal, pediatric, and adult ICU. Crit Care Med. 2017;45(1):103–28.
2. Rotondi AJ, Chelluri L, Sirio C, et al. Patients' recollections of stressful experiences while receiving prolonged mechanical ventilation in an intensive care unit. Crit Care Med. 2002;30(4):746–52.
3. Guttormson JL, Bremer KL, Jones RM. "Not being able to talk was horrid": a descriptive, correlational study of communication during mechanical ventilation. Intensive Crit Care Nurs. 2015;31(3):179–86.
4. Tembo AC, Higgins I, Parker V. The experience of communication difficulties in critically ill patients in and beyond intensive care: findings from a larger phenomenological study. Intensive Crit Care Nurs. 2015;31(3):171–8.
5. Karlsson V, Lindahl B, Bergbom I. Patients' statements and experiences concerning receiving mechanical ventilation: a prospective video-recorded study. Nurs Inq. 2012;19(3):247–58.
6. Khalaila R, Zbidat W, Anwar K, Bayya A, Linton DM, Sviri S. Communication difficulties and psychoemotional distress in patients receiving mechanical ventilation. Am J Crit Care. 2011;20(6):470–9.
7. Baumgarten M, Poulsen I. Patients' experiences of being mechanically ventilated in an ICU: a qualitative metasynthesis. Scand J Caring Sci. 2015;29(2):205–14.
8. Nelson JE, Meier DE, Litke A, Natale DA, Siegel RE, Morrison RS. The symptom burden of chronic critical illness. Crit Care Med. 2004;32(7):1527–34.
9. Nelson JE, Meier DE, Oei EJ, et al. Self-reported symptom experience of critically ill cancer patients receiving intensive care. Crit Care Med. 2001;29(2):277–82.
10. Pennock BE, Crawshaw L, Maher T, Price T, Kaplan PD. Distressful events in the ICU as perceived by patients recovering from coronary artery bypass surgery. Heart Lung. 1994;23(4):323–7.
11. Menzel LK. Factors related to the emotional responses of intubated patients to being unable to speak. Heart Lung. 1998;27(4):245–52.
12. Radtke JV, Tate JA, Happ MB. Nurses' perceptions of communication training in the ICU. Intensive Crit Care Nurs. 2012;28(1):16–25.
13. Holm A, Viftrup A, Karlsson V, Nikolajsen L, Dreyer P. Nurses' communication with mechanically ventilated patients in the intensive care unit: umbrella review. J Adv Nurs. 2020;76(11):2909–20.
14. Holm A, Dreyer P. Nurse-patient communication within the context of non-sedated mechanical ventilation: a hermeneutic-phenomenological study. Nurs Crit Care. 2018;23(2):88–94.
15. Yoo HJ, Lim OB, Shim JL. Critical care nurses' communication experiences with patients and families in an intensive care unit: A qualitative study. Plos one. 2020;15(7):e0235694.
16. Broyles LM, Tate JA, Happ MB. Use of augmentative and alternative communication strategies by family members in the intensive care unit. Am J Crit Care. 2012;21(2):e21–32.
17. Dziadzko V, Dziadzko MA, Johnson MM, Gajic O, Karnatovskaia LV. Acute psychological trauma in the critically ill: patient and family perspectives. Gen Hosp Psychiatry. 2017;47:68–74.
18. Shin JW, Happ MB, Tate JA. VidaTalk™ patient communication application "opened up" communication between nonvocal ICU patients and their family. Intensive Crit Care Nurs. 2021;66:103075.
19. Engstrom A, Soderberg S. Receiving power through confirmation: the meaning of close relatives for people who have been critically ill. J Adv Nurs. 2007;59(6):569–76. https://doi.org/10.1111/j.1365-2648.2007.04336.x.
20. Magnus VS, Turkington L. Communication interaction in ICU—patient and staff experiences and perceptions. Intensive Crit Care Nurs. 2006;22(3):167–80. https://doi.org/10.1016/j.iccn.2005.09.009.

21. Tolotti A, Bagnasco A, Catania G, et al. The communication experience of tracheostomy patients with nurses in the intensive care unit: a phenomenological study. Intensive Crit Care Nurs. 2018;46:24–31.
22. Al-Mutair AS, Plummer V, O'Brien A, Clerehan R. Family needs and involvement in the intensive care unit: a literature review. J Clin Nurs. 2013;22(13–14):1805–17.
23. Alsharari AF. The needs of family members of patients admitted to the intensive care unit. Patient Prefer Adherence. 2019;13:465.
24. Høghaug G, Fagermoen MS, Lerdal A. The visitor's regard of their need for support, comfort, information proximity and assurance in the intensive care unit. Intensive Crit Care Nurs. 2012;28(5):263–8.
25. Fumis RRL, Nishimoto IN, Deheinzelin D. Families' interactions with physicians in the intensive care unit: the impact on family's satisfaction. J Crit Care. 2008;23(3):281–6.
26. Altschuler T, Santiago R, Gormley J. Ensuring communication access for all during the COVID-19 pandemic and beyond: supporting patients, providers, and caregivers in hospitals. Augment Altern Commun. 2021;37(3):155–67.
27. Marmo S, Milner KA. From open to closed: COVID-19 restrictions on previously unrestricted visitation policies in adult intensive care units. Am J Crit Care. 2023;32(1):31–41.
28. Hart JL, Turnbull AE, Oppenheim IM, Courtright KR. Family-centered care during the COVID-19 era. J Pain Symptom Manag. 2020;60(2):e93–7.
29. Liu K, Nakamura K, Katsukawa H, et al. ABCDEF bundle and supportive ICU practices for patients with coronavirus disease 2019 infection: an international point prevalence study. Crit Care Explor. 2021;3(3):e0353. https://doi.org/10.1097/cce.0000000000000353.
30. Pun BT, Badenes R, La Calle GH, et al. Prevalence and risk factors for delirium in critically ill patients with COVID-19 (COVID-D): a multicentre cohort study. Lancet Respir Med. 2021;9(3):239–50.
31. Chen C, Wittenberg E, Sullivan SS, Lorenz RA, Chang Y-P. The experiences of family members of ventilated COVID-19 patients in the intensive care unit: a qualitative study. Am J Hospice Palliat Med. 2021;38(7):869–76.
32. Amass T, Van Scoy LJ, Hua M, et al. Stress-related disorders of family members of patients admitted to the intensive care unit with COVID-19. JAMA Intern Med. 2022;182:624.
33. American Speech Language Hearing Association (ASHA). Augmentative and Alternative Communication American Speech-Language-Hearing Association. 2022. https://www.asha.org/public/speech/disorders/AAC/. Accessed 19 Dec 2022.
34. Happ MB, Miller ES, Tate JA, Shin J. Current applications of patient communication technologies in geriatric critical care. Indianapolis, IN: Gerontological Society of America; 2022.
35. Mooney B, Lawrence C, Johnson EG, Slaboden A, Ball K. How COVID-19 patients were moved to speak: a rehabilitation interdisciplinary case series. HSS J. 2020;16(1_Suppl):56–63.
36. Scibilia SJ, Gendreau SK, Towbin RT, Happ MB. Impact of COVID-19 on patient-provider communication in critical care. Crit Care Nurse. 2022;42:e1–9.
37. Shin JW, Choi J, Tate J. Interventions using digital technology to promote family engagement in the adult intensive care unit: an integrative review. Heart Lung. 2023;58:166–78.
38. Carlucci M, Carpagnano LF, Dalfino L, Dalfino L, Migliore G. Stand by me 2.0. Visits by family members at COVID-19 time. Acta Biomed. 2020;91(2):71–4. https://doi.org/10.23750/abm.v91i2.9569.
39. Sasangohar F, Dhala A, Zheng F, Ahmadi N, Kash B, Masud F. Use of telecritical care for family visitation to ICU during the COVID-19 pandemic: an interview study and sentiment analysis. BMJ Qual Saf. 2020;30:715. https://doi.org/10.1136/bmjqs-2020-011604.
40. Langer T, Depalo FC, Forlini C, et al. Communication and visiting policies in Italian intensive care units during the first COVID-19 pandemic wave and lockdown: a nationwide survey. BMC Anesthesiol. 2022;22(1):1–11.
41. Rose L, Cook A, Casey J, Meyer J. Restricted family visiting in intensive care during COVID-19. Intensive Crit Care Nurs. 2020;60:102896.

42. Kennedy NR, Steinberg A, Arnold RM, et al. Perspectives on telephone and video communication in the intensive care unit during COVID-19. Ann Am Thorac Soc. 2021;18(5):838–47.
43. Azoulay É, Curtis JR, Kentish-Barnes N. Ten reasons for focusing on the care we provide for family members of critically ill patients with COVID-19. Intensive Care Med. 2021;47(2):230–3.
44. Feder S, Smith D, Griffin H, et al. "Why couldn't I go in to see him?" Bereaved families' perceptions of end-of-life communication during COVID-19. J Am Geriatr Soc. 2021;69(3):587–92.
45. Bartoli D, Trotta F, Simeone S, et al. The lived experiences of family members of Covid-19 patients admitted to intensive care unit: a phenomenological study. Heart Lung. 2021;50(6):926–32.
46. Elma A, Cook D, Howard M, et al. Use of video technology in end-of-life care for hospitalized patients during the COVID-19 pandemic. Am J Crit Care. 2022;31(3):240–8.
47. Negro A, Mucci M, Beccaria P, et al. Introducing the video call to facilitate the communication between health care providers and families of patients in the intensive care unit during COVID-19 pandemia. Intensive Crit Care Nurs. 2020;60:102893.
48. Arabi YM, Azoulay E, Al-Dorzi HM, et al. How the COVID-19 pandemic will change the future of critical care. Intensive Care Med. 2021;47(3):282–91.
49. Shin JW, Tan A, Tate J, Balas M, Dabelko-Schoeny H, Happ MB. Preliminary efficacy of the vidatalk™ communication application on family psychological symptoms in the intensive care unit: A pilot study. Heart & Lung. 2025;70:14–22.
50. Happ M, Tate JA. Tips for communicating with your COVID-19 patients on mechanical ventilation. 2020. https://www.thoracic.org/about/ats-podcasts/tips-for-communicating-with-yourcovid-19-patients-on-mechanical-ventilation.php. Accessed 6 May 2021.
51. Happ MB. Giving voice: nurse-patient communication in the intensive care unit. Am J Crit Care. 2021;30(4):256–65.

Chapter 4
Strategies to Facilitate Communication with Families in the ICU

Andre Carlos Kajdacsy-Balla Amaral

Introduction: A Framework for Communication

Communication lies in the center of all sociocultural interactions [1]. Actions are a product of social interactions and are preceded by some sort of communication. Therefore, it follows that communication is a *necessary* component of systems composed of more than one subject, to initiate and guide actions towards achieving a goal.

To better understand strategies to improve communication it is helpful to consider a framework, such as the one based on the seminal work of Shannon [2], which describes communication as the flow of information between two points. This framework considers communication as a rational process, not taking into account social characteristics of the participants, limitations in memory, and how cognition influences communication [3]. However, it needs to be expanded to include these three elements that modulate the flow of information and underline why the same type of information sharing leads to different actions and outcomes in encounters with different parties.

For this chapter we define communication as the exchange of *information* and *meaning* between subjects, which is modulated by cognition, social aspects of the interaction and memory constraints [4].

A. C. K.-B. Amaral (✉)
Department of Critical Care Medicine, Sunnybrook Health Sciences Centre, Interdepartmental Division of Critical Care Medicine, University of Toronto, Toronto, ON, Canada
e-mail: andrecarlos.amaral@sunnybrook.ca

© The Author(s), under exclusive license to Springer Nature Switzerland AG 2025

A. J. Vance et al. (eds.), *Families in the Intensive Care Unit*,
https://doi.org/10.1007/978-3-031-83786-9_4

Cognitive Influences on Communication

Because individuals have different *cognitive processes*, people understand the same information and meaning in different ways. Clinicians interpret a statement of "do not resuscitate" (DNR) differently, depending on their cognitive background. In a recent survey, patients with a DNR orders would not be offered antibiotics or oxygen therapy by of 6% hospital physicians, 27% of nurses, and 30% of primary practice doctors ($p < 0.001$) [5]. Therefore, it is no surprise that discussion of a "no resuscitation" order with families is likely to lead to confusion. Many families will instinctively (and rightly so) believe it means "no more treatments."

Environmental factors influence cognition and understanding information. The same information is associated with different responses if received under (1) strenuous conditions (such as the family that was awake all night, or struggling to visit their loved one while working and taking care of their immediate family); (2) emotional distress (such as a family members being angry due to perceptions of unfairness, which leads to nonrational decisions [6]); or (3) time constraints.

For example, if a family member comes to visit their loved one after an entire day of work and family obligations, their cognitive and emotional capacities will be exhausted and they won't be able to fully engage and understand complex problems, increasing the likelihood of default decisions, such as no change in goals of care. This phenomenon of cognitive exhaustion is well described in other situations. For example, primary care clinicians prescribe more antibiotics for upper respiratory tract infections during late morning or late afternoon appointments [7].

Another important source of cognitive biases are the rules and norms of an institution. Local norms related to end-of-life practices are as influential on decision-making as patient characteristics. For example, admission to a hospital with high rates of DNR orders increases the chances of a DNR order to a similar magnitude that a diagnosis of metastatic cancer carries [8]. The explanation for this phenomenon was elegantly demonstrated in a high-fidelity simulation study. Researchers enrolled clinicians from two organizations within the same state, but on opposite ends of the spectrum of treatment intensity at end-of-life. When exposed to the same simulated patient with a known preference for no intubation or ICU admission clinicians from the hospital that usually provided higher intensity end-of-life care felt more conflict about not providing life supporting therapies [9].

The Role of Clinician's Emotional Response on Communication and Treatment Options

It's important to also consider that clinicians are human and affected by their own emotional responses, which may influence the quality of communication, clinical assessments and how treatment options are explored with families and patients.

In a qualitative study of primary care clinicians, the clinician's emotional response to a patient's request for antidepressants—frequently characterized by annoyance—influenced their assessment and led to changes in decision-making, a bias that was not recognized by clinicians [10].

Unrecognized emotions are frequently experienced by physicians [11] and may be associated with harmful behaviors, such as inappropriately interrupting the patient, changing the subject, avoiding patients' psychological issues, avoiding bonding with patients to prevent suffering, avoiding conducting certain medical procedures again, or avoiding patients altogether [12].

Emotions influence decision-making and outcomes as demonstrated in a simulation study of "rude" parents in pediatrics. The authors randomized teams to meet with simulated parents that would either provide rude comments unrelated to the team's performance or to a control group with neutral comments. Simulation scores for both treatment and team communication were lower in those teams exposed to rudeness demonstrating the significant impact on clinical performance of the emotional response to the parents' behavior. This effect was mitigated by a strategy to modify cognitive biases before the encounters [13].

Social Influences on Communication

Social characteristics of the participants—such as ethnicity, professional background, age, gender—will influence the amount, type, and quality of information sharing and understanding. These social determinants of communication can be divided into three social dimensions: *affinity, rank, and knowledge* [4]. Greater perceived distances in social dimensions limit shared understanding of problems and impair communication (Table 4.1).

Affinity between subjects is how similar they see each other. These similarities include gender, age, ethnicity, language, citizenship, and other characteristics. We use the term *affinity distance* to describe differences in these characteristics between parties involved in a conversation. Affinity distances influence communication, for example, in a study of perceived differences about health beliefs, patients cared by

Table 4.1 Social dimensions that influence communication

Social dimension	Definition	Example
Affinity	The degree to which participants perceive similarities between them	Race, gender, and cultural background influence decision-making [15, 16]
Ranking	The degree to which participants perceive hierarchical differences between them	Information sharing and acceptance of palliation at end-of-life are influenced by socioeconomic status [17, 18]
Specific knowledge	The degree to which participants have differences in knowledge in a specific domain (such as medicine)	Physicians overestimate medical literacy and tend to be more empathetic towards patients with higher educational background [20, 21]

clinicians of the same race were more likely to share health beliefs than patients cared by clinicians of a different race [14], similarly, matching patient to physician's gender improves the quality of patient-centered communication [15].

An interesting manifestation of the affinity distance is exemplified in a study about recent immigrants to Canada, suggesting that cultural background had an important influence on decisions at the end-of-life. Compared to long-term residents, immigrants to Canada had a higher relative risk of receiving ICU admission (RR 1.16), mechanical ventilation (RR 1.28) or tracheostomy (RR 1.61) at the end-of-life [16]. Interestingly, this effect was no longer observed for immigrants that had lived in Canada for longer than 10 years, suggesting an adaptation to the social values and norms.

Ranking is how individuals see themselves as "higher," "lower" or in the "same" rank as the other subject. For example, a soldier will recognize the higher rank of a lieutenant while in the army but may assign the same rank when they meet in a nonmilitary party. Greater rank distances impair communication. For example, socioeconomic status shapes communication encounters between patients and physicians. Patients from lower socioeconomic status experience a more directive and less participatory consultation, while those from higher classes receive more information from physicians [17], which may be one of the reasons underlying an increased willingness to accept palliation for patients on prolonged mechanical ventilation in families with higher income [18].

Specific knowledge is the amount of task-related knowledge that a subject has. More knowledgeable subjects will assume a more active role in communications, while less knowledgeable subjects will assume a more passive role. Greater knowledge distances impair communication [19]. This is an important implicit bias, demonstrated by physicians more frequently "mirroring" body language from patients with higher educational backgrounds [20]. Information should be discussed at the proper literacy level, but unfortunately physicians overestimate medical literacy in as many as 54% of patients [21].

In an attempt to improve families' understanding of key concepts in critically ill patients, Peigne and colleagues conducted an extensive mixed-methods study to identify key questions that families should ask clinicians [22], however a randomized trial where families received a copy of these questions to use during meetings was not successful in improving families' comprehension or satisfaction [23]. Although the results are disappointing, they may simply represent a failure of the method used to educate families and not necessarily of the concept. Clearly further research is necessary on how to best improve health literacy for patients and families.

The Effects of Memory on Communication

Memory capacity influences communication. In communications with families about diagnosis, treatments, and prognosis, most, if not all, the information is novel. Because we are able to deal with 7 (±2) items at a time cognitively [24], the amount of information that can be processed by families is limited and excess information will be forgotten or misunderstood. The implications for communication are clear, in complex cases multiple meetings and repetition of the information [25] are required to allow families to understand all relevant information, and in simpler cases the amount of information should be limited to allow for better understanding and decision-making.

Communication Moments in the Critical Care Environment

We meet family members both in formal and informal moments. The most recognized moments of communication with families are interprofessional rounds (IPR) and family meetings, however informal moments, such as bedside updates outside of IPR are common and considered very valuable by families [25].

IPR are key moments of patient-centered interprofessional communication, collaboration, and education. These moments can be used to engage patients and families in information-sharing and decision-making, effectively creating family- and patient-centered rounds (FCR) [26, 27]. Family presence at bedside rounds is advocated by various professional organizations in health care, but nowhere is the need for family-centered rounds greater than in intensive care units (ICUs), where many patients lack the capacity for medical decision-making [27].

Family inclusion in rounds is the least studied area within family-centered care, especially in adult ICUs. Data from two systematic reviews of family presence on rounds in neonatal, pediatric, adult ICUs, and medical wards reveal that family-centered rounds can lead to increased satisfaction among patients, families, and health care staff, enhance communication among them, and decrease family stress and anxiety while improving patient outcomes [26, 27].

If family-centered principles are not translated into practice, family-centered rounds may not have their intended results [28]. An international survey of rounding practices shows great variation in family presence during rounds, varying from 92% in North America to less than 40% in Latin America [29]. Barriers to include families on rounds include concerns about duration of discussions, appropriate teaching, and difficulties in discussing goals of care during rounds [30]. These concerns are not backed up by empirical data. Post-implementation data of family inclusion on rounds in a trauma center suggests that their presence may actually favor more discussions about goals of care, and reduces the need for family meetings (from 5 meeting/week to less than 1 meeting/week, $p < 0.01$) [31]. In a single-center observational study of rounding time and ICU strain, the presence of families on rounds did not influence the duration of individual patient's rounding time [32]. These results should be seen in the light of the potential unintended consequence of not providing families with enough time for questions and decision-making [33].

On the other end of the spectrum, scheduled family meetings cover a large spectrum of the current literature on communication with families of critically ill patients. Having a formal family meeting within a pre-specified timeframe is even considered by some to be an important marker of quality of care. However, it is important to recognize that the literature on family meetings for critically ill patients heavily emphasizes end-of-life care and relatively little effort is devoted to understanding the communication practices and gaps with family members of patients where a decision about end-of-life is not being sought. Therefore, the discussion around strategies to improve communication will also rely on data from other clinical settings. The integration of formal (family meetings and bedside rounds), informal communication moments (bedside updates) and the more recent practice of daily phone calls [34] is probably necessary to fully support the different communication and information needs of all patients and family members in an ICU [35].

Strategies to Improve Communication in the Critical Care Environment

Guidelines and Good Communication Practices

Several examples of good communication practices exist in the literature [27]. They are presented here for completeness, but the more in-depth discussion is limited to other strategies (Table 4.2) where relevant gaps exist and clinicians may not be aware of them.

Good communication practices in critical care include:

1. Establish early (less than 48 h) meetings with families/patients.
2. Use a "shared decision-making" model.
3. Have consistent staff for each patient.
4. Interprofessional team participates in communication.
5. Open visitation, including participation on rounds.

Increase Medical Literacy of Patients and Families

Tools and behaviors aimed at increasing medical literacy should improve communication by decreasing social distances, helping patients and families better understand treatment options. Better understanding leads to better decision-making. For example, in a study about surrogate decision-makers willingness to accept palliation for patients on prolonged mechanical ventilation, better knowledge of palliative care was associated with increases in acceptance of palliation [18].

However, families understand very little about critical illness. Only 50% of families can describe whether the patient is at risk of dying and they don't know which organs are failing or which treatments are being provided in the ICU [36]. Families' limited understanding of these issues makes it "*almost impossible*" to make informed decisions [37].

Table 4.2 Strategies to improve communication with families

Strategy	Mechanisms	Example
Increase medical literacy	Decreases knowledge distances	Video-assisted education on goals of care [38–41, 67]
Default options and clear recommendations	Decreases cognitive exhaustion of family members	Default option for "comfort care," when appropriate [42]
Explore and validate concerns	Decreases clinicians' cognitive fatigue and implicit social biases Decreases affinity distance Improves family recall of conversation	Clinician training on empathy [51, 53, 67] VALUE mnemonic [54] Engage palliative care in family meetings [56] Use tools to help families express their concerns [52]
Train emotional self-awareness	Decreases clinicians' implicit social biases	Reframe problems to consider alternative approaches [58, 59]
Avoid conflicting information	Decreases knowledge distance Decreases cognitive load	Nighttime communication bundle [61] Daily written communication [62]
Use strategies to mitigate implicit biases in communication	Decreases social distances	Pre-meet with translator prior to family meeting [64] Daily phone calls to families [34]

The systematic use of tools that cover knowledge gaps leads to changes in decision-making. In a randomized trial of 119 hospitalized patients, preference for a DNR order was 56% for those who watched a video about code status and cardiopulmonary resuscitation (CPR), versus 17% in a control group ($p < 0.01$) [38]. Similar effects of video-assisted education were seen for intubation preferences in hospitalized patients [39], and for prioritizing comfort care in outpatients with advanced heart failure [40] and elderly patients [41].

It is possible that these effects are mediated not solely by the improved knowledge (in this case about goals of care), but also by providing information in a standardized way and without emotional attachments (positive or negative) that may exist if the same information was provided by clinicians caring for the patient.

Consider the Use Default Options and Make Clear Recommendations When Medically Appropriate

When presenting therapeutic options, the format of presentation influences decision-making. For example, in a randomized controlled trial of advance directives, patients were randomized to three groups, and received the same advance directive document. However, one group received the document with "comfort care" as the default, a second received a "life extension" default, and a third received it without a default.

Patients were allowed to choose their option and if it differed from the default, they would cross it out and choose their preference. Patients with a default of "comfort care" chose comfort care more frequently than those randomized to "life extension" (77% vs. 41%, $p < 0.01$) [42]. Similarly, the manner of presenting a preferred medical treatment influences understanding of prognosis. In a simulated study that compared a direct and clear response to a question on prognosis versus indirect responses or redirection of the discussion led to a clearer understanding of a poor prognosis when the response was direct [43].

However, institutions' cultural aspects influence how clinicians present and discuss care plans at the end-of-life. In a study of four US hospitals with distinct approaches and cultures towards autonomy and best interests, the training environment influenced trainees' attitudes regarding decision-making, and on their willingness to discuss and suggest limitations in goals of care [44]. Those trained in hospitals with a strong patient autonomy culture had an unreflective attitude about autonomy and would offer treatments at the end-of-life even when their medical expertise would suggest otherwise. Default options and teaching clarity of language help in solving this problem as they institutionalize the suggested "norm" for certain conditions, while empowering patients and families to make different decisions.

These results strongly suggest that framing decisions and answers influences choice. Therefore, when clinicians communicate and propose plans of care, the plan that is medically preferred should be suggested. While patient autonomy for decision-making is pivotal in communication, it should not be used as an excuse to avoid making medical recommendations when a preferred approach exists. Professional guidance is relevant for medical decision-making and should be used to help families.

Explore and Validate Concerns

Exploring and validating patient's concerns leads to in-depth understanding of patient's symptoms, feelings, expectations, and ideas. When patients/families ask questions or make assertive statements/requests in a meeting, exploring these concerns can influence outcomes of the discussion. In fact, the emotional content of family meetings in the ICU is associated with increased family satisfaction: (1) assurance that the patient will not be abandoned, (2) assurance that the patient will be comfortable and won't suffer, and (3) support for decisions about end-of-life, whether to withdrawal or not [45].

In an ideal situation, these concerns would prompt clinicians to further investigate the subject and come to better-informed decisions; on the other hand, said concerns may also lead to premature closure when taken at face value, leading to poorly-informed decisions. However, clinicians respond less frequently (28% vs. 72%) to patients' emotional cues compared to informational cues during an assessment [46], which is an important gap in communication as responding to those increases patient's recall of information [47]. Moreover, clinicians not only don't respond, but they also react to these emotional cues by reducing communication space (topic changing for example) instead of acknowledging the patient's emotional distress. For example, neurologists reacted to patient emotions by reducing space (changing subject, taking no notice, giving medical advice) for 58% of emotional cues and 76% of concerns [48]. This common behavior impairs communication and decision-making; for example, a clinician is ten times more likely to prescribe an antidepressant if emotional concerns are not explored during an appointment [49].

Responding to these cues in an empathetic way leads to greater family satisfaction [50]. The authors suggested the following recommendations for empathetic behaviors:

1. Take a moment at the beginning of a family conference to inquire into the families' emotional state.
2. Acknowledge both verbal and nonverbal expressions of emotion. Use these expressions of emotion as opportunities to support family members.
3. Create empathic opportunities by acknowledging that most families face a significant emotional burden when a loved one is critically ill or dying.

Clinicians can be trained to recognize and respond to these emotional cues [51] and patients can use tools, such as the interactive tailored patient assessment, to increase their expression of cues and concerns [52]. Strategies that include training clinicians on empathy and emotional support can lead to improved perception of the quality of communication and shorter ICU length-of-stay for dying patients [53]. Exploring concerns may also improve outcomes for family members. In a multicentric randomized trial in France, the use of a structured approach to family meetings at the end-of-life, which included several strategies directed to exploring and validating concerns (VALUE [54], Table 4.3), family member's symptoms of anxiety (67% vs. 45%, $p = 0.02$) and depression (56% vs. 29%, $p = 0.003$) decreased significantly in the intervention group [55].

Another potential strategy to improve response to emotional cues is to conduct combined meetings with palliative care. In combined meetings, the intensivist tends to provide clinical information, while the palliative care specialist would frequently focus on quality of life and provide families with emotional support, thus providing a balanced approach to communication [56]. However, it's worth noting that in one

Table 4.3 VALUE mnemonic to approach family meetings [54]

Item	Description
V	Value and appreciate what family members say
A	Acknowledge family members' emotions
L	Listen
U	Understand the patient as a person by asking questions
E	Elicit questions from family members

trial the systematic addition of palliative care-led meeting did not improve outcomes [57]. These results may have been influenced by the limited nature of the intervention which consisted of two structured meetings with the palliative team without mandatory presence of the ICU team, and the already very high perception of quality of communication, emotional support, and family satisfaction in the control group.

Train Emotional Self-Awareness

Because emotions interfere with clinician's responses to patients' and families' requests, increased self-awareness may lead to less biased assessments and treatments. Most aspects of social distances should be removed once the clinician practices self-awareness or consider the use of decision-rules that are clearly outlined. The act of removing these biases has also been termed *cognitive debiasing* and others have suggested several strategies to mitigate it [13, 58].

Consider self-reflection when in meetings with families. Self-reflection may help reframe problems and diagnosis to identify missing or incorrect information [59]. After, or ideally during an encounter, clinicians can ask themselves questions that may point towards biases and use these to reorient the discussion. Common questions that can help include:

1. Were there any points at which I wanted to end the visit prematurely?
2. If there were relevant data that I ignored, what might they be?
3. What would a trusted peer say about the way I managed this situation?
4. Were there any points at which I felt judgmental about the patient—in a positive or negative way?

Avoid Conflicting Information

Parents of hospitalized children most often attribute miscommunication to conflicting information from healthcare providers [60]. Families of critically ill patients are exposed to many different providers, increasing the chances of conflicting information, and decreasing trust in the team and satisfaction with care. As many of these encounters occur at night, strategies to improve nighttime communication may prove useful to increase family's experiences.

In a single-center pediatric study, a nighttime communication bundle led to improvements in parent-reported quality of communication [61]. The bundle included (1) an early nighttime interprofessional brief to discuss active patients and family concerns, (2) bedside team huddle on the two most active patients, and (3) a written family update sheet for the two most active patients written by the daytime team. A strategy commonly used by experienced clinicians to avoid the traps of conflicting information involves asking families to explain their understanding of the current situation, their expectations and what they have been told in previous encounters.

A novel strategy to provide clear and concise information is the use of daily written summaries. In a single-center, proof-of-concept study, families received a daily written communication summarizing the problems the patient experienced with a brief discussion of etiology, clinical trajectory, and ongoing investigations. This led to improvements in the quality of communication and in families' experience of depression and anxiety [62].

Use Strategies to Mitigate Implicit Biases in Communication

As discussed above under "Affinity," social distances will lead to implicit biases that are difficult to recognize and mitigate. These can further increase gaps in communication with families and patients of different social backgrounds and is a well-recognized source of conflict in the ICU [63].

Language barriers are one of the key elements of affinity distance. A study of end-of-life care for families with limited English proficiency identified several barriers to good communication, including limited ability to assess patient and family understanding, impaired relationship building, and limited ability for families to understand decision-making concepts. The authors suggested facilitators to improve communication such as pre-meeting between clinician and interpreter, and communication of different cultural perspectives [64].

The inclusion of clinicians of the same race, gender, and culture during family meetings can help discussions as it provides an opportunity for better understanding of concerns and issues [14, 15]. Similarly, facilitators trained to support communication between staff and families, adapt communication to each family's needs, and mediate conflicts can lead to a reduction in symptoms of depression in family members [65].

One important issue of equity and diversity is whether families can be available for rounds or informal discussions at the bedside during daytime. This is a barrier that will be encountered more frequently in families with limited economical resources and those who live further from the hospital, leading to further imbalances in communication with an already underprivileged population. Families that don't receive regular updates may feel panicky [66]. With the COVID-19 pandemic and restricted visitation policies a new practice of daily phone calls [34] or virtual visits [66] emerged, which should be considered as a standard of care for families that can't be in the unit during regular hours.

Conclusions

A framework for understanding communication beyond the simple concept of information sharing clarifies communication problems and potential solution. The role of emotions, cognition, social aspects, and memory in communication cannot be overlooked and may actually represent important variables that can help clinicians improve communication in difficult situations.

References

1. Eco U. A theory of semiotics. Indiana University Press; 1978. 354 p.
2. Shannon CE. A mathematical theory of communication. Bell System Tech J. 1948;27:379–423.
3. Kajdacsy-Balla Amaral AC. Facilitating interactions between healthcare providers in the ICU. In: Scales D, Rubenfeld G, editors. The organization of critical care, Respiratory medicine. New York: Humana; 2014. p. 109–25.
4. Kluver J, Kluver C. On communication: an interdisciplinary and mathematical approach. Dordrecht: Springer; 2007. 240 p
5. O'Brien H, Scarlett S, Brady A, Harkin K, Kenny RA, Moriarty J. Do-not-attempt-resuscitation (DNAR) orders: understanding and interpretation of their use in the hospitalised patient in Ireland. A brief report. J Med Ethics. 2017;44:201.
6. van't Wout M, Chang LJ, Sanfey AG. The influence of emotion regulation on social interactive decision-making. Emotion (Washington, DC). 2010;10(6):815–21.
7. Linder JA, Doctor JN, Friedberg MW, Reyes Nieva H, Birks C, Meeker D, et al. Time of day and the decision to prescribe antibiotics. JAMA Intern Med. 2014;174(12):2029–31.
8. Walkey AJ, Barnato AE, Rinne ST, Cooke CR, Shieh MS, Pekow PS, et al. Hospital variation in do-not-resuscitate orders and end-of-life healthcare use in the United States. Ann Am Thorac Soc. 2017;14(9):1485–9.
9. Barnato AE, Mohan D, Lane RK, Huang YM, Angus DC, Farris C, et al. Advance care planning norms may contribute to hospital variation in end-of-life ICU use: a simulation study. Med Decis Making. 2014;34(4):473–84.
10. Tentler A, Silberman J, Paterniti DA, Kravitz RL, Epstein RM. Factors affecting physicians' responses to patients' requests for antidepressants: focus group study. J Gen Intern Med. 2008;23(1):51–7.
11. Silva JV, Carvalho I. Physicians experiencing intense emotions while seeing their patients: what happens? Perm J. 2016;20(3):31–7.
12. Ely JW, Levinson W, Elder NC, Mainous AG III, Vinson DC. Perceived causes of family physicians' errors. J Fam Pract. 1995;40(4):337–44.
13. Riskin A, Erez A, Foulk TA, Riskin-Geuz KS, Ziv A, Sela R, et al. Rudeness and medical team performance. Pediatrics. 2017;139(2):e20162305.
14. Kennedy BM, Rehman M, Johnson WD, Magee MB, Leonard R, Katzmarzyk PT. Healthcare providers versus patients' understanding of health beliefs and values. Patient Exp J. 2017;4(3):29–37.
15. Sandhu H, Adams A, Singleton L, Clark-Carter D, Kidd J. The impact of gender dyads on doctor–patient communication: a systematic review. Patient Educ Couns. 2009;76(3):348–55.
16. Yarnell CJ, Fu L, Manuel D, Tanuseputro P, Stukel T, Pinto R, et al. Association between immigrant status and end-of-life care in Ontario, Canada. JAMA. 2017;318(15):1479–88.
17. Willems S, De Maesschalck S, Deveugele M, Derese A, De Maeseneer J. Socio-economic status of the patient and doctor-patient communication: does it make a difference? Patient Educ Couns. 2005;56(2):139–46.

18. Chen YC, Fan HY, Curtis JR, Lee OK, Liu CK, Huang SJ. Determinants of receiving palliative care and ventilator withdrawal among patients with prolonged mechanical ventilation. Crit Care Med. 2017;45(10):1625–34.
19. Boltey EM, Wright N, Mosley EA, White MR, Iwashyna TJ, Manojlovich M, et al. Exploring the process of information sharing in an adult intensive care unit: an ethnographic study. J Interprof Care. 2022;36(2):168–76.
20. Street R, Buller D. Patients characteristics affecting physician–patient nonverbal communication. Hum Commun Res. 1988;15:60–90.
21. Kelly PA, Haidet P. Physician overestimation of patient literacy: a potential source of health care disparities. Patient Educ Couns. 2007;66(1):119–22.
22. Peigne V, Chaize M, Falissard B, Kentish-Barnes N, Rusinova K, Megarbane B, et al. Important questions asked by family members of intensive care unit patients. Crit Care Med. 2011;39(6):1365–71.
23. Azoulay E, Forel JM, Vinatier I, Truillet R, Renault A, Valade S, et al. Questions to improve family-staff communication in the ICU: a randomized controlled trial. Intensive Care Med. 2018;44(11):1879–87.
24. Miller GA. The magical number seven plus or minus two: some limits on our capacity for processing information. Psychol Rev. 1956;63:81–97.
25. Kalocsai C, Amaral A, Piquette D, Walter G, Dev SP, Taylor P, et al. "It's better to have three brains working instead of one": a qualitative study of building therapeutic alliance with family members of critically ill patients. BMC Health Serv Res. 2018;18(1):533.
26. Cypress BS. Family presence on rounds: a systematic review of literature. Dimens Crit Care Nurs. 2012;31(1):53–64.
27. Davidson JE, Powers K, Hedayat KM, Tieszen M, Kon AA, Shepard E, et al. Clinical practice guidelines for support of the family in the patient-centered intensive care unit: American College of Critical Care Medicine Task Force 2004–2005. Crit Care Med. 2007;35(2):605–22.
28. Subramony A, Hametz PA, Balmer D. Family-centered rounds in theory and practice: an ethnographic case study. Acad Pediatr. 2014;14(2):200–6.
29. Amaral A, Vincent JL, Rose L, Mikkelsen ME, Webb S, Ramos GV, et al. An international perspective on the frequency, perception of utility, and quality of interprofessional rounds practices in intensive care units. J Crit Care. 2020;55:28–34.
30. Santiago C, Lazar L, Jiang D, Burns KE. A survey of the attitudes and perceptions of multidisciplinary team members towards family presence at bedside rounds in the intensive care unit. Intensive Crit Care Nurs. 2014;30(1):13–21.
31. Allen SR, Pascual J, Martin N, Reilly P, Luckianow G, Datner E, et al. A novel method of optimizing patient- and family-centered care in the ICU. J Trauma Acute Care Surg. 2017;82(3):582–6.
32. Brown SE, Rey MM, Pardo D, Weinreb S, Ratcliffe SJ, Gabler NB, et al. The allocation of intensivists' rounding time under conditions of intensive care unit capacity strain. Am J Respir Crit Care Med. 2014;190(7):831–4.
33. Jacobowski NL, Girard TD, Mulder JA, Ely EW. Communication in critical care: family rounds in the intensive care unit. Am J Crit Care. 2010;19(5):421–30.
34. Fritz C, Claude LA, Hamada S, Trosdorf M, de la Barre H, Yavchitz A, et al. Daily telephone call during the COVID-19 pandemic: perceptions of families and providers. Am J Crit Care. 2022;31(1):77–81.
35. Seaman JB, Arnold RM, Scheunemann LP, White DB. An integrated framework for effective and efficient communication with families in the adult intensive care unit. Ann Am Thorac Soc. 2017;14(6):1015–20.
36. Azoulay E, Chevret S, Leleu G, Pochard F, Barboteu M, Adrie C, et al. Half the families of intensive care unit patients experience inadequate communication with physicians. Crit Care Med. 2000;28(8):3044–9.
37. Nelson JEMDJD, Puntillo KAR, Pronovost PJM, Walker ASMA, McAdam JLR, Ilaoa DRN, et al. In their own words: patients and families define high-quality palliative care in the intensive care unit*. Crit Care Med. 2010;38(3):808–18.

38. Merino AM, Greiner R, Hartwig K. A randomized controlled trial of a CPR decision support video for patients admitted to the general medicine service. J Hosp Med. 2017;12(9):700–4.
39. El-Jawahri A, Mitchell SL, Paasche-Orlow MK, Temel JS, Jackson VA, Rutledge RR, et al. A randomized controlled trial of a CPR and intubation video decision support tool for hospitalized patients. J Gen Intern Med. 2015;30(8):1071–80.
40. El-Jawahri A, Paasche-Orlow MK, Matlock D, Stevenson LW, Lewis EF, Stewart G, et al. Randomized, controlled trial of an advance care planning video decision support tool for patients with advanced heart failure. Circulation. 2016;134(1):52–60.
41. Volandes AE, Paasche-Orlow MK, Barry MJ, Gillick MR, Minaker KL, Chang Y, et al. Video decision support tool for advance care planning in dementia: randomised controlled trial. BMJ. 2009;338:b2159.
42. Halpern SD, Loewenstein G, Volpp KG, Cooney E, Vranas K, Quill CM, et al. Default options in advance directives influence how patients set goals for end-of-life care. Health Affairs (Project Hope). 2013;32(2):408–17.
43. Oppenheim IM, Lee EM, Vasher ST, Zaeh SE, Hart JL, Turnbull AE. Effect of intensivist communication in a simulated setting on interpretation of prognosis among family members of patients at high risk of intensive care unit admission: a randomized trial. JAMA Netw Open. 2020;3(4):e201945.
44. Dzeng E, Colaianni A, Roland M, Chander G, Smith TJ, Kelly MP, et al. Influence of institutional culture and policies on do-not-resuscitate decision making at the end of life. JAMA Intern Med. 2015;175(5):812–9.
45. Stapleton RD, Engelberg RA, Wenrich MD, Goss CH, Curtis JR. Clinician statements and family satisfaction with family conferences in the intensive care unit. Crit Care Med. 2006;34(6):1679–85.
46. Butow PN, Brown RF, Cogar S, Tattersall MH, Dunn SM. Oncologists' reactions to cancer patients' verbal cues. Psychooncology. 2002;11(1):47–58.
47. Jansen J, van Weert JC, de Groot J, van Dulmen S, Heeren TJ, Bensing JM. Emotional and informational patient cues: the impact of nurses' responses on recall. Patient Educ Couns. 2010;79(2):218–24.
48. Del Piccolo L, Pietrolongo E, Radice D, Tortorella C, Confalonieri P, Pugliatti M, et al. Patient expression of emotions and neurologist responses in first multiple sclerosis consultations. PLoS One. 2015;10(6):e0127734.
49. Epstein RM, Shields CG, Franks P, Meldrum SC, Feldman M, Kravitz RL. Exploring and validating patient concerns: relation to prescribing for depression. Ann Fam Med. 2007;5(1):21–8.
50. Selph RB, Shiang J, Engelberg R, Curtis JR, White DB. Empathy and life support decisions in intensive care units. J Gen Intern Med. 2008;23(9):1311–7.
51. Blanch-Hartigan D. An effective training to increase accurate recognition of patient emotion cues. Patient Educ Couns. 2012;89(2):274–80.
52. Heyn L, Ruland CM, Finset A. Effects of an interactive tailored patient assessment tool on eliciting and responding to cancer patients' cues and concerns in clinical consultations with physicians and nurses. Patient Educ Couns. 2012;86(2):158–65.
53. White DB, Angus DC, Shields AM, Buddadhumaruk P, Pidro C, Paner C, et al. A randomized trial of a family-support intervention in intensive care units. N Engl J Med. 2018;378(25):2365–75.
54. Davidson JE, Aslakson RA, Long AC, Puntillo KA, Kross EK, Hart J, Cox CE, Wunsch H, Wickline MA, Nunnally ME, Netzer G, Kentish-Barnes N. Guidelines for family-centered care in the neonatal, pediatric, and adult ICU. Crit Care Med. 2017;45:103–28.
55. Lautrette A, Darmon M, Megarbane B, Joly LM, Chevret S, Adrie C, et al. A communication strategy and brochure for relatives of patients dying in the ICU. N Engl J Med. 2007;356(5):469–78.
56. Ciriello AG, Dizon ZB, October TW. Speaking a different language: a qualitative analysis comparing language of palliative care and pediatric intensive care unit physicians. Am J Hosp Palliat Care. 2018;35(3):384–9.

57. Carson SS, Cox CE, Wallenstein S, Hanson LC, Danis M, Tulsky JA, et al. Effect of palliative care-led meetings for families of patients with chronic critical illness: a randomized clinical trial. JAMA. 2016;316(1):51–62.
58. Croskerry P, Singhal G, Mamede S. Cognitive debiasing 2: impediments to and strategies for change. BMJ Qual Saf. 2013;22 Suppl 2:ii65–72.
59. Borrell-Carrio F, Epstein RM. Preventing errors in clinical practice: a call for self-awareness. Ann Fam Med. 2004;2(4):310–6.
60. Khan A, Furtak SL, Melvin P, Rogers JE, Schuster MA, Landrigan CP. Parent-provider miscommunications in hospitalized children. Hosp Pediatr. 2017;7(9):505–15.
61. Khan A, Baird J, Rogers JE, Furtak SL, Williams KA, Allair B, et al. Parent and provider experience and shared understanding after a family-centered nighttime communication intervention. Acad Pediatr. 2017;17(4):389–402.
62. Greenberg JA, Basapur S, Quinn TV, Bulger JL, Schwartz NH, Oh SK, et al. Daily written care summaries for families of critically ill patients: a randomized controlled trial. Crit Care Med. 2022;50(9):1296–305.
63. Czyż-Szypenbejl K, Mędrzycka-Dąbrowska W, Falcó-Pegueroles A, Lange S. Conflict sources and management in the ICU setting before and during COVID-19: a scoping review of the literature. Int J Environ Res Public Health. 2022;19(3):1875.
64. Barwise AK, Nyquist CA, Espinoza Suarez NR, Jaramillo C, Thorsteinsdottir B, Gajic O, et al. End-of-life decision-making for ICU patients with limited English proficiency: a qualitative study of healthcare team insights. Crit Care Med. 2019;47(10):1380–7.
65. Curtis JR, Treece PD, Nielsen EL, Gold J, Ciechanowski PS, Shannon SE, et al. Randomized trial of communication facilitators to reduce family distress and intensity of end-of-life care. Am J Respir Crit Care Med. 2016;193(2):154–62.
66. Krewulak KD, Jaworska N, Spence KL, Mizen SJ, Kupsch S, Stelfox HT, et al. Impact of restricted visitation policies during the first wave of the COVID-19 pandemic on communication between critically ill patients, families, and clinicians: a qualitative interview study. Ann Am Thorac Soc. 2022;19(7):1169–76.
67. Kentish-Barnes N, Chevret S, Valade S, Jaber S, Kerhuel L, Guisset O, et al. A three-step support strategy for relatives of patients dying in the intensive care unit: a cluster randomised trial. Lancet. 2022;399(10325):656–64.

Chapter 5
Intensive Care Unit Conflicts and the Family

Sheera F. Lerman and O. Joseph Bienvenu

Introduction

Conflicts are common in the intensive care unit (ICU) setting: between clinicians, between clinicians and families, and within families [1, 2]. This should not be surprising, as numerous factors contribute to a relatively stressful environment, including very vulnerable patients and the need for rapid and frequent patient-related decisions and activities, often incorporating input from consultants, in an evolving ethical and legal landscape [3]. The focus of this chapter is the nature and effects of conflicts in the ICU setting on families of adult patients in intensive care, as well as how clinicians might mitigate or resolve these conflicts.

Figure 5.1 illustrates, in a simplified form, some of the kinds of conflicts that can occur in ICU settings. For the purposes of the illustration, we assume that the patient's illness and/or medications incapacitate them cognitively (i.e., the patient is not shown). Second, we assume a simple team structure (ignoring the possibility of multiple physicians working together as a team, as well as consulting physicians, rotating nurses, social workers, rehabilitation specialists, respiratory therapists, chaplains, palliative care clinicians, and others who may meet with the patient and family). Third, we ignore the fact that families often include multiple persons, who may not be able to be present, and many patients have loved ones besides family members. One would hope that all parties represented in this simplified diagram are communicating, in some fashion, and that shared understanding is possible, though this may be naïve. However, even if these are the case, conflicts can occur.

S. F. Lerman · O. J. Bienvenu (✉)
Psychiatry and Behavioral Sciences, Johns Hopkins University School of Medicine, Baltimore, MD, USA
e-mail: szohar1@jhmi.edu; obienve1@jhmi.edu

© The Author(s), under exclusive license to Springer Nature Switzerland AG 2025
A. J. Vance et al. (eds.), *Families in the Intensive Care Unit*,
https://doi.org/10.1007/978-3-031-83786-9_5

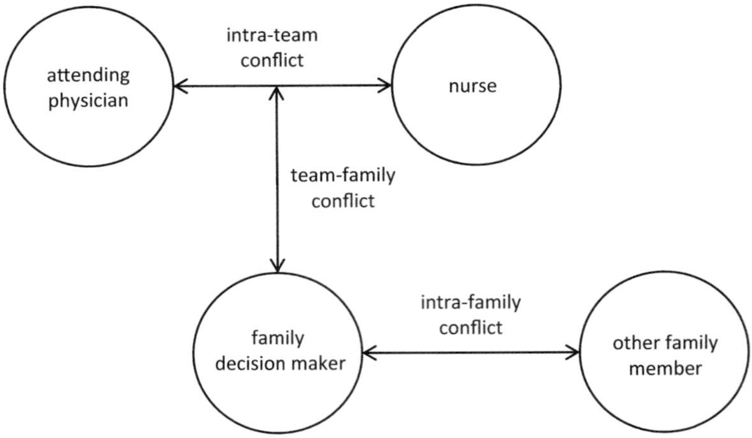

Fig. 5.1 Simplified diagram of the kinds of conflicts that can occur in ICUs

Conflict Between Groups

It may be useful to consider ways in which theories from social psychology may inform intergroup conflicts in the ICU. Such theories might illuminate conflicts between families and clinical teams, as well as conflicts between discipline groups (e.g., physicians vs. nurses).

Intergroup conflict can occur when groups perceive they are competing for limited resources, as opposed to working together toward a goal [4, 5]. An imperfect example would be competition for scarce ICU beds; this example is imperfect because conflict would typically occur between families and ICU clinicians, as opposed to directly between families. Nevertheless, families may perceive that ICU teams are discriminating against them and their loved ones because of race, socioeconomic status, etc., favoring patients and families like the ICU clinicians themselves [6]. Clinicians working together with families to help the patient recover or be comfortable with preserved dignity is the obvious preferred goal.

Conflicts in the ICU

In 2010, Fassier and Azoulay reviewed the literature on conflicts in adult ICUs [1]. They noted wide variability in the literature, in the definition of conflict, in its measurement, in patient settings, and in respondents among other factors [7–12] (Table 5.1). From the perspective of ICU clinicians [9, 10, 12], intra-team conflict was common, and end-of-life decision-making and communication were a common source of conflict. The authors noted that in-ICU conflict negatively affects patient safety and patient- and family-centered care. In addition, the authors noted that in-ICU conflict negatively affects team cohesion and morale, leading to staff burnout

Table 5.1 Brief summary of studies reviewed by Fassier and Azoulay [1], in chronological order

Burns and colleagues [7] prospectively identified patients with conflicts or at risk for decision-making conflicts as reported by clinical teams in seven Boston ICUs. Definition of positive screen for risk for decision-making conflicts: (a) the patient lacked decision-making capacity and a clearly identified surrogate, (b) the team perceived intra-team, team-family, or intra-family conflict, (c) the patient exceeded the 85th percentile of length of stay in that ICU, or (d) the patient was admitted to the ICU because of an iatrogenic event. In phase I, 21% of patients screened positive, and in phase II, 18% of patients screened positive. In phase II, social workers met with family members of patients who screened positive and provided feedback to the clinical team, and the team decided whether to take further action (e.g., a family meeting, regular family meetings, a social services consult, pastoral services, an ethics consult, a pain service consult, etc.). The intervention increased the likelihood of deliberative decision-making (deciding to forego resuscitation, to choose comfort-care only, or to pursue an aggressive-care treatment plan), though it was not associated with a change in patient or surrogate satisfaction with care
Abbott and colleagues [8] performed semi-structured interviews with next-of-kin family members of patients in Durham, NC ICUs who had faced decisions to forego life-sustaining treatment (>1 year afterward). Family members recalled conflicts in 46% of cases: intra-team 4%, team-family 40%, and intra-family 4%. Family members recalled conflicts with the team mainly about communication and perceived unprofessional behavior (e.g., not involving next-of-kin sufficiently in treatment discussions). Family members who had spoken with patients in advance about end-of-life decisions (63%) reported that treatment decisions were less burdensome, 48% of family members found the presence of chaplains reassuring, and 48% of family members preferred the attending physician ("doctor in charge") as their source of information. A total of 27% of family members mentioned a need for physical space to have conferences with physicians and family discussions
Breen and colleagues [9] performed semi-structured interviews with Durham, NC ICU physicians and nurses involved in the care of patients for whom decisions to forego life-sustaining therapy were considered. At least one team member perceived a conflict in 78% of patient cases: intra-team 48%, team-family 48%, and intra-family 24%. Clinicians attributed conflict to decisions regarding life-sustaining treatment, communication, pain control, and social issues
Studdert and colleagues [10] performed semi-structured interviews with Boston ICU physicians and nurses to learn about conflict regarding patients whose length of stay exceeded the 85th percentile for their unit. The clinicians reported conflicts in 32% of cases: intra-team 31%, team-family 57%, and intra-family 12%. The main perceived sources of conflict between teams and families included decisions regarding life-sustaining treatment, difficulties communicating effectively, inability or unavailability of surrogate decision-makers, and overwhelming emotions due to the patient's state. The main perceived source of intra-team conflict was disagreement about particulars of the care plan. The main perceived sources of intra-family conflict were decisions regarding life-sustaining treatment and other care. Nurses detected all conflicts more frequently, especially intra-team conflicts. Spousal presence was associated with less team-family conflict, especially disputes over life-sustaining treatment
Danjoux Meth and colleagues [11] performed semi-structured interviews with Ontario ICU clinicians, administrators, and bioethicists regarding in-ICU conflicts. Qualitative results focused on inter-team, intra-team, and team-family conflicts. Respondents perceived lack of communication, personnel (nursing shortage), experience, and goals of care as contributing to conflict
Azoulay and colleagues [12] conducted an international multicenter survey to measure the prevalence and correlates of conflict perceived by ICU physicians and nurses in the last week. A total of 72% of clinicians perceived at least one conflict: intra-team 85% and team-family 27%. Clinicians attributed conflict to personal behaviors and end-of-life decisions and noted that conflicts contributed to job strain

[13–15]. All team members and family members deserve to have a voice in a patient's care, not just a passive role. Team and family members need clear explanations and an opportunity to ask questions, as well as make suggestions, to facilitate a sense of mastery in what can be a stressful situation. The authors also noted that in-ICU conflict could increase healthcare costs, through delays in decision-making and even lawsuits. Fassier and Azoulay had several recommendations for the field [1]. First, the field could benefit from a more in-depth social science perspective on conflict, to address the ICU system of care as a whole. Second, the field could benefit from further studies of multimodal interventions to prevent and mitigate or resolve conflict. As shown in Table 5.1, only one study tested such an intervention [7], which relied heavily on the communication and psychosocial assessment skills of ICU social workers [16]. Third, the field could benefit from guidelines to address conflict. Finally, the authors opined that conflict prevention strategies should better incorporate family concerns and team communication [1]. As noted in Table 5.1, only one study sought family members' perspectives directly [8]. Table 5.2 lists common perceived sources of conflict for family members of patients in the ICU.

More recently, clinical investigators have addressed some of the issues raised by Fassier and Azoulay [1], particularly the perspective of family members:

- Schuster and colleagues assessed physician-surrogate conflict in San Francisco ICUs simultaneously in physicians (attendings or fellows) and surrogates (all patients were incapacitated) [17]. The authors reported that either the physician or a surrogate identified conflict in 63% of cases, though physicians were less likely to perceive conflict than surrogates were (28% vs. 43%). In addition, with some exceptions, physician and surrogate perceptions regarding the presence of any conflict were quite different (60% agreement, kappa = 0.14). Surrogates and physicians were less likely to perceive conflict if surrogates rated the physicians' bedside manner highly. Additionally, physicians perceived any conflict more frequently when surrogates reported discrimination in a healthcare setting in the last year.
- Huff and colleagues interviewed non-clinician caregivers at Duke and the Medical University of South Carolina to determine how relationships between caregivers and ICU clinicians affected a number of patient- and caregiver-centered outcomes [18]. Non-clinician caregivers who described a greater therapeutic alliance with the attending physician reported greater communication quality, trust, and patient-centeredness of care, as well as less decisional conflict.

Table 5.2 Common perceived sources of conflict for family members of patients in the ICU

Decisions to withdraw or withhold treatments
Adequacy of communication
Staff behavior (perceived lack of professionalism, disrespect, experimentation on loved ones)
Family members' strong emotional reactions, mistrust of staff, unavailability, and indecisiveness
Pain management

One might expect that therapeutic alliance, as measured in this study [18], might related to bedside manner in Shuster and colleagues' study [17].

- Chiarchiaro and colleagues surveyed surrogate decision-makers of patients with acute respiratory distress syndrome in the context of a multicenter prospective cohort study involving five American academic medical centers [19]. Nearly half of surrogates reported moderate to high levels of decisional conflict regarding foregoing life-sustaining treatments. Surrogate decision-makers who reported prior conversations with their ill loved ones regarding care preferences if incapacitated reported lower decisional conflict about whether to continue life support. These findings are reminiscent of those of Abbott and colleagues [8] (Table 5.1). The authors noted that, in addition to helping ensure that clinicians honor incapacitated patients' choices; advance care planning can reduce the burden on loved ones who must act as surrogates [19]. Such a burden can be substantial [20].
- Miller and colleagues assessed decision conflict in surrogate decision-makers of incapacitated patients on mechanical ventilation >96 h in the medical ICU at Wake Forest Baptist Medical Center [21]. Consistent with one of the authors' hypotheses, surrogates reported more decisional conflict with end-of-life decisions than other treatment decisions. Interestingly, surrogates expressed little decisional regret a month later.
- Olding and colleagues conducted a scoping review of patient and family involvement in adult critical care settings [22]. They noted two research gaps relevant to this chapter: (1) the broader sociocultural processes that shape patient and family involvement, and (2) potential bidirectional relationships between family involvement and ICU clinician teamwork.
- Mehter and colleagues interviewed Boston-area critical care physicians about their approach to and management of conflict with families in the context of end-of-life decision-making. The authors analyzed their data using qualitative techniques [23]. Physicians described this as a complex task, emphasizing the importance of tending to family members' emotional health. In the context of family resistance to physician recommendations for less aggressive care, physicians sometimes deferred to family surrogate decisions, while at other times they attempted to persuade families. The authors noted that attempting to manipulate families with biased information could backfire badly. Physicians were more comfortable deferring to families when families appeared to genuinely attempt to represent patients' wishes, while simultaneously addressing patients' pain and suffering.
- Ashana and colleagues assessed family and physician agreement regarding the presence of conflict between them in the context of a clinical trial testing a decision aid [24]. In this study, conflict was reported infrequently by family members or physicians, but, like in the study of Schuster and colleagues [17], agreement regarding the presence of conflict was poor ($K = 0.12$). Conflict was more likely when either families or physicians were minorities, and when there was substantial discordance between families' and physicians' prognostic assessments.

End-of-Life Decision-Making Conflict

End-of-life decision-making is a prominent source of conflict in the ICU setting. It is perhaps worth noting in what ways ethical and legal principles in end-of-life ICU care have developed over the years. In 2010, Luce provided a cogent account of this, from an American perspective [3]. He began by noting that, in the early days of ICU care in the 1950s and 1960s, beneficence and non-maleficence guided medical care in the ICU and elsewhere. Clinicians generally behaved more paternalistically than now, and "do not resuscitate" and "do not intubate" orders did not exist. In fact, clinicians considered withholding cardiopulmonary resuscitation (CPR) immoral (even homicide or, at least, euthanasia), and doing so was against hospitals' policies, though clinicians gradually realized the limits of CPR [25]. In the 1970s, family members began challenging these ideas, arguing in effect for increasing patient autonomy to refuse life-sustaining treatments, though the legal cases actually involved family members of unconscious patients. Over the years, shared decision-making became common practice, as did withholding and withdrawing life support in ICUs [26–28]. With the rise of patient and family autonomy, clinicians became increasingly uncomfortable with providing treatments that they did not see as beneficial [29]. This has been described as the rise and fall of the "futility" movement, which ebbed with increasing recognition of substantial variability in physicians' and families' values regarding life in particular circumstances. However, despite conflicts and sometimes-intense emotions, most families and physicians eventually agree on treatment plans [3].

Conflict Mitigation and Resolution Strategies

Employment of effective strategies for conflict mitigation and resolution depends on the type and source of the conflict. In a recent review [30], Kayser and Kaplan explored sources of conflict in the ICU and created a process map to identify resources to resolve conflict (Fig. 5.2). The early use of conflict management

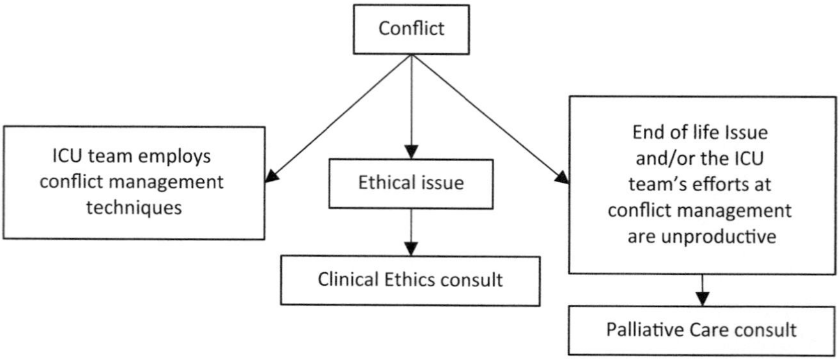

Fig. 5.2 A process map to engage resources to resolve conflict, inspired by Kayser and Kaplan [30]

techniques such as recognition, mediation, and de-escalation are important to prevent conflicts with family members of ICU patients.

Conflict Mediation Techniques

The mediation process includes a neutral third party that facilitates effective communication and creates conflict solutions [31]. Mediation can assist individuals from both sides of the conflict to communicate their interests and needs and improve understanding, compassion, and collaboration [32]. Prevention of full-blown conflicts can begin with the recognition of the moral emotions that underlay a conflict, such as anger or frustration. Then the use of de-escalation strategies such as the separation between positions and interests can be effectively used. A "position" is the declaration of what a person wants such as the family member's position on the type of care their loved one should receive. An "interest" is the reason behind the position stemming from values, motivations, and concerns. Finding shared interests, even with what appear to be opposite positions, can allow the different sides to engage in compromise and conflict resolution [33]. When these strategies are not sufficient, or ethical issues arise, the utilization of consultation services such as palliative care or clinical ethics can facilitate conflict resolution [30].

Consultative Services

Most hospital systems include team-based consultation services which can be an important resource to assist with conflict resolution. Palliative care and clinical ethics consultation services have unique roles in the process of conflict mediation.

Clinical ethics consultation is an important resource available to hospital staff, patients, and their family members to address ethical dilemmas, moral doubts, and conflicts [34]. In a systematic review Au et al. [35] summarized the results of studies assessing the impact of clinical ethics consultation on outcomes in adult ICUs and found that clinical ethics consultation decreased ICU length of stay and increased family and healthcare provider satisfaction. It is important to note that not all conflicts within the ICU involve an ethical dilemma; thus, in some cases a clinical ethics consultation is not warranted, and other conflict resolutions strategies are more appropriate [30].

Palliative Care Interventions in the ICU: Potential Role in Reducing In-ICU Conflict?

Aslakson and colleagues systematically reviewed studies of palliative care interventions in ICUs [36]. The authors defined palliative care relatively broadly, drawing on Robert Wood Johnson consensus group-identified domains for quality end-of-life care in the ICU [37]:

1. Patient- and family-centered decision-making
2. Communication
3. Continuity of care
4. Emotional and practical support
5. Symptom management and comfort care
6. Spiritual support
7. Emotional and organizational support for ICU clinicians

Notably, many of the above domains are relevant to any medical care, not just end-of-life care, and many of these interventions could reduce team-family conflict. The interventions included, e.g., intensive communication efforts (e.g., early multidisciplinary family meetings, informational brochures, etc.) [38, 39], ethics team consults [40], palliative care consults [41], and referral to a comprehensive supportive care team for hopelessly ill patients and their family members [42]. Perhaps not surprisingly, the authors found that most of the interventions decreased ICU and hospital length of stay. Importantly, though, most of the interventions were associated with, if anything, decreased mortality [36].

One of the studies reviewed by Aslakson and colleagues [36] deserves further mention, in that it addressed in-ICU conflict more directly. In addition, though not included in the review of Fassier and Azoulay [1], it is a multimodal intervention that seems to prevent and mitigate or resolve conflict by promoting its obverse-consensus.

Lilly and colleagues performed a before-and-after study of proactive multidisciplinary meetings within 72 h of critical care admission for patients who had a predicted ICU length of stay longer than 5 days, a predicted mortality of >25%, or a change in functional status that was potentially irreversible and sufficient to preclude eventual return home [38]. Meetings were led by attending physicians and included a nurse, house officer, the patient's family (including the healthcare proxy), and, whenever possible, the patient. Meetings had four objectives:

1. To review the medical facts and options for treatment
2. To discuss the patient's perspectives on death and dying, chronic dependence, loss of function, and the acceptability of the risks and discomforts of critical care
3. To agree on a care plan
4. To agree on criteria by which success or failure of the care plan would be judged (clinical milestones, with expected time frames)

The clinicians used the agreed-upon time frames to set up subsequent formal family meetings, or varied if patients and/or families needed more time to process difficult medical facts. The clinical teams educated and prepared patients and families for home care, rehabilitation, or chronic care, as appropriate. If clinical milestones were not achievable, patients and families learned the limits of advanced supportive technology, and the teams and families explored other alternatives, including palliative care. Attending physicians also held weekly multidisciplinary meetings with nurses, social workers, chaplains, and rehabilitation specialists to ensure a uniform understanding of the patient's wishes and care plan. Thus, clinical teams could provide consistent information to the patient and family and identify barriers to the care plan.

Attending physicians recorded disagreements within the team and between the team and family daily. During the intervention period, the average time of within-team non-consensus decreased from 0.56 to 0.02 days per patient, and the average time of team-family non-consensus decreased from 1.7 to 0.09 days per patient. The median length of stay decreased from 4 to 3 days, and mortality did not change.

An Example of Mitigation of Team-Family Conflicts Regarding Potentially Inappropriate Treatments

In 2015, the American Thoracic Society, the American Association of Critical Care Nurses, the American College of Chest Physicians, the European Society for Intensive Care Medicine, and the Society of Critical Care Medicine issued a joint statement regarding how clinicians should respond to requests for potentially inappropriate treatments in ICUs [43]. First, the committee recommended that hospitals employ strategies to prevent intractable treatment conflicts, including proactive communication and early involvement of ethics or palliative care consultants if needed. Second, the committee recommended using the term "potentially inappropriate," rather than "futile," when discussing treatments that might accomplish the effect sought by the patient/family, but about which clinicians have conflicting ethical concerns. In that case, ICU clinicians should explain and advocate for the treatment plan they believe appropriate. If conflicts remain intractable after thorough communication and negotiation, the committee recommends hospital review, attempts to find a willing provider at another institution, and an opportunity for external review. In cases in which there is insufficient time to follow these steps, and clinicians have a high degree of certainty that the requested treatment is outside the realm of accepted practice, the committee recommended that clinicians seek procedural oversight if possible but opined that clinicians need not provide the requested treatment. Third, the committee recommended against clinicians providing treatments that cannot accomplish a given physiologic goal, as well as legally proscribed (or discretionary) treatments. Fourth, the committee recommended that the medical profession engage the public and advocate for policies and laws regarding when life-prolonging treatments are appropriate.

Conclusions

In-ICU conflicts are common and tend to be less apparent to physicians than to nurses, who spend more time with patients and family members. Timely and clear communication, involving multiple voices, is necessary to prevent or mitigate conflict regarding patients with poor prognoses. Conflict recognition, conflict management, and de-escalation strategies as well as the utilization of ethics and palliative care consults can facilitate conflict resolution without increasing patient mortality or adding to team burden.

References

1. Fassier T, Azoulay E. Conflicts and communication gaps in the intensive care unit. Curr Opin Crit Care. 2010;16(6):654–65.
2. Wujtewicz M, Wujtewicz MA, Owczuk R. Conflicts in the intensive care unit. Anaesthesiol Intensive Ther. 2015;47(4):360–2.
3. Luce JM. A history of resolving conflicts over end-of-life care in intensive care units in the United States. Crit Care Med. 2010;38(8):1623–9.
4. Sherif M, Harvey OJ, White BJ, Hood WR, Sherif CW. Intergroup cooperation and competition: the Robbers Cave experiment. Norman, OK: University Book Exchange; 1961.
5. Jackson JW. Realistic group conflict theory: a review and evaluation of the theoretical and empirical literature. Psychol Rec. 1993;43(3):395–413.
6. Tajfel H, Turner JC. An integrative theory of intergroup conflict. In: Austin WG, Worchel S, editors. The social psychology of intergroup relations. Monterey, CA: Brooks/Cole; 1979. p. 33–47.
7. Burns JP, Mello MM, Studdert DM, Puopolo AL, Truog RD, Brennan TA. Results of a clinical trial on care improvement for the critically ill. Crit Care Med. 2003;31(8):2107–17.
8. Abbott KH, Sago JG, Breen CM, Abernethy AP, Tulsky JA. Families looking back: one year after discussion of withdrawal or withholding of life-sustaining support. Crit Care Med. 2001;29(1):197–201.
9. Breen CM, Abernethy AP, Abbott KH, Tulsky JA. Conflict associated with decisions to limit life-sustaining treatment in intensive care units. J Gen Intern Med. 2001;16(5):283–9.
10. Studdert DM, Mello MM, Burns JP, Puopolo AL, Galper BZ, Truog RD, et al. Conflict in the care of patients with prolonged stay in the ICU: types, sources, and predictors. Intensive Care Med. 2003;29(9):1489–97.
11. Danjoux Meth N, Lawless B, Hawryluck L. Conflicts in the ICU: perspectives of administrators and clinicians. Intensive Care Med. 2009;35(12):2068–77.
12. Azoulay E, Timsit JF, Sprung CL, Soares M, Rusinová K, Lafabrie A, et al. Prevalence and factors of intensive care unit conflicts: the Conflicus study. Am J Respir Crit Care Med. 2009;180(9):853–60.
13. Embriaco N, Azoulay E, Barrau K, Kentish N, Pochard F, Loundou A, et al. High level of burnout in intensivists: prevalence and associated factors. Am J Respir Crit Care Med. 2007;175(7):686–92.
14. Burghi G, Lambert J, Chaize M, Goinheix K, Quiroga C, Fariña G, et al. Prevalence, risk factors and consequences of severe burnout syndrome in ICU. Intensive Care Med. 2014;40(11):1785–6.
15. Bienvenu OJ. Is this critical care clinician burned out? Intensive Care Med. 2016;42(11):1794–6.
16. Hartman-Shea K, Hahn AP, Fritz Kraus J, Cordts G, Sevransky J. The role of the social worker in the adult critical care unit: a systematic review of the literature. Soc Work Health Care. 2011;50(2):143–57.
17. Schuster RA, Hong SY, Arnold RM, White DB. Investigating conflict in ICUs—is the clinicians' perspective enough? Crit Care Med. 2014;42(2):328–35.
18. Huff NG, Nadig N, Ford DW, Cox CE. Therapeutic alliance between the caregivers of critical illness survivors and intensive care unit clinicians. Ann Am Thorac Soc. 2015;12(11):1646–53.

19. Chiarchiaro J, Buddadhumaruk P, Arnold RM, White DB. Prior advance care planning is associated with less decisional conflict among surrogates for critically ill patients. Ann Am Thorac Soc. 2015;12(10):1528–33.
20. Wendler D, Rid A. Systematic review: the effect on surrogates of making treatment decisions for others. Ann Intern Med. 2011;154(5):336–46.
21. Miller JJ, Morris P, Files DC, Gower E, Young M. Decision conflict and regret among surrogate decision makers in the medical intensive care unit. J Crit Care. 2016;32:79–84.
22. Olding M, McMillan SE, Reeves S, Schmitt MH, Puntillo K, Kitto S. Patient and family involvement in adult critical and intensive care settings: a scoping review. Health Expect. 2016;19(6):1183–202.
23. Mehter HM, McCannon JB, Clark JA, Wiener RS. Physician approaches to conflict with families surrounding end-of-life decision-making in the intensive care unit. A qualitative study. Ann Am Thorac Soc. 2018;15(2):241–9.
24. Ashana DC, Jan A, Parish A, Johnson KS, Steinhauser KE, Olsen MK, et al. Interpersonal perception: family- and physician-reported conflict in the intensive care unit. Ann Am Thorac Soc. 2022;19(11):1937–42.
25. Bedell SE, Delbanco TL, Cook EF, Epstein FH. Survival after cardiopulmonary resuscitation in the hospital. N Engl J Med. 1983;309(10):569–76.
26. Smedira NG, Evans BH, Grais LS, Cohen NH, Lo B, Cooke M, et al. Withholding and withdrawal of life support from the critically ill. N Engl J Med. 1990;322(5):309–15.
27. Prendergast TJ, Luce JM. Increasing incidence of withholding and withdrawal of life support from the critically ill. Am J Respir Crit Care Med. 1997;155(1):15–20.
28. Prendergast TJ, Claessens MT, Luce JM. A national survey of end-of-life care for critically ill patients. Am J Respir Crit Care Med. 1998;158(4):1163–7.
29. Schneiderman LJ, Jecker NS, Jonsen AR. Medical futility: its meaning and ethical implications. Ann Intern Med. 1990;112(12):949–54.
30. Kayser JB, Kaplan LJ. Conflict management in the ICU. Crit Care Med. 2020;48(9):1349–57.
31. Moore C. The mediation process: practical strategies for resolving conflict. 3rd ed. New York: Wiley; 2003.
32. Gerardi D. Using mediation techniques to manage conflict and create healthy work environments. AACN Clin Issues. 2004;15(2):182–95.
33. Fiester A. Contentious conversation: using mediation techniques in difficult clinical ethics consultations. J Clin Ethics. 2015;26(4):324–30.
34. Picozzi M, Gasparetto A. Clinical ethics consultation in the intensive care unit. Minerva Anestesiol. 2020;86(6):670–7.
35. Au SS, Roze des Ordons A, Fiest KM, Lorenzetti DL, Jette N. Outcomes of ethics consultations in adult ICUs: a systematic review and meta-analysis. Crit Care Med. 2018;46(5):799–808.
36. Aslakson R, Cheng J, Vollenweider D, Galusca D, Smith TJ, Pronovost PJ. Evidence-based palliative care in the intensive care unit: a systematic review of interventions. J Palliat Med. 2014;17(2):219–35.
37. Clarke EB, Luce JM, Curtis JR, Danis M, Levy M, Nelson J, et al. Quality indicators for end-of-life care in the intensive care unit. Crit Care Med. 2003;31(9):2255–62.
38. Lilly CM, De Meo DL, Sonna LA, Haley KJ, Massaro AF, Wallace RF, et al. An intensive communication intervention for the critically ill. Am J Med. 2000;109(6):469–75.
39. Azoulay E, Pochard F, Chevret S, Jourdain M, Bornstain C, Wernet A, et al. Impact of a family information leaflet on effectiveness of information provided to family members of intensive care unit patients: a multicenter, prospective, randomized, controlled trial. Am J Respir Crit Care Med. 2002;165(4):438–42.
40. Dowdy MD, Robertson C, Bander JA. A study of proactive ethics consultation for critically and terminally ill patients with extended lengths of stay. Crit Care Med. 1998;26(2):252–9.
41. Campbell ML, Guzman JA. Impact of a proactive approach to improve end-of-life care in a medical ICU. Chest. 2003;123(1):266–71.

42. Carlson RW, Devich L, Frank RR. Development of a comprehensive supportive care team for the hopelessly ill on a university hospital medical service. JAMA. 1988;259(3):378–83.
43. Bosslet GT, Pope TMR, Rubenfeld GD, Lo B, Truog RD, Rushton CH, Curtis JR, et al. An official ATS/AACN/ACCP/ESICM/SCCM policy statement: responding to requests for potentially inappropriate treatments in intensive care units. Am J Respir Crit Care Med. 2015;191(11):1318–30.

Chapter 6
Family Role in Patient Safety in the Intensive Care Unit

Amelia Bowman and Sarah J. Beesley

Introduction

Family members feel a natural inclination to protect and provide for their loved ones. Unsurprisingly, this is only accentuated when their loved one is sick, yet it is at this critical time a family member may feel most helpless to provide aid [1]. During the recent pandemic, a dramatic shift in visitation policies was necessary while public health ramifications of the novel coronavirus were still being understood. Unfortunately, while the pandemic has eased, many ICUs have retained more restrictive policies [2].

As in prior chapters, the definition of family is broad and includes "spouses, blood relatives, in-laws, step-relatives, fiancés, significant others, friends, caring neighbors, colleagues, fellow congregants, and other people with a personal attachment to the person with advanced serious illness—in other words, the people 'for whom it matters'" [3]. Despite this, heteronormative biases and the gender binary paradigm permeate the United States medical system and have often led to exclusion of important family members from the bedside of their loved ones. To best involve families, providers must avoid assumptions and seek to treat each patient and family member with respect and dignity. The patient's values will be best represented by involving the patient-designated family members into their care.

A. Bowman
Division of Pulmonary and Critical Care, Department of Medicine, University of Utah School of Medicine, Salt Lake City, UT, USA

S. J. Beesley (✉)
Division of Pulmonary and Critical Care, Department of Medicine, University of Utah School of Medicine, Salt Lake City, UT, USA

Department of Critical Care, Intermountain Medical Center, Shock Trauma Intensive Care Unit, Murray, UT, USA
e-mail: sarah.beesley@imail.org

© The Author(s), under exclusive license to Springer Nature Switzerland AG 2025
A. J. Vance et al. (eds.), *Families in the Intensive Care Unit*, https://doi.org/10.1007/978-3-031-83786-9_6

Table 6.1 Family involvement in ICU patient safety

Family member role	Potential safety benefits
Participate in bedside care	Better preparation for discharge needs
Be present during procedures	Patient calmer and more cooperative, more vigilance by provider
Alert staff to changes in condition	More rapid response to clinical change
Represent patient values and wishes to team	Patient treated in the manner that best respects them

Because of varied legislation in the United States, it's also important to be sure that the patient's designated healthcare representative is formally established through an advance directive [4, 5].

As the personal representative of the patient, a family member can play a critical role in patient safety in the intensive care unit (ICU) [6]. However, family members have often been excluded from this role by policies that keep them away from the bedside (such as restricted visitation) and have not been traditionally included in creation of protocols and design of facilities. In order to include families in a way that can maximize patient safety, healthcare providers must encourage the following: (1) family members must be allowed to be present in the ICU and included during rounds, procedures, and bedside care; (2) family members need to be empowered to speak up if something is not going well with their loved one or if they are concerned about a potential error; and (3) family members need to be given a role to play in development of hospital safety policy and plans that would encourage these actions, such as through patient family advisory councils (PFACs). A sample of the roles a family member can play and the impact on safety is found in Table 6.1.

Emotional Safety

Emotional harms have been increasingly recognized as a preventable medical error [7, 8]. To many patients, these emotional harms are more distressing than other more traditional physical adverse events [9]. Emotional injury can include insults to a person's dignity or self-respect, including racism and other forms of discrimination [7, 10]. ICU patients are particularly susceptible to dehumanization due to their frequently impaired consciousness, limited agency, and the deindividuation and mechanization that are frequent in the ICU [11]. The psychological demands of ICU clinical practice may drive clinicians to dehumanize patients inadvertently through empathy reduction and moral disengagement [11]. The feeling of inadequate respect has not been shown to be tied to a patient's clinical characteristics but more to a lack of control [8]. At its root, family engagement works to maintain or reinstate the humanity of the patient by recognizing family members as full partners in care [12]. While much work is being done to further characterize the best way to engage with patients and families and help them retain a sense of control, inclusion of families as part of the team should not wait [13–15]. Families can provide independent knowledge of the patient's full identity, and empowering family members to be part of the team both combats dehumanization and encourages safety [16].

Necessity of Family Presence

Family members cannot participate in or contribute to safety in the ICU if they are not present. While many ICU's had moved towards open visitation, the recent pandemic led to reinstatement of restrictive visitor policies as a public health necessity. Unfortunately, many facilities have not returned to more open policies even as the public health threat of a novel virus has waned and the harms of restricting visiting are shown to affect not only patients and their families [17], but the healthcare team as well [2, 18, 19]. Family members want to be able to visit their loved ones on their own schedule and as much as they and the patient would like [20–23]. When family members are allowed unrestricted access, communication with staff and satisfaction with care is improved [20, 24–27]. Frequently exceptions are made to visiting hours by ICU staff; unfortunately, having informal and unregulated exceptions by ICU staff can lead to discrimination as the decision to restrict or liberalize visiting hours may be based on physical appearance, language, culture, race or religion [28]. This perpetuates clinician-centered, paternalistic approaches to medical care [29]. The presence of family members at the bedside may also directly benefit patients by reducing the incidence and duration of delirium [30, 31]. The first step to allowing family members to participate in and improve patient safety is to allow them to be present in the ICU.

Family Involvement in Daily Rounds

Beyond simple visitation, family members are increasingly joining daily ICU rounds which provides a potential opportunity to improve communication and family satisfaction [32–35]. Family presence during rounds may add to the discussion in ways that improves safety as family members are able to providing important history or insights impacting the plan of care. Additionally, if they are aware of the plan for the day, they may be able to help speak up when something changes.

Family Involvement in Bedside Care

Family members may also want to be part of routine bedside care in the ICU, participating in activities such as bathing, feeding, and suctioning [36, 37]. While not well studied, having family participate in care during the hospital stay may improve safety during the ICU stay and after discharge [38]. While their loved one is in the hospital, family members can facilitate bedside care—examples include holding an emesis bag up when the patient vomits or reorienting them when confused. Additionally, family members who are involved during an inpatient stay often become attuned to activities such as wound care, physical therapy, and keeping track of inputs and outputs. A program designed by nurses formally invited family members to help care for patients as they recovered from cardiothoracic surgical procedures. Participation in this program was associated with a reduction in 30-day hospital readmission among these selected patients, possibly indicating that safety after discharge was improved by involving the family members early in care [39]. Family involvement in care may also reduce emotional harms. In two randomized trials where families were educated and invited to participate in care in the Newborn Intensive Care Unit (NICU) [40, 41], family involvement led to improved satisfaction. Part of that satisfaction came from the increased amount of time mothers spent in the ICU [41, 42].

Family Presence During ICU Procedures

Families in adult ICUs are still frequently asked to leave the patient's room during procedures, including central line placement and intubation as well as cardiopulmonary resuscitation (CPR), regardless of whether the patient would prefer family to be present and family would like to stay [43–45]. Family presence during procedures may positively impact patient safety in a few important ways. Family presence in ICU during procedures provide an additional layer of supervision encouraging professionalism and best practices [46, 47]. As a physician prepares for a procedure, if she knows that a family member may be scrutinizing her sterile technique, she is more careful as she dons her gown. When family members are at the bedside to hold a hand or talk to their loved one, an agitated patient (from pain, delirium, fear, language barriers), can be calmed and safely taken through a procedure without sedating medications or the need for additional staff (Fig. 6.1). Communication and transparency improve when family members are included in care, including procedures [26]. This open relationship and transparent communication is associated with better family-team dynamics and may improve family members' sense of understanding and control [48–50].

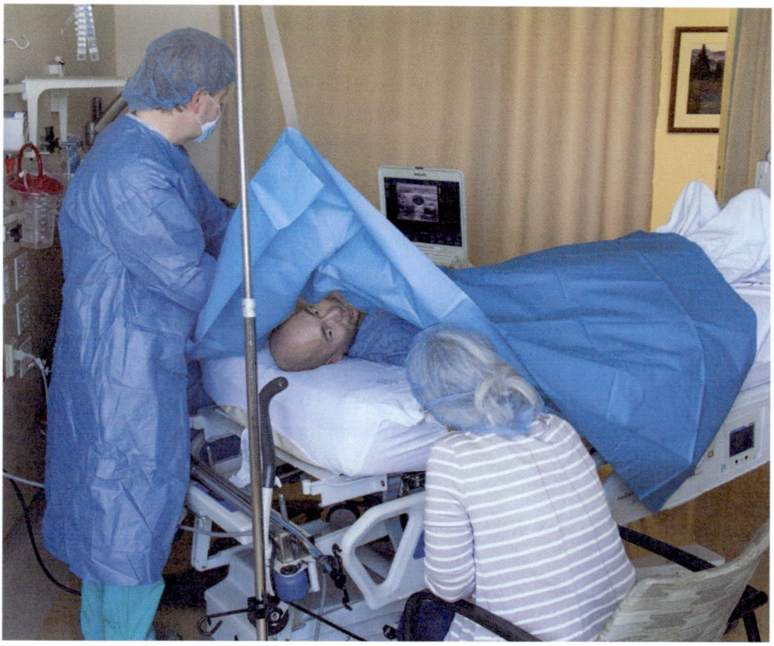

Fig. 6.1 Family present during ICU procedure

Medical Error and Adverse Events

In 2000, the Institute of Medicine, now the National Academy of Medicine, published the seminal report *To Err is Human* which identified the startling prevalence of medical errors and adverse events in the US Healthcare system. This report estimated 29% of hospitalizations in the USA were affected by an adverse event, costing the healthcare system tens of billions of dollars and resulting in an astonishing 44,000 excess deaths annually [51]. The subsequent report *Crossing the Quality Chasm* outlined specific steps to decrease medical errors and adverse events, including the statement, "In many cases the best window on the safety and quality of care is through the eyes of the patient" [6]. In the intervening decades, quality and safety have been prioritized, and patient and family engagement have served as an important component of this effort. Family members are invested in preventing errors that could harm their loved one, and can be recruited and encouraged to act as another gatekeeper at the bedside. For example, medication errors consistently make up more than 50% of medical errors and adverse events. When family members are informed about the medication plan and know their family member's allergies, they can serve an important role in ensuring accurate medication administration. Repeated studies have demonstrated that patients and families consistently identify medical errors and adverse events overlooked by hospital staff [52–54]. Importantly, physician review confirmed that a majority of these events were relevant [53]. While some of the medical errors and adverse events reported by families are identified after discharge from the ICU or hospital, a significant proportion go unidentified while the patient is hospitalized [54]. This finding highlights the need for active engagement of patients and family members in the care team.

In addition, family members represent a consistent member of the patient's care team present during each stage of their hospital stay. Transitions in care (from one level of care to another, or from one care team to another) are a high-risk time for medical errors. Family presence offers another slice in the "swiss cheese model" to keep a mistake from leading to harm [55]. A recent case in a tertiary care hospital intensive care unit illustrated this. A patient had a complicated abdominal surgery, resulting in a partial gastrectomy and discontinuity of the alimentary track. Despite an order to only use a jejunal tube for feeds, the feeds were connected to a nasogastric tube and started. The patient's spouse arrived soon after and noticed the error, notifying the medical team immediately. The feeds were switched to the jejunal tube and a serious adverse event was prevented. While the medical team cannot count on family members to prevent errors and should be as vigilant as possible, the reality is that medical errors are terrifyingly common and family members may help reduce these.

In a recent study in the United States, family members participated in semi-structured interviews to identify errors that occurred during the admission. The family member reporting yielded 16% more errors and 10% more adverse events than hospital incident reports completed solely by staff. By including families in safety surveillance, the group identified otherwise unrecognized errors and adverse events [52]. Medical teams should encourage family members to know what is happening with their loved one's treatment, to be involved in care and when they see something, to say something.

Family Role in Hand Hygiene

Healthcare-associated infections represent another important safety issue for hospitalized patients, and a concerning contributor to the spread of infections in the hospital remains hand hygiene non-compliance among healthcare workers. In response, the World Health Organization has developed a five-step strategy to improve hand hygiene. One of the steps includes instituting a "safety climate, with active and visible participation from healthcare workers, manages, and when feasible, patients" [56]. One strategy to implement this recommendation has been to educate patients on the importance of asking healthcare workers to wash their hands, with an average improvement in hand hygiene of 34% [56]. Unfortunately, patients in the intensive care unit are often not well enough to educate about hand hygiene, or to reliably prompt healthcare workers. However, family members can assume this role for the patient if they feel comfortable asking healthcare workers to wash their hands [56, 57]. Several reasons for this hesitation have been identified; patients and their family members do not want to bother an already busy care team, they are unsure who to direct their comment towards, they do not want to cause problems, and they fear that their lack of medical knowledge makes it inappropriate for them to speak up [58]. Of note, having a lower education level, belonging to a minority group and being older makes patients and their family members less likely to speak up about hand hygiene, as well as concern for medical errors and adverse events in general [59]. This fact puts already marginalized groups at even greater risk of harm during their hospital stay. Importantly, a single explicit invitation from healthcare workers to ask about hand hygiene increased the likelihood that patients and their families would do so [60]. This finding highlights the role of open communication between healthcare staff and patients and their families in creating a culture of quality and safety.

Family Activated Rapid Response Teams

A primary benefit of hospitalization for an ill patient is to allow for close monitoring of clinical status, but despite this, there are frequently unanticipated events and clinical deterioration may not immediately be recognized by staff. Rapid identification and interventions improve outcome for such patients, and as a result early warning scores and rapid response teams have been developed to alert providers and promptly react to clinical deterioration. In some cases, patients may worsen prior to hospital staff recognition. To help decrease the delay in recognition and treatment, early warning scores and rapid response teams have been developed to alert care providers to early signs of clinical deterioration. One additional step to improve this response has been the integration of family members. Family members are often acutely aware of changes to their family members' clinical status. There is evidence that when patients and family members are empowered to alert care team members or activate a rapid response team themselves, they almost always do so appropriately [61]. In fact, the addition of family activated rapid response teams decreased the number of non-ICU codes in one observational study without having excessive false positive alerts [62]. Family members can be an important ally for patient safety in this way.

Speaking Up

If family members are present and have a concern regarding patient care or safety, there is no benefit if the family member doesn't inform the team. However, family members must feel that the team will be receptive to feedback and concerns from a layperson. Concerns about fear of abandonment or reprisal from the medical team have been expressed by family members as reasons for not wanting to speak up if they see something concerning [63]. In particular, for family members marginalized by education, cultural or language barriers, this can be particularly challenging [64]. Additionally, when concerns are raised by family members, they often do not feel that they are being adequately understood and addressed [65]. Family members must be respected when they bring concerns to the table, and some institutions have begun including the patient and family perspective in analysis of adverse events [66]. When asked about medical error, family members are able to identify factors contributing to the error and possible recommendations for addressing these [67]. While the structure of family and patient involvement in medical error discussions continues to evolve, including patient and family members when able could help improve safety for future patients.

Patient-Family Advisory Councils

Another way for family members to have a venue to speak up and influence care for patients is in the form of Patient-Family Advisory Councils (PFACs) (see Fig. 6.2). The first PFAC was started in 1998 at Dana Farber Cancer Center and these councils have become increasingly common over the past decade [68]. PFACs are usually formed from prior patients or family members who are interested in more engagement, sometimes following invitation from the medical team who has interacted with them. These groups have varied formats but in general meet together periodically with ICU or hospital leadership to provide patient and family perspective to ICU operations, design and safety procedures. The PFAC can also identify issues that were not apparent to the ICU staff, such as the way certain care transitions are stressful and how signage appears to family to be unwelcoming or confusing. Family involvement in designing ICU layout provides a unique perspective that can improve the environment, making it more patient- and family-centered [69].

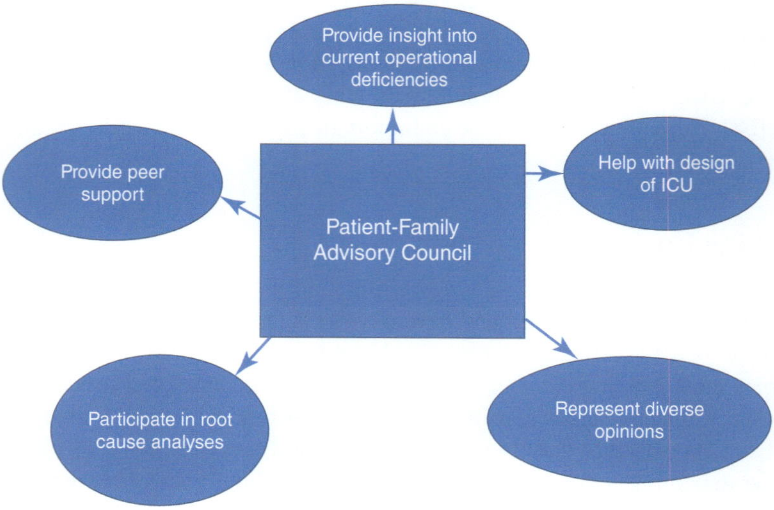

Fig. 6.2 Roles of patient family advisory councils

In particular, PFACs can provide a voice for vulnerable populations. When an advisory board included family members with limited-English proficiency Latina mothers, the board members reported that their participation was an important way to improve the clinic services. Additionally, board membership countered the negative experiences of discrimination and marginalization [70].

PFAC members may be motivated to reach out to other family members and provide peer support. In a pediatric ICU in Utah, PFAC members spend time with family members of current ICU patients to answer questions as well as help with expectations for life beyond the ICU. Formal peer support groups are also being studied for the impact on PICS-F more broadly.

Beyond having family members represented on PFACs, some institutions have included them on safety or quality committees where direct input on hospital policy and procedure is sought [6]. Family member involvement in hospital or ICU policy is critical as they can represent diverse viewpoints to change clinical practice, making care more patient- and family-friendly, as well as safer. However, for a PFAC to be an effective voice in an institution, the PFAC must be included in decision-making processes, and the institution must be open to change based on PFAC feedback [71]. Advice for forming and utilizing a PFAC can be found from multiple sources online, including a helpful handbook from the Agency for Healthcare Research and Quality [72].

Conclusion

Family members want to be a part of loved ones care, and can help to protect their loved one from both emotional and physical harms [20, 26, 73, 74]. Severe visitor restrictions during the COVID-19 pandemic resulted in significant psychological distress for both patients and families [17]. As the healthcare system equilibrates, it is essential to re-prioritize patient and family engagement as a cornerstone of culture of quality and safety. Including those who have the most invested in good outcomes for a patient can improve vigilance at the bedside and may lead to reduced errors and better overall safety for patients in these critical and tenuous situations. Family members should be involved in patient safety design and implementation, including PFACs.

Acknowledgments We appreciate the insights and advice on this chapter from the following: Intermountain Medical Center Patient Family Advisory Council members, nursing staff of the Shock Trauma Intensive Care Unit at Intermountain Medical Center, and the Center for Humanizing Critical Care led by Samuel Brown, MD and Elliotte Hirshberg, MD.

Financial Support and Conflicts of Interest No disclosures.

References

1. Davidson JE. Family-centered care: meeting the needs of patients' families and helping families adapt to critical illness. Crit Care Nurse. 2009;29(3):28–34; quiz 35.
2. Marmo S, Milner KA. From open to closed: COVID-19 restrictions on previously unrestricted visitation policies in adult intensive care units. Am J Crit Care. 2023;32(1):31–41.
3. Pizzo P, Walker D, Bomba P. Dying in America: improving quality and honoring individual preferences near the end of life. Washington, DC: Insitute of Medicine; 2015.
4. Lawton A, White J, Fromme EK. End-of-life and advance care planning considerations for lesbian, gay, bisexual, and transgender patients #275. J Palliat Med. 2014;17(1):106–8.
5. DeMartino ES, Dudzinski DM, Doyle CK, Sperry BP, Gregory SE, Siegler M, Sulmasy DP, Mueller PS, Kramer DB. Who decides when a patient can't? Statutes on alternate decision makers. N Engl J Med. 2017;376(15):1478–82.
6. National Patient Safety Foundation's Lucian Leape Institute. Safety is personal: partnering with patients and families for the safest care. Boston, MA: Foundation NPS; 2014.
7. Sokol-Hessner L, Folcarelli PH, Sands KE. Emotional harm from disrespect: the neglected preventable harm. BMJ Qual Saf. 2015;24(9):550–3.
8. Law AC, Roche S, Reichheld A, Folcarelli P, Cocchi MN, Howell MD, Sands K, Stevens JP. Failures in the respectful care of critically ill patients. Jt Comm J Qual Patient Saf. 2019;45(4):276–84.
9. Masso Guijarro P, Aranaz Andres JM, Mira JJ, Perdiguero E, Aibar C. Adverse events in hospitals: the patient's point of view. Qual Saf Health Care. 2010;19(2):144–7.
10. Johnstone MJ, Kanitsaki O. The neglect of racism as an ethical issue in health care. J Immigr Minor Health. 2010;12(4):489–95.
11. Haque OS, Waytz A. Dehumanization in medicine: causes, solutions, and functions. Perspect Psychol Sci. 2012;7(2):176–86.
12. Brown SM, Rozenblum R, Aboumatar H, Fagan MB, Milic M, Lee BS, Turner K, Frosch DL. Defining patient and family engagement in the intensive care unit. Am J Respir Crit Care Med. 2015;191(3):358–60.
13. Haines KJ, Kelly P, Fitzgerald P, Skinner EH, Iwashyna TJ. The untapped potential of patient and family engagement in the organization of critical care. Crit Care Med. 2017;45(5):899–906.
14. Olding M, McMillan SE, Reeves S, Schmitt MH, Puntillo K, Kitto S. Patient and family involvement in adult critical and intensive care settings: a scoping review. Health Expect. 2016;19(6):1183–202.
15. Xyrichis A, Fletcher S, Brearley S, Philippou J, Purssell E, Terblanche M, Rafferty AM, Reeves S. Interventions to promote patients and families' involvement in adult intensive care settings: a protocol for a mixed-method systematic review. Syst Rev. 2019;8(1):185.
16. Spruce L. Back to basics: patient and family engagement. AORN J. 2015;102(1):34–37; quiz 38–39.
17. Digby R, Manias E, Haines KJ, Orosz J, Ihle J, Bucknall TK. Family experiences and perceptions of intensive care unit care and communication during the COVID-19 pandemic. Austral Crit Care. 2022;36:S7.
18. Moss SJ, Krewulak KD, Stelfox HT, Ahmed SB, Anglin MC, Bagshaw SM, Burns KEA, Cook DJ, Doig CJ, Fox-Robichaud A, et al. Restricted visitation policies in acute care settings during the COVID-19 pandemic: a scoping review. Crit Care. 2021;25(1):347.
19. McPeake J, Kentish-Barnes N, Banse E, Anderson L, Cuzco C, Azoulay E, Quasim T, Castro P, Puxty K. Clinician perceptions of the impact of ICU family visiting restrictions during the COVID-19 pandemic: an international investigation. Crit Care. 2023;27(1):33.
20. Davidson JE, Powers K, Hedayat KM, Tieszen M, Kon AA, Shepard E, Spuhler V, Todres ID, Levy M, Barr J, et al. Clinical practice guidelines for support of the family in the patient-centered intensive care unit: American College of Critical Care Medicine Task Force 2004–2005. Crit Care Med. 2007;35(2):605–22.

21. Nurses AAoCC. AACN practice alert: family presence during resuscitation and invasive procedures. 2010.
22. Fulbrooke P, Latour J, Albarran J, de Graaf W, Lyng F, Devictor D, Norekval T, The Presence of Family Members During Cardiopulmonary Resuscitation Working group. The Presence of Family Members During Cardiopulmonary Resuscitation: European Federation of Critical Care Nursing Associations, Europena Society of Paediatric and Neonatal Intensive Care and European Society of Cardiology Council on Cardiovascular Nursing and Allied Profressions Joint Position Statement. Connect: The World of Critical Care Nursing. 2007;5(4):86–8.
23. Jacob M, Horton C, Rance-Ashley S, Field T, Patterson R, Johnson C, Saunders H, Shelton T, Miller J, Frobos C. Needs of patients' family members in an intensive care unit with continuous visitation. Am J Crit Care. 2016;25(2):118–25.
24. Barratt F, Wallis DN. Relatives in the resuscitation room: their point of view. J Accid Emerg Med. 1998;15(2):109–11.
25. Brown SM. We still lack patient centered visitation in intensive care units. BMJ. 2015;350:h792.
26. Carman KL, Dardess P, Maurer M, Workman T, Ganachari D, Pathak-Sen E. A roadmap for patient and family engagement in healthcare practice and research. Prepared by the American Institutes for Research under a grant from the Gordon and Betty Moore Foundation, Dominick Frosch, Project Officer and Fellow; Susan Baade, Program Officer; 2014.
27. Chapman DK, Collingridge DS, Mitchell LA, Wright ES, Hopkins RO, Butler JM, Brown SM. Satisfaction with elimination of all visitation restrictions in a mixed-profile intensive care unit. Am J Crit Care. 2016;25(1):46–50.
28. Netzer G, Iwashyna TJ. Fair is fair: preventing the misuse of visiting hours to reduce inequities. Ann Am Thorac Soc. 2017;14:1744.
29. Simon SK, Phillips K, Badalamenti S, Ohlert J, Krumberger J. Current practices regarding visitation policies in critical care units. Am J Crit Care. 1997;6(3):210–7.
30. Rosa RG, Tonietto TF, da Silva DB, Gutierres FA, Ascoli AM, Madeira LC, Rutzen W, Falavigna M, Robinson CC, Salluh JI, et al. Effectiveness and safety of an extended ICU visitation model for delirium prevention: a before and after study. Crit Care Med. 2017;45(10):1660–7.
31. Wu Y, Wang G, Zhang Z, Fan L, Ma F, Yue W, Li B, Tian J. Efficacy and safety of unrestricted visiting policy for critically ill patients: a meta-analysis. Crit Care. 2022;26(1):267.
32. Stickney CA, Ziniel SI, Brett MS, Truog RD. Family participation during intensive care unit rounds: attitudes and experiences of parents and healthcare providers in a tertiary pediatric intensive care unit. J Pediatr. 2014;164(2):402–6.e401–4.
33. Calderone A, Debay V, Goldfarb MJ. Family presence on rounds in adult critical care: a scoping review. Crit Care Explor. 2022;4(11):e0787.
34. Jacobowski NL, Girard TD, Mulder JA, Ely EW. Communication in critical care: family rounds in the intensive care unit. Am J Crit Care. 2010;19(5):421–30.
35. Davidson JE. Family presence on rounds in neonatal, pediatric, and adult intensive care units. Ann Am Thorac Soc. 2013;10(2):152–6.
36. Azoulay E, Pochard F, Chevret S, Adrie C, Bollaert PE, Brun F, Dreyfuss D, Garrouste-Orgeas M, Goldgran-Toledano D, Jourdain M, et al. Opinions about surrogate designation: a population survey in France. Crit Care Med. 2003;31(6):1711–4.
37. Wyskiel RM, Weeks K, Marsteller JA. Inviting families to participate in care: a family involvement menu. Jt Comm J Qual Patient Saf. 2015;41(1):43–6.
38. Wyskiel RM, Chang BH, Alday AA, Thompson DA, Rosen MA, Dietz AS, Marsteller JA. Towards expanding the acute care team: learning how to involve families in care processes. Fam Syst Health. 2015;33(3):242–9.
39. Van De Graaff M, Beesley SJ, Butler J, Benuzillo J, Poll JB, Oniki T, Francis M, Cable D, Hopkins RO, Lappe DL, et al. Partners in healing: postsurgical outcomes after family involvement in nursing care. Chest. 2018;153(2):572–4.
40. Franck LS, Oulton K, Nderitu S, Lim M, Fang S, Kaiser A. Parent involvement in pain management for NICU infants: a randomized controlled trial. Pediatrics. 2011;128(3):510–8.

41. Bastani F, Abadi TA, Haghani H. Effect of family-centered care on improving parental satisfaction and reducing readmission among premature infants: a randomized controlled trial. J Clin Diagn Res. 2015;9(1):SC04–8.
42. Skoog M, Milner KA, Gatti-Petito J, Dintyala K. The impact of family engagement on anxiety levels in a cardiothoracic intensive care unit. Crit Care Nurse. 2016;36(2):84–9.
43. Mortelmans LJ, Cas WM, Van Hellemond PL, De Cauwer HG. Should relatives witness resuscitation in the emergency department? The point of view of the Belgian Emergency Department staff. Eur J Emerg Med. 2009;16(2):87–91.
44. McClenathan BM, Torrington KG, Uyehara CF. Family member presence during cardiopulmonary resuscitation: a survey of US and international critical care professionals. Chest. 2002;122(6):2204–11.
45. Jakab M, Day AZ, Kraguljac A, Brown M, Mehta S. Family presence in the adult ICU during bedside procedures. J Intensive Care Med. 2019;34(7):587–93.
46. Haley KJ, Fessler DMT. Nobody's watching: subtle cues affect generosity in an anonymous economic game. Evol Hum Behav. 2005;26(3):245–56.
47. Sevransky JE, Nicholl B, Nicholl JB, Buchman TG. Patient- and family-centered care: first steps on a long journey. Crit Care Med. 2017;45(5):757–8.
48. Teutsch C. Patient-doctor communication. Med Clin North Am. 2003;87(5):1115–45.
49. Mello MM, Studdert DM, Kachalia A. The medical liability climate and prospects for reform. JAMA. 2014;312(20):2146–55.
50. Boothman RC, Imhoff SJ, Campbell DA Jr. Nurturing a culture of patient safety and achieving lower malpractice risk through disclosure: lessons learned and future directions. Front Health Serv Manag. 2012;28(3):13–28.
51. Committee on Quality of Health Care in America IoM. To err is human: building a safer health system. National Academics Press; 2000.
52. Khan A, Coffey M, Litterer KP, Baird JD, Furtak SL, Garcia BM, Ashland MA, Calaman S, Kuzma NC, O'Toole JK, et al. Families as partners in hospital error and adverse event surveillance. JAMA Pediatr. 2017;171(4):372–81.
53. Khan A, Furtak SL, Melvin P, Rogers JE, Schuster MA, Landrigan CP. Parent-reported errors and adverse events in hospitalized children. JAMA Pediatr. 2016;170(4):e154608.
54. Weissman JS, Schneider EC, Weingart SN, Epstein AM, David-Kasdan J, Feibelmann S, Annas CL, Ridley N, Kirle L, Gatsonis C. Comparing patient-reported hospital adverse events with medical record review: do patients know something that hospitals do not? Ann Intern Med. 2008;149(2):100–8.
55. Reason J. Human error: models and management. BMJ. 2000;320(7237):768–70.
56. McGuckin M, Govednik J. Patient empowerment and hand hygiene, 1997–2012. J Hosp Infect. 2013;84(3):191–9.
57. McGuckin M, Waterman R, Porten L, Bello S, Caruso M, Juzaitis B, Krug E, Mazer S, Ostrawski S. Patient education model for increasing handwashing compliance. Am J Infect Control. 1999;27(4):309–14.
58. Bell SK, Roche SD, Mueller A, Dente E, O'Reilly K, Sarnoff Lee B, Sands K, Talmor D, Brown SM. Speaking up about care concerns in the ICU: patient and family experiences, attitudes and perceived barriers. BMJ Qual Saf. 2018;27:928.
59. Fisher K, Smith K, Gallagher T, Burns L, Morales C, Mazor K. We want to know: eliciting hospitalized patients' perspectives on breakdowns in care. J Hosp Med. 2017;12(8):603–9.
60. Longtin Y, Sax H, Allegranzi B, Hugonnet S, Pittet D. Patients' beliefs and perceptions of their participation to increase healthcare worker compliance with hand hygiene. Infect Control Hosp Epidemiol. 2009;30(9):830–9.
61. McKinney A, Fitzsimons D, Blackwood B, McGaughey J. Patient and family-initiated escalation of care: a qualitative systematic review protocol. Syst Rev. 2019;8(1):91.
62. Gerdik C, Vallish RO, Miles K, Godwin SA, Wludyka PS, Panni MK. Successful implementation of a family and patient activated rapid response team in an adult level 1 trauma center. Resuscitation. 2010;81(12):1676–81.

63. Mazor KM, Roblin DW, Greene SM, Lemay CA, Firneno CL, Calvi J, Prouty CD, Horner K, Gallagher TH. Toward patient-centered cancer care: patient perceptions of problematic events, impact, and response. J Clin Oncol. 2012;30(15):1784–90.
64. Delbanco T, Bell SK. Guilty, afraid, and alone—struggling with medical error. N Engl J Med. 2007;357(17):1682–3.
65. Fisher KA, Ahmad S, Jackson M, Mazor KM. Surrogate decision makers' perspectives on preventable breakdowns in care among critically ill patients: a qualitative study. Patient Educ Couns. 2016;99(10):1685–93.
66. Etchegaray JM, Ottosen MJ, Burress L, Sage WM, Bell SK, Gallagher TH, Thomas EJ. Structuring patient and family involvement in medical error event disclosure and analysis. Health Aff. 2014;33(1):46–52.
67. Etchegaray JM, Ottosen MJ, Aigbe A, Sedlock E, Sage WM, Bell SK, Gallagher TH, Thomas EJ. Patients as partners in learning from unexpected events. Health Serv Res. 2016;51(Suppl 3):2600–14.
68. Niehaus K. Using a patient and family advisory council as a mechanism to hear the patient's voice. J Oncol Pract. 2017;13(8):509–11.
69. Bazuin D, Cardon K. Creating healing intensive care unit environments: physical and psychological considerations in designing critical care areas. Crit Care Nurs Q. 2011;34(4):259–67.
70. DeCamp LR, Polk S, Chrismer MC, Giusti F, Thompson DA, Sibinga E. Health care engagement of limited English proficient Latino families: lessons learned from advisory board development. Prog Community Health Partnersh. 2015;9(4):521–30.
71. Niehaus K: A patient and family advisory council for quality; making its voice heard at Memorial Sloan Kettering Cancer Center. NEJM Catal. 2017.
72. Strategy 1: working with patients and families as advisors. http://www.ahrq.gov/professionals/systems/hospital/engagingfamilies/strategy1/index.html.
73. Azoulay E, Pochard F, Chevret S, Lemaire F, Mokhtari M, Le Gall JR, Dhainaut JF, Schlemmer B, French FG. Meeting the needs of intensive care unit patient families: a multicenter study. Am J Respir Crit Care Med. 2001;163(1):135–9.
74. Chapman D, Collingridge DS, Mitchell LA, Wright ES, Hopkins RO, Butler JM, Brown SM. Family and nurse satisfaction with elimination of all visitation restrictions in a mixed-profile intensive care unit, a prospective observational study. Am J Crit Care. 2015;25:46.

Chapter 7
Personalized Interventions to Support Families in the Intensive Care Unit

Christopher E. Cox

Background

Clinical interventions in the field of critical care are increasingly focused on building the evidence base for individualizing management. Ideal positive end-expiratory pressure (PEEP) targeting, echocardiography-targeted volume resuscitation, and biomarker-guided antibiotics reflect our desire to better personalize and possibly amplify the effects initially observed with interventions applied relatively rigidly. It seems that the tension entailed between one clinician's concern about "cookbook medicine" and a manager's concern about high inter-clinician variability is in no danger of receding anytime soon.

In this spirit, it is worth considering ways in which one could conduct replicable family-focused interventions that permit at least a moderate amount of individualization—all within the limitations of the clinical setting itself. The rationale for this approach is strong:

1. The gold standard of medical care is to center it on the patient and their family.
2. Families often feel as though their role is ill-defined in the clinical encounter, which limits engagement.
3. Families commonly have information and comprehension deficits that prevent full participation in care and may limit their own well-being.
4. Few systems can actually assist clinicians in understanding if family members have specific needs—and if so, what types or severity exist.

C. E. Cox (✉)
Division of Pulmonary & Critical Care Medicine, Department of Medicine, Duke University, Durham, NC, USA

Program to Support People and Enhance Recovery, Duke University, Durham, NC, USA
e-mail: christopher.cox@duke.edu

© The Author(s), under exclusive license to Springer Nature Switzerland AG 2025

A. J. Vance et al. (eds.), *Families in the Intensive Care Unit*,
https://doi.org/10.1007/978-3-031-83786-9_7

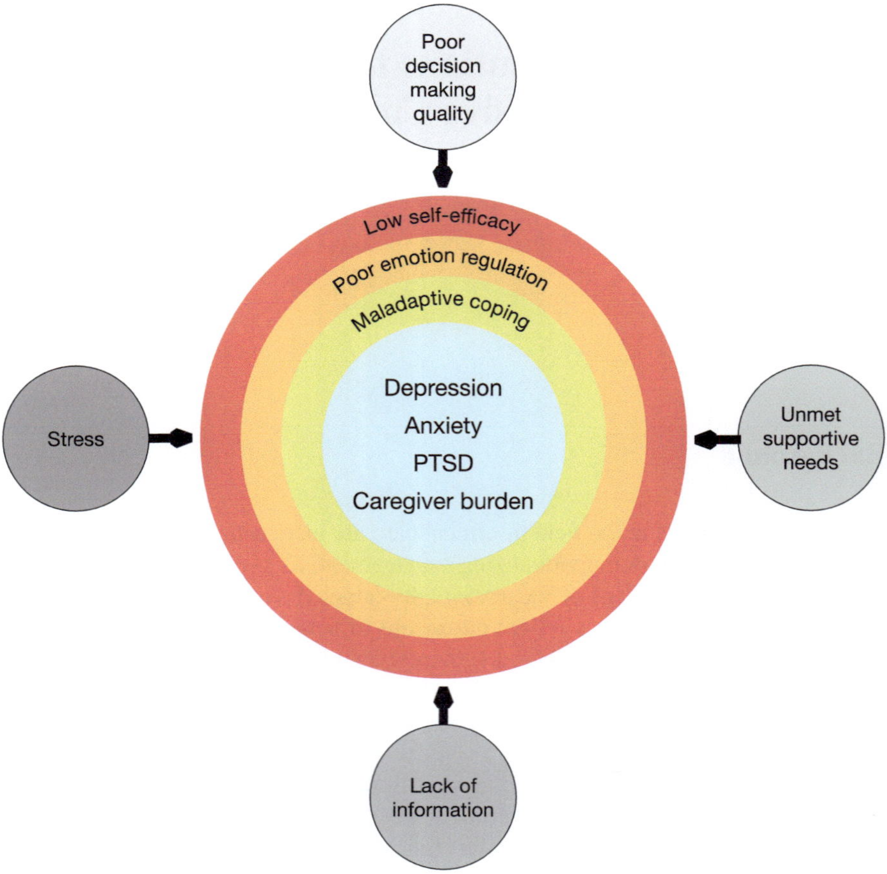

Fig. 7.1 Conceptual model

5. Few interventions are able to be adapted to the specific needs of families which could vary tremendously based on age, health literacy level, language skills, and cultural background.

As shown in the conceptual model in Fig. 7.1, the end result of these factors may be a set of serious missed opportunities that define the family intensive care unit syndrome [1].

In this chapter, we offer three examples of how these different missed opportunities could be transformed into "wins." These examples include lessons learned from our own mistakes, unlucky decisions, and difficult-to-swallow outcomes—but successes as well. We focus on our own interventions not because we think they are comparatively exceptional to the work of others, but because we can be intensely critical of their conception and conduct. It is our hope that these lessons learned can help others to move the field forward just a little bit quicker.

Example 1: Providing Personalized Information to Assist in Decision-Making

Decision-making is central to the practice of medicine. Observational studies have shown that ICU clinicians make over 100 decisions a day, nearly ten per patient [2]. Yet some of the most crucial decisions involve patients' surrogates—that is, their family caregivers. There is reason to believe that the quality of this decision-making process is suboptimal. In fact, one observational study found that half of family members did not adequately understand the diagnosis, treatments, or prognosis of their critically ill loved one [3].

It can be easy for clinicians to lose sight of just how overwhelming it can be for surrogate decision-makers to navigate a loved one's critical illness and the high-stakes decisions involved. Although we often focus interventions and attention on the decision itself, it is important to emphasize that the process of decision-making includes information gathering, decision-making, operationalizing the decision, and understanding the impact of the decision [4]. The evidence suggests that ICU clinicians may conduct the process of shared decision-making with family caregivers incompletely [5, 6]. Another barrier to high-quality decision-making is poor numeracy among family caregivers [7].

With this in mind, we developed a written decision aid for family caregivers of patients with prolonged mechanical ventilation that included individualized 1-year estimates of prognosis [8]. The aim of this intervention was to provide a template for shared decision-making, including stages from information gathering to values elicitation to the decision itself. When administered to family members and their ICU clinicians on day 10 of ventilation, we observed that there were sizable differences in key outcomes in comparison to a usual care control condition. The level of prognostic discordance was reduced from 47% to 7% with the decision aid, while it changed little in control. Similarly, the quality of communication reported by family members, their comprehension of relevant medical factors related to the decision about life support prolongation, and the amount of decisional conflict improved. Equally important were the impact on the likelihood that ICU teams discussed what to expect long term for survival and functional status.

Next, we adapted the decision aid to a digital version able to guide family members through the exercise of goals of care elicitation, viewing of individual-level prognosis based on a prediction model with a tailored data visualization, and matching with a general treatment plan. Although highly personalized, when compared to usual care in a multicenter randomized trial the picture became more complicated. In contrast to the pilot, we observed no difference between groups in prognostic concordance during hospitalization as well as symptoms of depression, anxiety, and post-traumatic stress disorder (PTSD) at 6 months [9]. Though there was a significant reduction in decisional conflict and improvement in understanding of the ICU physicians' prognostic estimate by among family member intervention recipients, there were few other outcomes that moved.

What happened? For one thing, the decision aid was mentioned by ICU physicians in post-decision aid viewing family meetings less than 30% of the time. Secondly, family members' baseline estimates of prognosis were incredibly high. In fact, the median expected 1-year patient survival reported by family members at baseline was greater than 90%—a surprisingly skewed estimate that changed little with the intervention. Even more bracing was that the majority of intervention recipients actually chose a treatment option that was even more aggressive than that suggested by their responses to the decision aid's patient preference elicitation feature. Third, we likely underestimated the power of the clinical momentum built into the clinical scenario of prolonged mechanical ventilation, in which decisions to date had probably self-selected family members who were committedly optimistic and resistant to recalibration of expectations. Last, we did not fully anticipate the potential power of different sources of information that families drew on as clinical planning was conducted. That is to say, it is possible that family members' optimistic prognostic estimates were intended more to express a positive attitude or their faith, to act as pushback to what they may have perceived as pessimism from the clinical team, or even to safeguard against what may have been a fear that the quality of medical care for their loved one would worsen should they disclose their concern about prognosis. This was a humbling experience that showed complex situations can overwhelm even interventions built with great care and intended patient-centeredness.

Since this trial, more has been learned about decision-making and communication in the context of race. For example, using recorded interviews from the decision aid trial's family meeting researchers noted differences in the largely White clinicians' shared decision-making behaviors. Compared to meetings with White family members, clinicians meeting with family members who identified as Black were more likely to provide limited emotional support, fail to acknowledge trust and gratitude expressed by family members, share medical information, and challenge family members preferences for restorative care [10]. As the field of health equity evolves in pulmonary and critical care, we urge investigators to pay close attention to known disparities in ICU-based communication and care among persons minoritized by race, ethnicity, and language.

Example 2: Providing Personalized Support to Reduce Psychological Distress

Many researchers have described the psychological sequelae of critical illness among both patients and family caregivers [11–14]. Although this distress is common and persistent, few interventions have reliably improved these symptoms. We recently tested two novel interventions designed to reduce patient and family member distress that are worth discussing as touchpoints for future research.

Because psychological distress can persist for months to years, we aimed to target the post-discharge timeframe. After a development and testing pilot study [15], we evaluated a telephone- and web-based coping skills training program among ICU survivors and their family members [16]. The six-session coping skills intervention did not reduce symptoms of depression, anxiety, or post-traumatic stress disorder (PTSD) at 3 months. However, among patients with elevated levels of baseline distress, the intervention reduced depression at a statistically and clinically significant difference at 6 months.

A number of somewhat painful lessons were learned from the coping skills trial that are important for future researchers to consider. First, focusing interventions on those with clinically important symptoms at baseline is critical. We greatly overestimated the rate of incident distress developing during follow-up. Second, starting the intervention quickly after discharge can reduce attrition. Unfortunately, waiting weeks to months for those transferred to nursing homes or rehabilitation facilities does not translate into good policy. Third, we need better metrics to identify those who are neither too well to benefit nor too ill to adhere to post-discharge interventions. A sad postscript of the study was that the most vulnerable participants with low education and great financial distress were the most likely to drop out from the study.

We tried to learn from our many mistakes by subsequently adapting our coping skills intervention to a self-directed, month-long program delivered by a mobile app platform [17]. I drove around central North Carolina to interview ICU survivors discussing their own strategies for successful adaptive coping on video, later editing for inclusion in the app. Several other patient suggestions made their way into the intervention including more visuals, a tie-in workbook, videos of clinicians normalizing the sometimes slow process of recovery, and timed reminders to complete tasks. In a randomized pilot trial [17], we found that depression, anxiety, and quality of life were improved compared to control, while adherence was extremely high—81% for activity in all 4 weeks and 96% in at least 3.

We also conducted a multicenter pilot trial of a self-directed mobile app-based mindfulness intervention, comparing it to a standard telephone intervention and an education program control [18]. Based on a pilot that could be described most generously as moderately successful [19], we aimed to try a different approach to distress that focused less on didactics and more on mastering just a couple key techniques. Though this trial was unable to include lessons learned from the coping trial such as excluding those without elevated baseline distress, we were able to relax inclusion criteria beyond just those who received mechanical ventilation. Also, we used patient and family feedback from the coping skills trial to build an intervention that was self-directed and shorter (four weekly sessions). Interestingly, we found that the mobile app group experienced the greatest reduction in 3-month symptoms of depression, anxiety, and physical symptoms. The differences were even more pronounced when analyses were restricted to those with elevated baseline distress. Importantly, adherence and retention were substantially better than that observed in the coping skills trial. Because it is unclear to what extent the different component pieces of the intervention may be important in modulating distress, we recently conducted a multicenter trial that tested eight different versions to see which is the optimal build [20]. We found that a simple version—one that included an app-based introduction (instead of therapist), twice-daily guided meditation, and app-based management of increasing depression symptoms (instead of therapist)—was optimal considering effects on psychological distress symptoms, adherence, and feasibility [21].

Throughout much of our digital intervention work, we are consistently struck by how often we are completely wrong about what content or features patients actually use frequently and find most helpful. Many times these turn out to be elements on which we spend the least amount of time developing! Perhaps the single thread that has kept us moving mostly forward is how much time we spend testing out new ideas with patients, listening to their feedback, and constantly iterating. Yes, there are conceptual models and all of that, but there are also the realities of how best to fit something new into another person's daily routine. Where next? We anticipate that building an automated digital system wherein distress screening and intervention deployment can be feasibly performed after discharge, possibly through electronic health record patient portals, will be key to the broader application of interventions such as this.

Example 3: Using Family Caregiver-Reported Information to Power Smart Systems of Care

Palliative care aims to address the needs of patients and their family members, and by so doing, improve quality of life. In different populations and care settings palliative care has reduced suffering, aligned treatment with values, and enhanced physical, spiritual, and emotional well-being [22]. Yet, in the ICU setting, there is evidence that the quality of palliative care is highly variable across the spectrum of care from hospital systems to the level of the individual patient or family member [23].

There are two types of barriers to efficiently, reliably, and effectively delivering ICU-based palliative care. First, there are structural barriers to effective care delivery related to the small palliative care specialist workforce and the common deficiencies among intensivists in communication, shared decision-making, and recognition of symptoms. Clearly structural barriers are difficult to change. Second, there are process barriers related to issues such as identifying which patients and families need help, engaging family members in palliative care, and promoting efficient collaboration between palliative care specialists and ICU clinicians. Because process barriers are a more feasible intervention target, we have focused on these as a way to improve care quality.

At the ground level, there are significant challenges. First, although studies suggest that at least a quarter of patients and families likely have notable unmet palliative care needs [24], it is difficult to identify them—and even more challenging to do so in an efficient, automated manner. On average intensivists order palliative care consults for 5–9% of patients, suggesting that they may either fail to recognize needs or feel that they are adequately addressing them. However, while hospitals that use specific diseases or conditions to "trigger" consultation can reliably increase specialist utilization, this may either overwhelm the specialist service or direct care away from others who may need it more. Importantly, there is no strong evidence that the presence of a trigger correctly reflects a greater burden of unmet need than its absence [25].

To address these challenges in different ways, we developed two distinctly different digital approaches to the problems inherent in the delivery of both primary (i.e., ICU teams) and specialty (i.e., specialist palliative care) palliative care. The first intervention (ICUconnect) was designed as digital infrastructure for care delivery for a primary palliative care model. This app platform allows families to report their palliative care needs directly, displaying them by domain for rapid review by clinicians (see Fig. 7.2). The app provides tips for clinicians to address each need and automatically texts them a link to new needs reported over time by family members. In a recent randomized trial, we found that family members who received the intervention had a greater reduction in unmet needs over time compared to usual care control [26].

The second app-based system (PCplanner) provides a centralized structure for the delivery of palliative care for both specialists and ICU clinicians that is largely automated, easily visible, and acceptable. Guided by our previously published conceptual model, extensive pilot work, and past trial experiences, the intervention is an electronic health record (EHR) system-integrated app platform that identifies high-risk patient phenotypes, assesses family-reported needs, and promotes collaborative care delivered by palliative care specialists and ICU clinicians using a logic-driven process rooted in person-centered metrics [27, 28]. Our pilot trial demonstrated that the EHR-integrated app platform reduced unmet needs substantially among family members, improved the patient-centeredness of care, expedited the delivery of palliative care, reduced hospital length of stay, and increased the receipt of hospice care—in comparison to standard palliative care specialist controls [29]. Currently the intervention is being tested versus usual care control in a randomized clinical trial [30].

These digital interventions possess several attractive features that became especially useful during the COVID-19 pandemic. During times of hospital visitation restriction, self-reported needs because a sort of "cheat sheet" for ICU clinicians pressed for time while conducting daily telephone updates with family members after rounds. Many noted that having a list of needs, or talking points, ranked by severity allowed them to quickly direct the conversation toward peoples' greatest concerns—instead of using valuable time searching for the same information. A second realization was feedback from clinicians that the systematic process of reviewing needs with family members standardized their approach to communication and gave them additional confidence in quickly navigating to what mattered most. Last, family members reported that even though they were not physically present in the hospital, they felt more reassured that they were still able to some

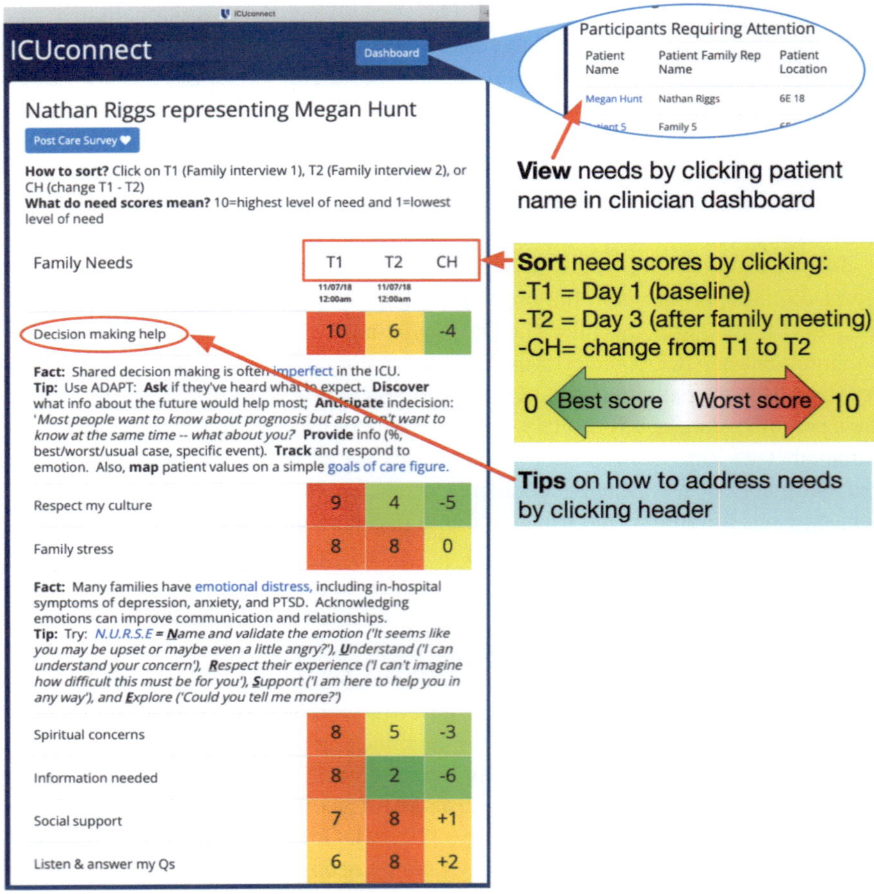

Fig. 7.2 Screenshot from palliative care app

extent to provide their loved one's voice through their reporting of needs via the mobile apps.

However, we concede that these interventions, though very much person-centered from conception to buildout, are imperfect. While some of these findings are compelling, these systems' limitations are worth discussing. First, while some patient populations targeted by the EHR-integrated app system may have specific interest for administrators (e.g., chronic critical illness), it is likely that this distinction may be unimportant at the ground level for clinicians and family members alike. Second, a focus on unmet need is more practical than triggers (which coincidentally are not correlated with the presence or severity of actual family-reported need) [31], though it is unclear how to define what constitutes an elevated level of need that is actionable—and whether there is an optimal needs score cutoff that should prompt the involvement of a specialist. Third, knowledge of various domains of need could allow non-physicians (e.g., chaplains, social workers, nurses) to address needs, though operationalizing this is an entirely different challenge with no clear guidebook. Last, it cannot be emphasized enough that these interventions' impacts depend almost entirely on the actions of ICU clinicians—the same group noted earlier that rarely mentioned the decision aid in family meetings that were part of the intervention itself. While we have tried to tailor every possible element of intervention delivery to clinicians' workflows, we often feel at the mercy of clinicians' workload, interest in the topic, philosophy on research, and sympathy for the research team. Yet we recognize that this is a tradeoff of "light touch," automated interventions that were inspired by the needs of low-resourced settings that may have no access to palliative care specialists. It is possible that for many situations, highly orchestrated interventions that incorporate dedicated research team members in all elements of the intervention may be a better path for some institutions and settings.

Summary

These practical examples of how we can empower ICU family members with information, therapeutic resources, and systems through which to directly report their needs. Though these examples represent different approaches and areas of impact, they are united by a goal of giving family members greater leverage and purpose within the dyadic clinician-family relationship. Focusing on approaches through which to better level this interaction may not only help to simplify interventions, but possibly increase their efficacy.

Conflicts of Interest Dr. Cox has neither competing financial or non-financial interests in this research.

References

1. Netzer G, Sullivan DR. Recognizing, naming, and measuring a family intensive care unit syndrome. Ann Am Thorac Soc. 2014;11(3):435–41. https://doi.org/10.1513/AnnalsATS.201309-308OT.
2. McKenzie MS, Auriemma CL, Olenik J, Cooney E, Gabler NB, Halpern SD. An observational study of decision making by medical intensivists. Crit Care Med. 2015;43(8):1660–8. https://doi.org/10.1097/CCM.0000000000001084.
3. Azoulay E, Chevret S, Leleu G, et al. Half the families of intensive care unit patients experience inadequate communication with physicians. Crit Care Med. 2000;28(8):3044–9.
4. Longo DR, Woolf SH. Rethinking the information priorities of patients. JAMA. 2014;311(18):1857–8. https://doi.org/10.1001/jama.2014.3038.
5. White DB, Braddock CH III, Bereknyei S, Curtis JR. Toward shared decision making at the end of life in intensive care units: opportunities for improvement. Arch Intern Med. 2007;167(5):461–7. https://doi.org/10.1001/archinte.167.5.461.

6. Cox CE, Martinu T, Sathy SJ, et al. Expectations and outcomes of prolonged mechanical ventilation. Crit Care Med. 2009;37(11):2888–94; quiz 2904. https://doi.org/10.1097/CCM.0b013e3181ab86ed.
7. Leiter N, Motta M, Reed RM, et al. Numeracy and interpretation of prognostic estimates in intracerebral hemorrhage among surrogate decision makers in the neurologic ICU. Crit Care Med. 2018;46(2):264–71. https://doi.org/10.1097/CCM.0000000000002887.
8. Cox CE, Lewis CL, Hanson LC, et al. Development and pilot testing of a decision aid for surrogates of patients with prolonged mechanical ventilation. Crit Care Med. 2012;40(8):2327–34. https://doi.org/10.1097/CCM.0b013e3182536a63.
9. Cox CE, White DB, Hough CL, et al. Effects of a personalized web-based decision aid for surrogate decision makers of patients with prolonged mechanical ventilation: a randomized clinical trial. Ann Intern Med. 2019;170(5):285–97. https://doi.org/10.7326/M18-2335.
10. Ashana DC, Welsh W, Preiss D, et al. Racial differences in shared decision-making about critical illness. JAMA Intern Med. 2024;184(4):424–32. https://doi.org/10.1001/jamainternmed.2023.8433.
11. Huang M, Parker AM, Bienvenu OJ, et al. Psychiatric symptoms in acute respiratory distress syndrome survivors: a 1-year national multicenter study. Crit Care Med. 2016;44(5):954–65. https://doi.org/10.1097/CCM.0000000000001621.
12. Bienvenu OJ, Colantuoni E, Mendez-Tellez PA, et al. Cooccurrence of and remission from general anxiety, depression, and posttraumatic stress disorder symptoms after acute lung injury: a 2-year longitudinal study. Crit Care Med. 2015;43(3):642–53. https://doi.org/10.1097/CCM.0000000000000752.
13. Rabiee A, Nikayin S, Hashem MD, et al. Depressive symptoms after critical illness: a systematic review and meta-analysis. Crit Care Med. 2016;44(9):1744–53. https://doi.org/10.1097/CCM.0000000000001811.
14. Jackson JC, Pandharipande PP, Girard TD, et al. Depression, post-traumatic stress disorder, and functional disability in survivors of critical illness in the BRAIN-ICU study: a longitudinal cohort study. Lancet Respir Med. 2014;2(5):369–79. https://doi.org/10.1016/S2213-2600(14)70051-7.
15. Cox CE, Porter LS, Hough CL, et al. Development and preliminary evaluation of a telephone-based coping skills training intervention for survivors of acute lung injury and their informal caregivers. Intensive Care Med. 2012;38(8):1289–97. https://doi.org/10.1007/s00134-012-2567-3.
16. Cox CE, Hough CL, Carson SS, et al. Effects of a telephone- and web-based coping skills training program compared with an education program for survivors of critical illness and their family members. A randomized clinical trial. Am J Respir Crit Care Med. 2018;197(1):66–78. https://doi.org/10.1164/rccm.201704-0720OC.
17. Cox CE, Kelleher SA, Parish A, et al. Feasibility of mobile app-based coping skills training for cardiorespiratory failure survivors: the Blueprint pilot randomized controlled trial. Ann Am Thorac Soc. 2023;20:861. https://doi.org/10.1513/AnnalsATS.202210-890OC.
18. Cox CE, Hough CL, Jones DM, et al. Effects of mindfulness training programmes delivered by a self-directed mobile app and by telephone compared with an education programme for survivors of critical illness: a pilot randomised clinical trial. Thorax. 2019;74(1):33–42. https://doi.org/10.1136/thoraxjnl-2017-211264.
19. Cox CE, Porter LS, Buck PJ, et al. Development and preliminary evaluation of a telephone-based mindfulness training intervention for survivors of critical illness. Ann Am Thorac Soc. 2014;11(2):173–81. https://doi.org/10.1513/AnnalsATS.201308-283OC.
20. Cox CE, Olsen MK, Gallis JA, et al. Optimizing a self-directed mobile mindfulness intervention for improving cardiorespiratory failure survivors' psychological distress (LIFT2): design and rationale of a randomized factorial experimental clinical trial. Contemp Clin Trials. 2020;96:106119. https://doi.org/10.1016/j.cct.2020.106119.

21. Cox CE, Gallis JA, Olsen MK, et al. Mobile mindfulness intervention for psychological distress among intensive care unit survivors: a randomized clinical trial. JAMA Intern Med. 2024;184:749. https://doi.org/10.1001/jamainternmed.2024.0823.
22. Kelley AS, Morrison RS. Palliative care for the seriously ill. N Engl J Med. 2015;373(8):747–55. https://doi.org/10.1056/NEJMra1404684.
23. Aslakson RA, Reinke LF, Cox CE, Kross EK, Benzo RP, Curtis JR. Developing a research agenda for integrating palliative care into critical care and pulmonary practice to improve patient and family outcomes. J Palliat Med. 2017;20(4):329–43. https://doi.org/10.1089/jpm.2016.0567.
24. Hua MS, Li G, Blinderman CD, Wunsch H. Estimates of the need for palliative care consultation across United States intensive care units using a trigger-based model. Am J Respir Crit Care Med. 2014;189(4):428–36. https://doi.org/10.1164/rccm.201307-1229OC.
25. Creutzfeldt CJ, Engelberg RA, Healey L, et al. Palliative care needs in the neuro-ICU. Crit Care Med. 2015;43(8):1677–84. https://doi.org/10.1097/CCM.0000000000001018.
26. Cox CE, Ashana DC, Riley IL, et al. Mobile application-based communication facilitation platform for family members of critically ill patients: a randomized clinical trial. JAMA Netw Open. 2024;7(1):e2349666. https://doi.org/10.1001/jamanetworkopen.2023.49666.
27. Carson SS, Cox CE, Wallenstein S, et al. Effect of palliative care-led meetings for families of patients with chronic critical illness: a randomized clinical trial. JAMA. 2016;316(1):51–62. https://doi.org/10.1001/jama.2016.8474.
28. Wysham NG, Hua M, Hough CL, et al. Improving ICU-based palliative care delivery: a multicenter, multidisciplinary survey of critical care clinician attitudes and beliefs. Crit Care Med. 2017;45(4):e372–8. https://doi.org/10.1097/CCM.0000000000002099.
29. Cox CE, Jones DM, Reagan W, et al. Palliative care planner (PCplanner): a pilot study to evaluate acceptability and usability of an electronic health records system-integrated, needs-targeted app platform. Ann Am Thorac Soc. 2017;15(1):59–68.
30. Cox CE, Olsen MK, Casarett D, et al. Operationalizing needs-focused palliative care for older adults in intensive care units: design of and rationale for the PCplanner randomized clinical trial. Contemp Clin Trials. 2020;98:106163. https://doi.org/10.1016/j.cct.2020.106163.
31. Cox CE, Ashana DC, Haines KL, et al. Assessment of clinical palliative care trigger status vs actual needs among critically ill patients and their family members. JAMA Netw Open. 2022;5(1):e2144093. https://doi.org/10.1001/jamanetworkopen.2021.44093.

Chapter 8
Training Clinicians in Family-Centered Care

Jared Chiarchiaro, Erin K. Kross, and Catherine L. Hough

Introduction

Each year, over 30,000 medical trainees begin their journey as clinicians, learning their trade by actively providing care to millions of patients each year in the United States alone [1]. Training adult and pediatric critical care clinicians to provide family-centered care is essential both in the present—given the large footprint of graduate medical education—and in the future of medical practice. In this chapter, we will discuss key aspects of training clinicians in family-centered care. We will begin with a review of studies of directed educational programs intended to promote family-centered care. Next, we will consider impact of the care environments in which we practice and train clinicians. Third, we will explore the importance of self-care and programs that incorporate clinician wellness into training. We will present published guidelines relevant to training. And finally, we will discuss opportunities to improve the evidence-base regarding training clinicians in family-centered care.

J. Chiarchiaro (✉)
Division of Pulmonary and Critical Care Medicine, School of Medicine, Oregon Health & Sciences University, Portland, OR, USA
e-mail: chiarchi@ohsu.edu

E. K. Kross
Division of Pulmonary, Critical Care and Sleep Medicine, UW Medicine, Seattle, WA, USA

C. L. Hough
Oregon Health & Science University, Portland, OR, USA

© The Author(s), under exclusive license to Springer Nature Switzerland AG 2025
A. J. Vance et al. (eds.), *Families in the Intensive Care Unit*,
https://doi.org/10.1007/978-3-031-83786-9_8

Directed Educational Activities

Direct training and educational activities are effective in teaching clinicians how to respond to family needs and provide family-centered care. Given the importance of high-quality family communication to family-centered care and family-centered outcomes, communication training programs are an appealing intervention to improve the quality of communication in adult and pediatric intensive care units (ICUs). In the ICU setting, a family conference is a key event which often defines the goals of care for the patient, facilitates shared decision-making between the ICU team and surrogate decision-makers, and shapes the experience of the family involved in a patient's care [2, 3]. Several approaches are available that teach clinicians how to lead an ICU family conference, including the use of simulation and/or structured feedback from faculty [4, 5]. Advantages to integrating didactics and simulation with direct observation and feedback into existing critical care rotations include the ability to use internal resources with less interruption to the clinical schedule.

There are several key features that should be ensured when developing a training program to provide a safe environment for learning (Table 8.1; [5]). Some of these include having faculty champions and buy-in from program directors and other leaders in the training program, creating space and time for learner reflection, and creating ground rules for learner-centered expectations and faculty evaluator feedback. Communication training programs should consider including elements of narrative medicine. Narrative medicine is defined as the ability to acknowledge, absorb, interpret, and act on the stories and plights of others [6]. This may not only assist in the care of patients and their families but also serve as a component of self-care, particularly for clinicians who face a high mental and emotional toll in their work [7]. Finally, elements of diversity, equity, and inclusion have an important role in communication training programs. These may include components of implicit bias training and active bystander training. Improving health equity is an important way to meaningfully engage patients, families, and communities, which is essential in the implementation of communication skills training programs [8].

Table 8.1 Key strategies for ensuring a safe environment for communication skills training

Have dedicated faculty champion(s) who focus on developing rapport with learners, setting the tone for simulation encounters, and debriefing with faculty and with learners after simulation encounters
Ensure buy-in from program directors and other clinical leaders in the training program
Ensure learners have space and time for reflection before and after the simulation encounter
Clinician learners with ground rules to help set expectations, emphasizing learner-centered aspects of the activity, the role of the faculty evaluator, and provide learners with mechanisms to respond to intrasimulation crisis
Provide faculty evaluators with ground rules about feedback and debriefing, including specific, learner-specific feedback with active listening and elicitation of reflections from learners

Several different types of communication skills training programs are described in the literature. The critical care fellowship training program at the Montefiore Medical Center at Albert Einstein College of Medicine used family meeting simulation training along with a didactic lecture and case series of discussions and showed that their training program increased trainee level of comfort and performance of specific communication tasks including agenda setting, provision of meeting summary and creation of follow-up plans [5]. A different type of training program has been described by a multidisciplinary group at Scripps Mercy Hospital where they sought to train interdisciplinary teams of ICU clinicians in communication with families of critically ill patients to improve staff confidence in communicating with families and improve family satisfaction with their experiences in the ICU. This program trained a group of multidisciplinary staff (including resident physicians, nurses, social workers, chaplains, and case managers) through guided readings about communication techniques, brief didactics, and case simulation exercises (role play) and found that participants had improvement in self-reported confidence but there did not find differences in overall family satisfaction in the ICU before and after the intervention [9]. Despite investigators detecting no change in overall satisfaction, family members did report higher satisfaction after the intervention in several important domains, including decision-making in the ICU, increased frequency of communication with nurses and doctors, and increased honesty of information.

Opportunity exists to expand a procedural-training framework in innovative ways to teach clinicians to respond to family needs and provide family-centered care through the family conference. Evidence supports the use of competency-based modules and simulation in teaching invasive procedures [10]. Many training programs currently use this learning approach for procedures such as central line placement by providing learners with specific structured components and gradually increasing responsibility. The University of Washington has developed an approach to family conference training for internal medicine residents during their medical ICU rotation that combines didactic training, observation of others, supervised practice with feedback, and determination of competency [11]. The five components of this ICU family conference learning module are: (1) residents view a brief instructional video created by VitalTalk [12] with an overview of seven components of a family conference; (2) residents conduct at least two supervised family conferences; (3) supervisors use a standardized teaching and evaluation form; (4) residents document the family conference in a procedure log; and (5) residents document the family conference in the electronic medical record using a note template.

Programs developed to teach effective, evidence-based strategies for family communication should evaluate both learner-specific outcomes and patient- and family-outcomes. Communication training programs have consistently shown feasibility and acceptability of the training as well as improvement in clinician-reported communication skills [4, 5, 9, 13–18]. One study has demonstrated improvement in intensive care unit team relational coordination surrounding goals of care, which may be described as team-based communication skills training and important in multidisciplinary environments such as the intensive care unit [19]. A prospective before-and-after cohort study showed that a communication skills training program increased goals of care documentation, an important quality metric [20]. However, few have examined patient- or family-centered assessments or outcomes. Trainee self-assessments of competence do not correlate with family ratings of quality of communication [21]. One randomized trial examined an educational program for residents and nurse practitioner students using didactic teaching, skills practice using simulation, and reflective discussion and found that the skills-based intervention did improve trainee self-assessments and standardized patient evaluations, but this improvement in self-assessment came without any change in the primary outcome which was patient and family ratings of quality of communication. They also found no change in patient or family ratings of quality of end-of-life care and found a slight increase in patient-reported symptoms of depression [22]. This study highlights the importance of not relying on trainee self-assessment outcomes alone when studying these types of educational interventions.

The COVID-19 pandemic led to a need for rapid scaling of virtual learning environments, including for communication skills training. One study compared learner perceptions of a hybrid virtual/in-person version of a well-established communication skills training course to historic in-person-only versions and found that learners rated the hybrid version similarly to the traditional in-person version [23]. There are other examples of successful implementation of virtual learning more broadly in medical education. One study of a medical and pharmacy undergraduate biomedical science course showed no difference in exam scores between the virtual format and the hybrid format utilized the year prior [24]. In graduate medical education, the incorporation of virtual learning with lessons learned has reshaped how learners receive medical training [25]. There is much to learn about how to meaningfully integrate virtual technology with existing communication skills training and measure its efficacy.

The Influence of Environment

While didactics, group discussions, simulation, and role play all contribute to a clinician's education, training programs are intense experiences governed by hands-on-learning. Training environments are more like a crucible than a vacuum; a great many influences come together to form the culture and the hidden curriculum [26] which shape many aspects of both training and patient care. Trainee clinicians may be most influenced by their peers—others in training with whom they spend most of their time. The attitudes, behaviors, and language used by attending physicians and other faculty may have a disproportionate impact, as may the views and actions of other clinicians, such as nurses, respiratory and physical therapists. Incorporation of supportive care services which focus on the family's role during acute and chronic illness, such as palliative care and social work, into the workflow of residents likely promotes more family-centered care.

Beyond the impact of individuals, processes of care and hospital policies can have a profound influence. There are a multitude of reasons that a patient's loved ones may not be present for rounds, visiting hours, and family meetings. For example, people may be geographically distant or have additional caregiving responsibilities at home, financial constraints, or restrictive work hours. Hospital policy that promotes family presence conveys a strong message about its importance for patient care. Qualitative evidence demonstrates that institutional culture and policy may impact the development of professional attitudes, particularly for trainees [27]. It may be that the most effective educational approach is to actively work to promote initiatives to advance family-centered care within hospitals and healthcare systems. Similarly, it is likely that the policies and priorities of individual training programs have a significant impact on the importance of family-centered care for clinicians in training. For example: Are there faculty champions within the training program who model and advocate high-quality family-centered care? Are trainees routinely evaluated on their ability to provide family-centered care? Is the family conference specifically evaluated as an entrustable professional activity for trainees on specific rotations such as the medical ICU? Finally, the provision of hospital policy to afford families equal opportunity to see their loved ones and participate in shared decision-making is a health equity issue. One way to potentially overcome some of the above barriers is to support virtual technologies that ensure timely and meaningful meetings are taking place.

The Importance of Self-Care

Perhaps even more important than the external is the internal environment, the well-being of our trainees. The impact of emotional health on the job satisfaction and the quality of care by clinicians has become clearer over time, with effects including burnout and even suicide [28, 29]. In one large sample of resident physicians, nearly 13% of suffered from major depression and nearly 10% from suicidal ideation [30]. Resident physicians are at especially high risk of burnout, a syndrome of emotional exhaustion, depersonalization, and sense of low personal accomplishment, with a prevalence higher than 75% among internal medicine trainees [31, 32]. Imposterism has been shown to be an independent risk factor for both anxiety and burnout [33] and may be mitigated through improving self-efficacy with skills training [34]. Another likely contributor to burnout risk are maladaptive coping strategies that resident physicians have been shown to use in times of distress [35]. While it is likely that the provision of patient and family-centered care may prevent burnout by creating purpose and opportunities for human interactions within training, it is even more likely that an emotionally exhausted and depersonalized clinician will not be able to fully engage in this care [27]. Mindfulness, yoga, the creative arts [36] and other stress-reduction techniques have the potential to combat burnout and build resilience if offered as part of comprehensive wellness programs, which are becoming common in medical centers and universities. Indeed, there appears to be a growing recognition that the highest quality medical care requires clinicians to be in touch with their own humanity, a feat only possible if patient care is complemented by self-care [37, 38].

The intellectual and emotional intensity of critical care medicine may be a particular risk for burnout, and residents may need additional support during their ICU rotations. The ICU curriculum can incorporate opportunities for reflection and group support, also reinforcing the concept that self-care is as important as other educational topics. One such example is "Death Rounds," a facilitated discussion about experiences with the care of dying patients [39]. Beginning at the University of Washington's Harborview Medical Center in 2000, internal medicine residents rotating through the medical ICU attended Death Rounds together near the end of the rotation to discuss specific patients who had died that month under their care. The goal of the conference was to provide the residents with a chance to share their thoughts and feelings about the difficulty of caring for dying patients, and to reflect on opportunities to improve the quality of end-of-life care for both patients and their families. A survey conducted in 2002 indicated that Death Rounds was a valuable experience that improved residents' ability to cope with and care for dying patients. Indeed, Death Rounds has become a key part of the MICU experience, providing a much-needed "diastole" for residents and attending physicians alike. The format has allowed evolution and flexibility to accommodate the needs of the medical team, including peer support and a time to remind each other to practice "intensive self-care." The success of Death Rounds and greater need for such an opportunity to support each other as a care community is reflected in its permanent spot in the curriculum in the medical ICU rotation, nearly 20 years later, and its spread to other ICU services (such as neurocritical care [40]) and other institutions [39, 41]. Lastly, the rise of the Schwartz Rounds program, an interdisciplinary discussion of the psychological and emotional aspects of patient care, at healthcare centers around the world provides a growing example of the importance of community and conversation in improving clinician's ability to cope and deal with stress. Schwartz Rounds participants have endorsed the positive impact on patient and family-centered care at the individual and institutional level [42].

Evidence-Based Guidelines and Knowledge Gaps

While a growing body of evidence suggests methods we can use to better support training of house staff in the delivery of family-centered care in the ICU, many knowledge gaps persist. In 2017, the Society of Critical Care Medicine published updated guidelines for family-centered care in the ICU [43], endorsed by many other professional societies and groups. As one of several domains of

Table 8.2 Approaches to address knowledge gaps on the education of trainees in provision of family-centered care

Increase use of family-reported outcomes as the standard for quality of family communication, with cautious use of self-assessment tools
Collect data on cost of implementing communication training programs
Develop more long-term follow-up studies as skills may dissipate over time
Compare different communication teaching modalities such as didactic training versus role play versus simulation in both in-person and virtual environments
Measure the impact of educations/training programs on family member outcomes and ICU length of stay and costs, including assessment of potential unintended consequences

family-centered care, these evidence-based guidelines included examination of whether communication-training programs in the ICU for clinicians, including education or simulation, improve family psychological symptoms, family rating of quality of dying, patient- or family-rated quality of communication, family satisfaction with communication, clinician self-efficacy, or clinician psychological symptoms. They also examined the impact of family presence in a variety of settings and experiences within the ICU. The guidelines conclude that based on the existing evidence, including the known burdens to patients and families when there is poor communication and demonstrated improvements in clinician-reported skills and comfort following communication training, that ICU clinicians should receive family-centered communication training as one element of critical care training. However, the current evidence does not support one specific type of training program and further research is needed to understand whether and how training programs can be implemented to improve family-centered outcomes. Similarly, further research is needed to better understand the impacts on clinicians, patients, and families, as policies are adapted in support of family presence and engagement in the ICU (Table 8.2).

Conclusion

Opportunities to train clinicians in family-centered care are present throughout the hospital—not only in lecture halls and simulation suites, but also in our team rooms, our family meeting areas, our ICU hallways, and at our patients' bedsides. Additionally, facilitating our trainees' focus on self-care inside and outside the hospital is likely to enhance both provision of family-centered care and the ability to be emotional present and able to engage in the deeply human aspects of medicine which offer sustenance and satisfaction in our chosen profession (Fig. 8.1).

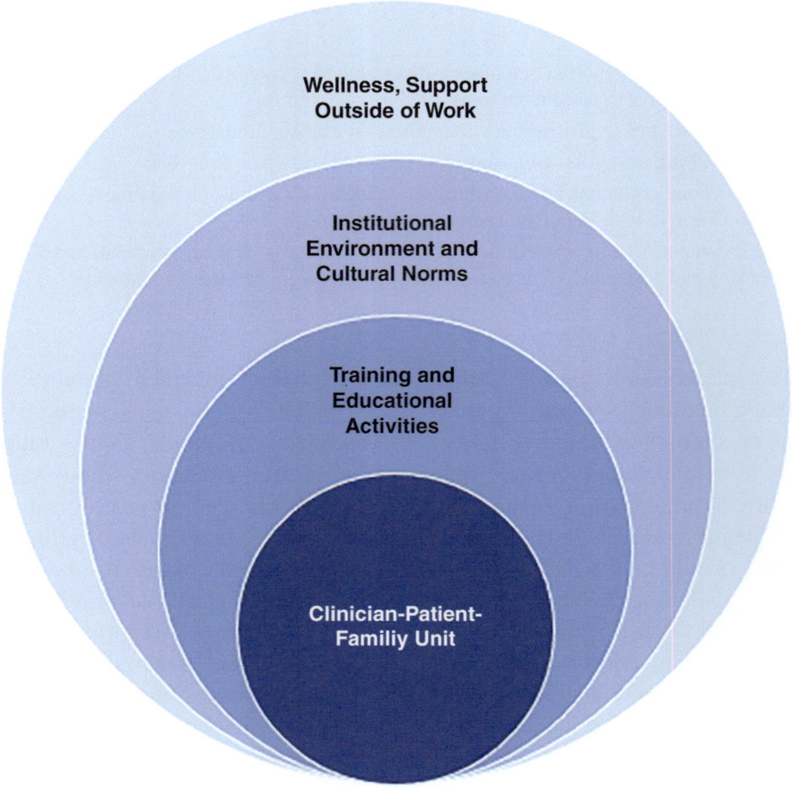

Fig. 8.1 Socio-ecological model [44] supporting clinicians in the delivery of family-centered care. Socio-Ecological Model [44] describing a set of systems and settings that influence the delivery of family centered care

References

1. Jena AB, DePasse JW, Prasad V. The declining demand for hospital care as a rationale for duty hour reform. J Gen Intern Med. 2014;29(10):1400–3.
2. Hurd CJ, Curtis JR. The intensive care unit family conference. Teaching a critical intensive care unit procedure. Ann Am Thorac Soc. 2015;12(4):469–71.
3. Curtis JR, White DB. Practical guidance for evidence-based ICU family conferences. Chest. 2008;134(4):835–43.
4. McCallister JW, Gustin JL, Wells-Di Gregorio S, Way DP, Mastronarde JG. Communication skills training curriculum for pulmonary and critical care fellows. Ann Am Thorac Soc. 2015;12(4):520–5.
5. Hope AA, Hsieh SJ, Howes JM, Keene AB, Fausto JA, Pinto PA, et al. Let's talk critical. Development and evaluation of a communication skills training program for critical care fellows. Ann Am Thorac Soc. 2015;12(4):505–11.
6. Charon R. The patient-physician relationship. Narrative medicine: a model for empathy, reflection, profession, and trust. JAMA. 2001;286(15):1897–902.

7. Awdish RLA, Hayes MM, Cooper AZ, Hosey MM, Trainor A, Weatherston R, et al. A way forward in the COVID-19 pandemic: making the case for narrative competence in pulmonary and critical care medicine. ATS Sch. 2022;3(2):188–96.
8. Simon M, Baur C, Guastello S, Ramiah K, Tufte J, Wisdom K, et al. Patient and family engaged care: an essential element of health equity. NAM Perspect. 2020; https://doi.org/10.31478/202007a.
9. Shaw DJ, Davidson JE, Smilde RI, Sondoozi T, Agan D. Multidisciplinary team training to enhance family communication in the ICU. Crit Care Med. 2014;42(2):265–71.
10. Huang GC, McSparron JI, Balk EM, Richards JB, Smith CC, Whelan JS, et al. Procedural instruction in invasive bedside procedures: a systematic review and meta-analysis of effective teaching approaches. BMJ Qual Saf. 2016;25(4):281–94.
11. Whitaker K, Kross EK, Hough CL, Hurd C, Back AL, Curtis JR. A procedural approach to teaching residents to conduct intensive care unit family conferences. J Palliat Med. 2016;19(10):1106–9.
12. www.vitaltalk.org [Internet]. [cited 2022 Nov 8]. www.vitaltalk.org.
13. Bays AM, Engelberg RA, Back AL, Ford DW, Downey L, Shannon SE, et al. Interprofessional communication skills training for serious illness: evaluation of a small-group, simulated patient intervention. J Palliat Med. 2014;17(2):159–66.
14. Boss RD, Urban A, Barnett MD, Arnold RM. Neonatal Critical Care Communication (NC3): training NICU physicians and nurse practitioners. J Perinatol. 2013;33(8):642–6.
15. Downar J, Knickle K, Granton JT, Hawryluck L. Using standardized family members to teach communication skills and ethical principles to critical care trainees. Crit Care Med. 2012;40(6):1814–9.
16. Hales BM, Hawryluck L. An interactive educational workshop to improve end of life communication skills. J Contin Educ Heal Prof. 2008;28(4):241–8; quiz 249–55.
17. Meyer EC, Sellers DE, Browning DM, McGuffie K, Solomon MZ, Truog RD. Difficult conversations: improving communication skills and relational abilities in health care. Pediatr Crit Care Med. 2009;10(3):352–9.
18. Lamiani G, Mistraletti G, Moreschi C, Andrighi E, Vegni E. Cultivating empathy and soft skills among intensive care residents: effects of a mandatory, simulation-based, experiential training. Ann Transplant. 2021;26:e931147.
19. Fettig L, Tang Q, Newton E, Rosario R, Matthias MS, Torke AM. A communication skills training workshop to improve ICU team relational coordination about goals of care: a pilot study. Am J Hosp Palliat Care. 2022;39(10):1157–64.
20. Orford NR, Milnes S, Simpson N, Keely G, Elderkin T, Bone A, et al. Effect of communication skills training on outcomes in critically ill patients with life-limiting illness referred for intensive care management: a before-and-after study. BMJ Support Palliat Care. 2019;9(1):e21.
21. Dickson RP, Engelberg RA, Back AL, Ford DW, Curtis JR. Internal medicine trainee self-assessments of end-of-life communication skills do not predict assessments of patients, families, or clinician-evaluators. J Palliat Med. 2012;15(4):418–26.
22. Curtis JR, Back AL, Ford DW, Downey L, Shannon SE, Doorenbos AZ, et al. Effect of communication skills training for residents and nurse practitioners on quality of communication with patients with serious illness: a randomized trial. JAMA. 2013;310(21):2271–81.
23. Chiarchiaro J, Arnold RM, Ernecoff NC, Claxton R, Childers JW, Schell JO. Serious illness communication skills training during a global pandemic. ATS Sch. 2022;3(1):64–75.
24. Nilaad SD, Lin E, Bailey J, Truong C, Gaboyan S, Mittal A, et al. Learning outcomes in a live virtual versus in-person curriculum for medical and pharmacy students. ATS Sch. 2022;3(3):399–412.
25. Almarzooq ZI, Lopes M, Kochar A. Virtual learning during the COVID-19 pandemic. J Am Coll Cardiol. 2020;75(20):2635–8.
26. Downar J. Resources for educating, training, and mentoring all physicians providing palliative care. J Palliat Med. 2018;21(S1):S57–62.
27. Dzeng E, Colaianni A, Roland M, Chander G, Smith TJ, Kelly MP, et al. Influence of institutional culture and policies on do-not-resuscitate decision making at the end of life. JAMA Intern Med. 2015;175(5):812–9.

28. Pulcrano M, Evans SRT, Sosin M. Quality of life and burnout rates across surgical specialties: a systematic review. JAMA Surg. 2016;151(10):970–8.
29. Devi S. Doctors in distress. Lancet. 2011;377(9764):454–5.
30. Bai S, Chang Q, Yao D, Zhang Y, Wu B, Shan L. The prevalence and risk factors for major depression and suicidal ideation in medical residents based on a large multi-center cross-sectional study using the propensity score-matched method. Soc Psychiatry Psychiatr Epidemiol. 2022;57(11):2279–91.
31. Dyrbye LN, West CP, Satele D, Boone S, Tan L, Sloan J, et al. Burnout among U.S. medical students, residents, and early career physicians relative to the general U.S. population. Acad Med. 2014;89(3):443–51.
32. Shanafelt TD, Bradley KA, Wipf JE, Back AL. Burnout and self-reported patient care in an internal medicine residency program. Ann Intern Med. 2002;136(5):358–67.
33. Liu RQ, Davidson J, van Hooren TA, van Koughnett JAM, Jones S, Ott MC. Impostorism and anxiety contribute to burnout among resident physicians. Med Teach. 2022;44(7):758–64.
34. Darban F, Balouchi A, Narouipour A, Safarzaei E, Shahdadi H. Effect of communication skills training on the burnout of nurses: a cross-sectional study. J Clin Diagn Res. 2016;10(4):IC01–4.
35. Burns KEA, Moss M, Lorens E, Jose EKA, Martin CM, Viglianti EM, et al. Wellness and coping of physicians who worked in ICUs during the pandemic: a multicenter cross-sectional North American survey. Crit Care Med. 2022;50:1689.
36. Reed K, Cochran KL, Edelblute A, Manzanares D, Sinn H, Henry M, et al. Creative arts therapy as a potential intervention to prevent burnout and build resilience in health care professionals. AACN Adv Crit Care. 2020;31(2):179–90.
37. Bodenheimer T, Sinsky C. From triple to quadruple aim: care of the patient requires care of the provider. Ann Fam Med. 2014;12(6):573–6.
38. Linzer M, Levine R, Meltzer D, Poplau S, Warde C, West CP. 10 bold steps to prevent burnout in general internal medicine. J Gen Intern Med. 2014;29(1):18–20.
39. Hough CL, Hudson LD, Salud A, Lahey T, Curtis JR. Death rounds: end-of-life discussions among medical residents in the intensive care unit. J Crit Care. 2005;20(1):20–5.
40. Khot S, Billings M, Owens D, Longstreth WT. Coping with death and dying on a neurology inpatient service: death rounds as an educational initiative for residents. Arch Neurol. 2011;68(11):1395–7.
41. Kitzes JA, Kalishman S, Kingsley DD, Mines J, Lawrence E. Palliative medicine death rounds: small group learning on a vital subject. Am J Hospice Palliat Med. 2009;25(6):483–91.
42. Lown BA, Manning CF. The Schwartz Center Rounds: evaluation of an interdisciplinary approach to enhancing patient-centered communication, teamwork, and provider support. Acad Med. 2010;85(6):1073–81.
43. Davidson JE, Aslakson RA, Long AC, Puntillo KA, Kross EK, Hart J, et al. Guidelines for family-centered care in the neonatal, pediatric, and adult ICU. Crit Care Med. 2017;45(1):103–28.
44. Bronfenbrenner U. Toward an experimental ecology of human development. Am Psychol. 1977;32(7):513–31.

Chapter 9
Cognitive Barriers to Effective Surrogate Decision-Making

Joanna L. Hart

Introduction

Family members of critically ill patients are routinely asked to participate in medical decision-making. Commonly, they adopt the role of surrogate decision-maker, or the individual advocating for and speaking on behalf of an incapacitated patient. In doing so, these surrogates are charged with sharing responsibility for complex medical decisions with uncertain risks, benefits, and outcomes. Participation in such shared decision-making leads to later psychological distress among family members of both surviving patients and those who die from their illnesses [1–3]. Additionally, when surrogates struggle to both interpret the information they receive and represent patients' wishes, the result may include care that is intolerable to patients or misaligned with their values [4–7]. Understanding the cognitive processes involved in decision-making is crucial to identifying and responding to these known ways in which the realities of shared decision-making deviate from their imagined ideals.

An economically "rational" decision may be defined as a complete consideration of possible courses of action, followed by the selection of a choice that will maximize potential benefits while minimizing possible risks [8]. However, within the intensive care unit (ICU) setting, decision-making processes fundamentally diverge from this rational model. Complex, preference-sensitive ICU care decisions are made in the context of key features of the choice environment that influence the

J. L. Hart (✉)
Division of Pulmonary, Allergy, and Critical Care and the Palliative and Advanced Illness Research Center, Department of Medicine, University of Pennsylvania School of Medicine, Philadelphia, PA, USA

Department of Medical Ethics and Health Policy, University of Pennsylvania School of Medicine, Philadelphia, PA, USA
e-mail: Joanna.Hart@pennmedicine.upenn.edu

© The Author(s), under exclusive license to Springer Nature Switzerland AG 2025
A. J. Vance et al. (eds.), *Families in the Intensive Care Unit*,
https://doi.org/10.1007/978-3-031-83786-9_9

process of decision-making. Family members acting as surrogates are faced with time pressures, threats of mortality, emotional and physical stress, and prognostic uncertainties. Therefore, decision-makers often have insufficient time, personal resources, and information available to engage in a rational decision-making process that adds additional demands on surrogates' time, cognitive burdens, and self-regulation.

In addition, scientific, structural, and skill barriers often limit whether the necessary decision-making information is available to surrogates. Prognostic data relevant to the decision often does not exist or, when available, lacks applicability to a particular patient given the heterogeneity of critical illness syndromes. The potential benefits and risks of the available treatment options are often undefined due to a lack of evidence and are always imbued with at least some degree of medical uncertainty. Further, clinicians may not present surrogates with the full array of potential options and the probabilities of these options' likely outcomes during collaborative or shared decision-making. Clinicians may limit discussion of options for reasons that include clinicians' own biases, clinical judgment, or lack of awareness. Finally, the known risks and benefits of each option must be integrated with patients' values, which are frequently unknown even to close family members. Therefore, the choice environments in which surrogate decision-makers are operating contribute to foreseeable missteps in the decision-making process, and may be centrally related to the known psychological burden carried by family members of critically ill patients [1]. In this chapter, we focus on the cognitive barriers to effective decision-making and associated ways in which critical care decision-makers may predictably deviate from rational decision-making. For this discussion, we define effective decision-making as choosing health care options that maximize the benefits to patients based on their own values and goals.

Heuristics and Biases

All people use heuristics, or cognitive shortcuts, when making decisions [9]. This includes when we face both low-stake decisions (e.g., what to eat for breakfast) and high-stake decisions (e.g., whether to undergo a potentially life-saving but highly morbid surgical procedure). We employ heuristics to reduce the cognitive load of decision-making and could hardly get through a day without them. Heuristics allow us to ignore or simplify certain pieces of information that we might otherwise need to process as we evaluate options. The result is a decreased burden of information integration as we make a decision, making decisions faster and with less effort (Fig. 9.1). Indeed, the burdens of decision fatigue are well documented [10, 11], highlighting the theological value of heuristics. Understanding how heuristics influence decision-makers and their choices is essential to building supportive and relevant decision environments for family members of critically ill patients.

Consider choosing a new television. A quick search on a major Internet retailer returns over 1000 options. A purely rational decision might require a comparative

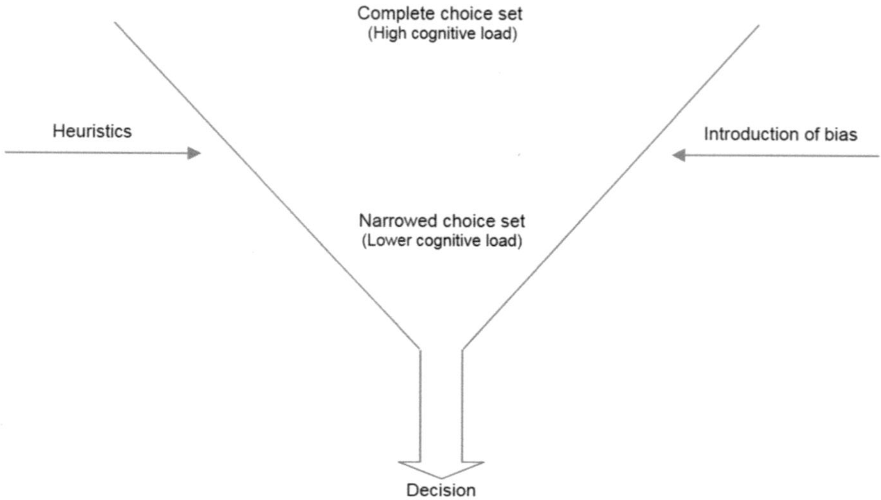

Fig. 9.1 Heuristics decrease cognitive load of decision-making and introduce bias

evaluation of each of these televisions, weighing the trade-offs of price, size, picture quality, Internet connectivity, parental controls, anticipated malfunction, and other features. Realistically, you would narrow this "choice set" of televisions down using past experiences, brand recognition, what size televisions are typical in your social network, a specific recommendation from a tech savvy friend or a trusted expert in television purchasing, or simply the television options that appear first in the search results. In this way, you no longer have to consider all 1000 options and your decision becomes easier. Easing that cognitive load and effort required is the function of heuristics.

Two classical explanations exist for why we use heuristics. First, decision-makers may make a rational trade-off between the quality of the decision-making process and the effort involved in making the decision, electing to sacrifice a comprehensive process for speed and frugality. For our example, a rational actor may recognize that a *better* decision process would be to evaluate each television, but instead decide that's not worth her time or effort to do so. Using a shortcut may degrade decision process quality, but this is recognized and acceptable to the decision-maker. Alternatively, decision-makers may not have the cognitive capacity to engage in the lengthy process of ideal decision-making. Therefore, employing heuristics reflects the limitations in our judgment. We don't choose to use shortcuts; we are simply incapable of comparing all 1000 television options, and so make suboptimal judgments.

Rejecting both of these theories, more recent views instead approach heuristics as a decision-maker's adaptive responses to a particular choice environment in order to meet his or her functional goals [9]. In other words, the use of heuristics represents neither an inherent loss of decision quality nor the necessary introduction of judgment errors, but instead a useful tool that decision-makers may use to simplify decisions in precise ways based on the particular situation at hand [12]. In this way, using shortcuts as you select your television means that you have narrowed the field systematically based on values important to you and successfully selected a television with time left over to eat dinner with your family, which you prefer to creating spreadsheets of television features.

While the use of heuristics should "confer no shame" [13], since we all use them, these tools often introduce error into the decision-making process or prevent corrections for error once introduced. These errors are known as bias, or the systematic deviation away from making choices that promote one's own goals or interests. And in the context of surrogate decision-making in the ICU, such bias may lead to undesired outcomes for critically ill patients and their family members. Because heuristics are particularly useful during times of cognitive strain, they are common in the critical care setting while also being inextricably linked to the formation and perpetuation of bias.

Biases in the ICU

Identifying when heuristics or resulting biases may be harmful in the context of critical care decision-making is a key first step in efforts to prevent them from causing actual harm to patients or surrogates. While evidence to date is limited in measuring the presence of these cognitive shortcuts in critical care decisions, clinicians guiding shared decision-making in the ICU would be helped by a working knowledge of how common heuristics and biases may influence decision-making [12, 14]. This includes recognizing clinicians' own risk of similar cognitive biases. During times of clinical strain, such as during the COVID-19 pandemic, the added cognitive stress on clinicians likely leads to increased reliance on the cognitive shortcuts of heuristics, thereby increasing the likelihood of harmful bias [15]. Such conditions may exacerbate failures in providing high-quality shared decision-making, tailored communication, and clinicians' attention to the choice environments families of critically ill patients face [14]. The separation of family members and surrogates from the hospitalized patient, as occurs during pandemic conditions or due to hospital policy, further increases surrogates' reliance on heuristics and biases and adds complexity to the high-stakes decision-making environment of the ICU [16]. We explore several well-described heuristics and biases that may be particularly relevant to the critical care setting as examples (Table 9.1).

Optimism and Impact Biases

Medical decision-makers must develop expectations of potential health outcomes when considering the available options. These expectations are then used to compare and weigh the relative risks and benefits of each potential path. Patients and

Table 9.1 Selected biases relevant to critical care decision-making

Bias	Definition	Implications for critical care decision-making
Optimism bias	The tendency to overestimate the likelihood of desirable outcomes	May improve coping with unfavorable prognoses May prevent adaptation to negative outcomes and impair risk-benefit analysis of treatment decisions
Impact bias	The systematic overestimation of the impact an event will have on an individual's life	May lead to avoidance of potentially beneficial therapies or elect for treatments that leave decision-makers unsatisfied
Commission bias	The tendency to regard a harmful outcome from action to be *more desirable* than the same harmful outcome following inaction	May lead to decisions to act despite unfavorable risk-benefit ratios May lead to negative surrogate outcomes if they feel an increased personal responsibility for a negative outcome
Omission bias	The tendency to regard a harmful outcome from inaction to be *more desirable* than the same harmful outcome following action	May lead to avoidance of potentially beneficial treatments
Status quo bias	The tendency to maintain the current or previous choice rather than making a different choice	May cause a continuation of unwanted treatments because comfort-oriented goals of care in the ICU requires deviating from the status quo
Availability bias	The tendency to infer the likelihood of a future event by relying on whether they have any experience with such an event	May cause decision-makers to rely on their own prior experiences rather than objective data shared by clinicians

surrogates seek to make health care choices that maximize their well-being [17–22]. Yet, the difficulties of predicting future mortality, illness burden, and accompanying emotions may limit their abilities to accomplish this goal [14, 23, 24]. These difficulties also make such prospection, or future-thinking, cognitively burdensome. To offset this cognitive burden, patients and surrogates may rely on heuristics that make individuals susceptible to associated biases. Indeed, errors in prospection may arise through systematic errors, such as failing to assess or accurately interpret the risks and benefits of treatment options [25, 26].

One such systematic error is optimism bias, or the tendency to overestimate the likelihood of desirable outcomes [27]. Forming overly optimistic expectations may help some individuals cope with unfavorable prognoses or likely outcomes, such as death or prolonged disability in the setting of critical illness. However, unrealistic optimism may also mean that individuals' avoidance of likely or possible negative outcomes may prevent them from fully considering the risks of a given choice, adapting to hardships [28–30], or selecting treatments that mitigate harm when all the likely outcomes are undesired. In this way, decision-makers may fail to choose an option that maximizes the future benefit to themselves and their family members.

Surrogates of critically ill patients are known to demonstrate high rates of optimism bias [31, 32]. In one demonstration of this, White and colleagues asked surrogates of ICU patients to interpret prognostic statements [7]. Although these statements were unrelated to their own loved one's condition, surrogates overwhelmingly demonstrated optimism bias in their interpretations. They reported that a physician statement of "90% chance of surviving" did not differ from the actual meaning while they interpreted a physician statement of "5% chance of surviving" as likely to result in a median of 15% survival with high variability in their responses (interquartile range, 5–40%) [7]. Wide ranges or deviation from the provided numerical estimate for both of these extremes would have suggested limited numeracy or mistrust of physician-provided estimates as a primary driver of these different interpretations. In contrast, the surrogates clearly responded differently to a poor prognosis when compared to a good one—the bias only emerged when a defense mechanism, such as optimism, was needed. This finding has since been replicated among parents when considering the communication of prognosis in critically ill neonates [33].

Impact bias is another well-recognized cause of prospective errors. When considering a health event or outcome, people systematically overestimate the impact that event will have on their life. Individuals may overestimate the beneficial effects that positive occurrences will have on their life or underestimate their ability to adapt to negative conditions [23]. For example, Smith and colleagues interviewed patients before and after kidney transplants [34]. Prior to transplant, the patients predicted how improved their quality of life would be after the transplant. Indeed, after transplant the patients did rate their quality of life as improved since pretransplant, but the magnitude of improvement was not nearly as dramatic as they had predicted.

In addition to overestimating the potential good to come from an event, human beings also underestimate our ability to adapt to negative situations. In a classic example, patients living with colostomies,[1] patients with reversed colostomies, and the general public indicated how many months of life they would give up in order to have normal bowel function rather than living with a colostomy. While all groups reported they would trade some months of life for normal bowel function, patients living with colostomies would give up 19 months of life on average while those without a colostomy would be willing to give up over 40 months of life. Therefore, although many patients who have not experienced colostomies rate bowel or bladder incontinence as states worse than death [35], those living with such conditions often find it more tolerable due their own likely unrecognized ability to adapt to a new health state.

[1] A colostomy is a surgical procedure that brings one end of the large intestine out through an opening made in the abdominal wall. Stool moves through the intestine and drains through the skin into a bag attached to the outside of the abdomen. This may be required due to blockage of or damage to the intestines and may be permanent or reversible. If reversed, the bowel is reconnected and stool no longer drains through the skin.

Unrealistic optimism and overestimates of impact may lead to systematic errors in medical decision-making, possibly in competing or conflicting directions. Optimism on the part of surrogate decision-makers may lead to preventable patient distress; excessive use of intensive measures near the end of life; and foreseeable, yet unforeseen, poor outcomes. In fact, critically ill patients are more likely to have longer ICU and hospital stays without any improvement in survival when their surrogates demonstrate optimism bias, even when adjusting for the patient's age and severity of illness [36]. Similarly, inaccurate expectations of impact may lead patients or surrogates to forgo potentially beneficial therapies or elect for treatments that leave them unsatisfied. Thus, these biases lead directly to care decisions that have been informed by inaccurate perceptions of future outcomes and are unlikely to maximize the benefit to patients.

Commission and Omission Biases

In the ICU, some seasoned clinicians will, somewhat cheekily, extoll less experienced clinicians to "don't just *do* something, *stand there*." In doing so, this phrase intends to combat the tendencies of individuals—particularly those with less experience—to feel compelled to act, otherwise known as commission bias. This bias may contribute to the overuse of diagnostics and interventions that ultimately do not benefit the patient simply because to do so is to act rather than to be a passive observer, and action may be favorable to some decision-makers. For example, Fagerlin and colleagues presented hypothetical scenarios to members of the public and asked them to consider treatment for a cancer diagnosis [37]. When faced with this hypothetical diagnosis, people were more likely to elect for cancer treatment that carried a *higher* risk of harm than living with the cancer itself! That is, they felt the need to act despite the fact that doing so carried an objectively unfavorable risk-benefit ratio. Similar situations undoubtedly play out in the critical care setting among patients and surrogates as well as clinicians. One possible explanation is that people feel the need to respond to a crisis rather than "standing by doing nothing," even if that response is more harmful than the crisis itself. Additionally, some may feel an increased personal responsibility for a negative outcome if the decision-maker makes no attempt to overcome the crisis.

However, omission bias may be even more common than commission bias. Individuals displaying omission bias regard a harmful outcome from *not* intervening (inaction) to be *more desirable* than the same harmful outcome following an active intervention. In an extreme but obvious form, allowing a person to die is viewed as preferable to actively killing. Evidence of this omission bias is apparent among physicians [38] and surrogates. For example, even prior to widespread misinformation about vaccines, some parents chose not to vaccinate their children with standard vaccines even while recognizing that the known risks of vaccination are smaller than the known risks associated with the disease the vaccine could prevent [17, 39, 40]. This omission bias may be due to decreased perceived personal responsibility for a poor outcome that follows from allowing the "natural progression" of disease.

While commission and omission biases oppose each other, together they provide the insight that medical decision-makers care not just about the outcomes of their decisions, but also the *manner* in which those outcomes arise. The implications of omission and commission bias in the ICU have yet to be well described. In theory, a patient's or surrogate's susceptibility to the biases of omission or commission would alter his or her treatment elections independent of the probabilities of predicted outcomes. For example, consider a surrogate choosing between electing for a life-supporting therapy or forgoing such a therapy. Rather than evaluating these options based on the patient's likely outcomes, the surrogate may instead base the decision on the perspective that electing for or against such a treatment alters his or her personal responsibility over undesirable outcomes that may follow. As such, the biases of omission and commission may not only influence the care a patient may receive, but also the surrogate's well-being afterwards [2, 3].

Status Quo Bias

Distinct from these concepts but closely related is status quo bias, or the tendency to maintain the current or previous choice rather than making a different choice [41]. Among several putative mechanisms underlying status quo bias is the possibility that people prefer to keep things the same lest they feel regret in the future over a choice they made that turned out poorly. Although decision-makers who maintain the status quo are also making a decision, they tend to experience less anticipated regret than those who choose against the status quo, as well as less actualized regret should a poor outcome result. This phenomenon suggests that decision-makers feel less personal responsibility for the outcome when they choose to remain with the existing status quo [42]. Therefore, decision-makers are again basing their choices on how large their personal role in outcomes would be rather than on the risks and benefits of each option.

In the critical care setting, nearly all individuals who enter the ICU do so with restorative goals [43]. Therefore, electing for comfort-oriented goals of care in the ICU requires deviating from the status quo. Interviews with surrogates of critically ill patients confirm their attention to regret management and desire to minimize personal responsibility for patients' death or poor outcomes [5], suggesting that status quo bias may have a large impact on patients' care.

The biases of commission, omission, and status quo together provide a framework for understanding how the process of decision-making may systematically introduce decision-making errors in the ICU. Patients and surrogates making decisions incorporate their own sense of personal responsibility into their choices, leading predictably to choices that seem to preserve future options and minimize regret, even when those choices differ from those that would be made in objective efforts to promote patients' goals.

Availability Bias

The availability bias is a heuristic that allows decision-makers to infer the likelihood of a future event by relying on whether they have any experience with such an event [44]. This is useful to decision-makers, as predicting future likelihoods requires considerable cognitive effort and, again, heuristics reduce the required cognitive load. One way to operationalize the availability bias is as *availability-by-recall*. This indicates that decision-makers rely on memory and experience to inform current decisions, often selecting the most available, or easily recalled, option [45].

Of particular interest within the context of critical care is the finding that the availability bias clearly influences risk perceptions. For example, when a person is asked whether death from leukemia or death from suicide is more common, the answer depends on his or her own experiences within his or her social network. That is, an individual with a family member who has died of leukemia will overestimate the risk of leukemia-associated deaths while an individual with a friend who has died from suicide will overestimate the risk of suicide-associated deaths [45]. Similar effects can be seen after exposure to media coverage of noteworthy but rare events, which leads people to overestimate the risk of such events [45].

These findings suggest that when patients or surrogates participate in high-stakes shared decision-making, they may rely on their own prior experiences rather than objective data shared by clinicians. Although this may reduce surrogates' cognitive load in an adaptive manner, the result may be predictable and systematic miscalculation of risk and subsequent errors in judgment.

We observed this phenomenon in interviewing individuals at high risk of adverse pulmonary conditions. When we asked patients and surrogates to consider the risks and benefits of management options for those conditions, some respondents relied on "available" but unrepresentative prior experiences [25]. As one respondent considered a bronchoscopy with transbronchial "biopsies," he equated the risks with his prior experience with a punch biopsy of the skin. Although they are both procedures with biopsies, the former is an invasive procedure requiring sedation and carrying the risk of a collapsed lung or hemorrhage while the latter is a performed under local anesthetic and carries minimal risk. In this way, availability bias may lead that patient to bypass sufficient evaluation of the risks and benefits of the options. In that case, rather than helping the decision-maker, the heuristic has introduced error into the decision-making process.

Overcoming Biases

Strategies to overcome biases introduced by the use of well-recognized heuristics may improve decision quality. These strategies can generally be grouped as those that avoid bias by circumventing the heuristic shortcuts to decisions, and those that directly harness the power of heuristics.

To date, much of the work in health care has focused on the avoidance of heuristics. By attempting to improve the quality and content of communication and information provided by clinicians to patients and their surrogates, these interventions have been based on the assumption that education would surmount the use of heuristics. In theory, strategies to improve decision-makers' knowledge may help overcome biases by slowing down the decision-making process, or helping the decision-maker become aware of the decision, the available options, and the key features or considerations. Increasing such awareness, decreasing time pressures, and making the task of decision-making easier through facilitation of information acquisition are all meaningful ways of reducing the tendency to rely on heuristics [46]. Metacommunication, or drawing attention to the decision-making process and the heuristics employed, may have a similar impact. Thus, surrogates may be more likely to engage in rational decision-making, ultimately choosing options that would have the highest chance of a desirable outcome.

Unfortunately, this approach has largely failed in the realm of serious illness decision-making [47–49]. The Study to Understand Prognoses and Preferences for Outcomes and Risks of Treatments (SUPPORT) Trial, a 2-year trial of clinician-focused and family-focused interventions to improve communication in the ICU, failed to improve patient care or outcomes [50]. More recently tested communication interventions have improved knowledge and awareness, but generally without changing treatment decisions or the care patients receive [51, 52].

By contrast, strategies that harness the use of heuristics recognize that it may be easier to redirect bias in constructive directions rather than to avoid bias altogether. Clinicians often act as *choice architects*, or the individuals responsible for designing choice environments for patients and surrogates [14]. Clinicians therefore have both the opportunity and great responsibility to influence choice environments in ways that maximize the likelihood that decision-makers choose options leading to good outcomes [53–55]. This approach uses insights from psychology, cognitive science, behavioral science, and economics, collectively termed *behavioral economics*. For example, simulation of treatments or outcomes and peer support may capitalize on the availability bias and the impact bias to allow the decision-maker to feel familiar with an otherwise unfamiliar choice or outcome. Scalable interventions that harness the default effect, or our tendency to opt for preselected choices, maintain autonomy while increasing the likelihood that a decision-maker will choose the option we have preselected for him or her [56–59]. Clinicians as choice architects have the opportunity to use these insights to help patients and surrogates overcome cognitive barriers to making choices that maximize benefit [53, 60].

However, the evidence base supporting use of these strategies in the ICU is still quite nascent. Used bluntly and without understanding the potential impact of such strategies is likely to harm patients and surrogates [14, 59]. Foundational work is therefore needed to identify the heuristics used most frequently by patients and surrogates, and to quantify the varying degrees of impact each has on patient and family outcomes. Developing, testing, and implementing scalable interventions to overcome these frequent and highly influential heuristics would then follow.

Conclusion

Shared decision-making is one of the most important roles of family members in the ICU. As surrogates, they are asked to understand often unfamiliar treatment options, weigh complex risks and benefits, predict patients' and their own responses to future health status, and assume the voice of their loved ones. The difficulties they encounter while engaging in decision-making and the errors that they make when selecting the best option are not personal shortcomings, but rather predictable and systematic nuances of human behavior. If clinicians are able to guide patients and their surrogates past these cognitive barriers, the resulting health care choices would more accurately reflect and promote patients' true preferences and goals.

References

1. Wendler D, Rid A. Systematic review: the effect on surrogates of making treatment decisions for others. Ann Intern Med. 2011;154(5):336–46. Epub 2011/03/02. https://doi.org/10.7326/0003-4819-154-5-201103010-00008.
2. Gries CJ, Engelberg RA, Kross EK, Zatzick D, Nielsen EL, Downey L, et al. Predictors of symptoms of posttraumatic stress and depression in family members after patient death in the ICU. Chest. 2010;137(2):280–7. https://doi.org/10.1378/chest.09-1291.
3. Kose I, Zincircioglu C, Ozturk YK, Cakmak M, Guldogan EA, Demir HF, et al. Factors affecting anxiety and depression symptoms in relatives of intensive care unit patients. J Intensive Care Med. 2016;31(9):611–7. https://doi.org/10.1177/0885066615595791.
4. Nelson JE, Hanson LC, Keller KL, Carson SS, Cox CE, Tulsky JA, et al. The voice of surrogate decision makers: family responses to prognostic information in chronic critical illness. Am J Respir Crit Care Med. 2017;196:864. https://doi.org/10.1164/rccm.201701-0201OC.
5. Schenker Y, Crowley-Matoka M, Dohan D, Tiver GA, Arnold RM, White DB. I don't want to be the one saying 'we should just let him die': intrapersonal tensions experienced by surrogate decision makers in the ICU. J Gen Intern Med. 2012;27(12):1657–65. Epub 2012/09/27. https://doi.org/10.1007/s11606-012-2129-y.
6. White DB, Ernecoff N, Buddadhumaruk P, Hong S, Weissfeld L, Curtis JR, et al. Prevalence of and factors related to discordance about prognosis between physicians and surrogate decision makers of critically ill patients. JAMA. 2016;315(19):2086–94. Epub 2016/05/18. https://doi.org/10.1001/jama.2016.5351.
7. Zier LS, Sottile PD, Hong SY, Weissfield LA, White DB. Surrogate decision makers' interpretation of prognostic information: a mixed-methods study. Ann Intern Med. 2012;156(5):360–6. Epub 2012/03/07. https://doi.org/10.7326/0003-4819-156-5-201203060-00008.
8. Hamilton JG, Lillie SE, Alden DL, Scherer L, Oser M, Rini C, et al. What is a good medical decision? A research agenda guided by perspectives from multiple stakeholders. J Behav Med. 2017;40(1):52–68. https://doi.org/10.1007/s10865-016-9785-z. Epub 2016/08/28.
9. Gigerenzer G, Gaissmaier W. Heuristic decision making. Annu Rev Psychol. 2011;62:451–82. https://doi.org/10.1146/annurev-psych-120709-145346.
10. Linder JA, Doctor JN, Friedberg MW, et al. Time of day and the decision to prescribe antibiotics. JAMA Intern Med. 2014;174(12):2029–31. https://doi.org/10.1001/jamainternmed.2014.5225.
11. Danziger S, Levav J, Avnaim-Pesso L. Extraneous factors in judicial decisions. Proc Natl Acad Sci. 2011;108(17):6889–92.

12. Blumenthal-Barby JS, Krieger H. Cognitive biases and heuristics in medical decision making: a critical review using a systematic search strategy. Med Decis Making. 2015;35(4):539–57. Epub 2014/08/26. https://doi.org/10.1177/0272989x14547740.
13. McDonald CJ. Medical heuristics: the silent adjudicators of clinical practice. Ann Intern Med. 1996;124(1 Pt 1):56–62. Epub 1996/01/01.
14. Malik L, Li C, Summer A, Ogunduyile L, Steingrub J, Lo B, Zlatev J, White DB. Clinicians' Use of Choice Framing in ICU Family Meetings. Crit Care Med. 2024;52(10):1533–1542. https://doi.org/10.1097/CCM.0000000000006360. Epub 2024 Jun 24. PMID: 38912880. PMC10663971.
15. Coen M, Sader J, Junod-Perron N, Audétat M-C, Nendaz M. Clinical reasoning in dire times. Analysis of cognitive biases in clinical cases during the COVID-19 pandemic. Intern Emerg Med. 2022;17(4):979–88. https://doi.org/10.1007/s11739-021-02884-9.
16. Moss SJ, Krewulak KD, Stelfox HT, Ahmed SB, Anglin MC, Bagshaw SM, et al. Restricted visitation policies in acute care settings during the COVID-19 pandemic: a scoping review. Crit Care. 2021;25(1):347. https://doi.org/10.1186/s13054-021-03763-7.
17. Chapman GB, Coups EJ. Emotions and preventive health behavior: worry, regret, and influenza vaccination. Health Psychol. 2006;25(1):82–90. https://doi.org/10.1037/0278-6133.25.1.82.
18. Connolly T, Zeelenberg M. Regret in decision making. Curr Dir Psychol Sci. 2002;11(6):212–6.
19. Nea J-W. The importance and complexity of regret in the measurement of 'good' decisions: a systematic review and content analysis of existing assessment instruments. Health Expect. 2010;14:59–83.
20. Reb J. Regret aversion and decision process quality: effects of regret salience on decision process carefulness. Organ Behav Hum Decis Process. 2008;105(2):169–82. https://doi.org/10.1016/j.obhdp.2007.08.006.
21. Summerville A. Counterfactual seeking: the scenic overlook of the road not taken. Pers Social Psychol Bull. 2011;37(11):1522–33. Epub 2011/07/08. https://doi.org/10.1177/0146167211413295.
22. Zeelenberg M, Beattie JM, Van der Pligt J, de Vries NK. Consequences of regret aversion: effects of expected feedback on risky decision making. Organ Behav Hum Decis Process. 1996;65(2):148–58.
23. Ubel PA, Loewenstein G, Schwarz N, Smith D. Misimagining the unimaginable: the disability paradox and health care decision making. Health Psychol. 2005;24(4 Suppl):S57–62. https://doi.org/10.1037/0278-6133.24.4.S57.
24. Halpern J, Arnold RM. Affective forecasting: an unrecognized challenge in making serious health decisions. J Gen Intern Med. 2008;23(10):1708–12. https://doi.org/10.1007/s11606-008-0719-5.
25. Hart JL, Pflug E, Madden V, Halpern SD. Thinking forward: future-oriented thinking among patients with tobacco-associated thoracic diseases and their surrogates. Am J Respir Crit Care Med. 2016;193(3):321–9. Epub 2015/10/06. https://doi.org/10.1164/rccm.201505-0882OC.
26. Weinstein ND. Unrealistic optimism about future life events. J Pers Soc Psychol. 1980;39(5):806–20. https://doi.org/10.1037/0022-3514.39.5.806.
27. Shepperd JA, Klein WM, Waters EA, Weinstein ND. Taking stock of unrealistic optimism. Perspect Psychol Sci. 2013;8(4):395–411. Epub 2013/07/01. https://doi.org/10.1177/1745691613485247.
28. Liberman N, Trope Y. Construal level theory of intertemporal judgment and decision. In: Loewenstein G, Read D, Baumeister RF, editors. Time and decision. New York: Russell Sage Foundation; 2003. p. 245–76.
29. Schacter DL, Addis DR, Buckner RL. Episodic simulation of future events: concepts, data, and applications. Ann N Y Acad Sci. 2008;1124:39–60. Epub 2008/04/11. https://doi.org/10.1196/annals.1440.001.
30. Mischel W, Ayduk O, Mendoza-Denton R. Sustaining delay of gratification over time: a hot-cool systems perspective. In: Loewenstein G, Read D, Baumeister RF, editors. Time and decision. New York: Russell Sage Foundation; 2003. p. 175–200.

31. Leiter N, Motta M, Reed RM, Adeyeye T, Wiegand DL, Shah NG, et al. Numeracy and interpretation of prognostic estimates in intracerebral hemorrhage among surrogate decision makers in the neurologic ICU. Crit Care Med. 2018;46(2):264–71. https://doi.org/10.1097/ccm.0000000000002887.
32. White DB, Carson S, Anderson W, Steingrub J, Bird G, Curtis JR, et al. A multicenter study of the causes and consequences of optimistic expectations about prognosis by surrogate decision-makers in ICUs. Crit Care Med. 2019;47:1184. https://doi.org/10.1097/CCM.0000000000003807.
33. Nayak B, Moon J-Y, Kim M, Fischhoff B, Haward MF. Optimism bias in understanding neonatal prognoses. J Perinatol. 2021;41(3):445–52. https://doi.org/10.1038/s41372-020-00773-1.
34. Smith D, Loewenstein G, Jepson C, Jankovich A, Feldman H, Ubel P. Mispredicting and misremembering: patients with renal failure overestimate improvements in quality of life after a kidney transplant. Health Psychol. 2008;27(5):653–8. Epub 2008/10/01. https://doi.org/10.1037/a0012647.
35. Rubin EB, Buehler AE, Halpern SD. States worse than death among hospitalized patients with serious illnesses. JAMA Intern Med. 2016;176(10):1557–9. Epub 2016/08/02. https://doi.org/10.1001/jamainternmed.2016.4362.
36. White DB, Hough CL, Carson SS, Anderson W, Peterson MW, Steingrub J, et al. Is optimism bias about prognosis by surrogate decision makers associated with more health care utilization at the end of life? Am J Respir Crit Care Med. 2015;191:A3774.
37. Fagerlin A, Zikmund-Fisher BJ, Ubel PA. Cure me even if it kills me: preferences for invasive cancer treatment. Med Decis Making. 2005;25(6):614–9. Epub 2005/11/12. https://doi.org/10.1177/0272989x05282639.
38. Aberegg SK, Haponik EF, Terry PB. Omission bias and decision making in pulmonary and critical care medicine. Chest. 2005;128(3):1497–505. Epub 2005/09/16. https://doi.org/10.1378/chest.128.3.1497.
39. Meszaros JR, Asch DA, Baron J, Hershey JC, Kunreuther H, Schwartz-Buzaglo J. Cognitive processes and the decisions of some parents to forego pertussis vaccination for their children. J Clin Epidemiol. 1996;49(6):697–703. Epub 1996/06/01.
40. Ritov I, Baron J. Reluctance to vaccinate: omission bias and ambiguity. J Behav Decis Mak. 1990;3:263–77.
41. Samuelson W, Zeckhauser R. Status quo bias in decision making. J Risk Uncertain. 1988;1(1):7–59.
42. Nicolle A, Fleming SM, Bach DR, Driver J, Dolan RJ. A regret-induced status quo bias. J Neurosci. 2011;31(9):3320.
43. Hart JL, Harhay MO, Gabler NB, Ratcliffe SJ, Quill CM, Halpern SD. Variability among US intensive care units in managing the care of patients admitted with preexisting limits on life-sustaining therapies. JAMA Intern Med. 2015;175(6):1019–26. . Epub 2015/03/31. https://doi.org/10.1001/jamainternmed.2015.0372.
44. Tversky A, Kahneman D. Judgment under uncertainty: heuristics and biases. Science. 1974;185(4157):1124.
45. Pachur T, Hertwig R, Steinmann F. How do people judge risks: availability heuristic, affect heuristic, or both? J Exp Psychol Appl. 2012;18(3):314–30. https://doi.org/10.1037/a0028279.
46. Croskerry P. The importance of cognitive errors in diagnosis and strategies to minimize them. Acad Med. 2003;78(8):775–80.
47. Curtis JR, Treece PD, Nielsen EL, Gold J, Ciechanowski PS, Shannon SE, et al. Randomized trial of communication facilitators to reduce family distress and intensity of end-of-life care. Am J Respir Crit Care Med. 2016;193(2):154–62. https://doi.org/10.1164/rccm.201505-0900OC.
48. Lautrette A, Darmon M, Megarbane B, Joly LM, Chevret S, Adrie C, et al. A communication strategy and brochure for relatives of patients dying in the ICU. N Engl J Med. 2007;356(5):469–78. https://doi.org/10.1056/NEJMoa063446.

49. Davidson JE, Aslakson RA, Long AC, Puntillo KA, Kross EK, Hart J, et al. Guidelines for family-centered care in the neonatal, pediatric, and adult ICU. Crit Care Med. 2017;45(1):103–28. Epub 2016/12/17. https://doi.org/10.1097/ccm.0000000000002169.
50. Connors AF Jr, Dawson NV, Desbiens NA, et al. A controlled trial to improve care for seriously ill hospitalized patients: the study to understand prognoses and preferences for outcomes and risks of treatments (support). JAMA. 1995;274(20):1591–8. https://doi.org/10.1001/jama.1995.03530200027032.
51. Austin CA, Mohottige D, Sudore RL, Smith AK, Hanson LC. Tools to promote shared decision making in serious illness: a systematic review. JAMA Intern Med. 2015;175(7):1213–21. https://doi.org/10.1001/jamainternmed.2015.1679.
52. Oczkowski SJW, Chung H-O, Hanvey L, Mbuagbaw L, You JJ. Communication tools for end-of-life decision-making in the intensive care unit: a systematic review and meta-analysis. Crit Care. 2016;20:97. https://doi.org/10.1186/s13054-016-1264-y.
53. Milkman KL, Chugh D, Bazerman MH. How can decision making be improved? Perspect Psychol Sci. 2009;4(4):379–83. https://doi.org/10.1111/j.1745-6924.2009.01142.x.
54. Swindell JS, McGuire AL, Halpern SD. Shaping patients' decisions. Chest. 2011;139(2):424–9. Epub 2011/02/03. https://doi.org/10.1378/chest.10-0605.
55. Gorin M, Joffe S, Dickert N, Halpern S. Justifying clinical nudges. Hast Cent Rep. 2017;47(2):32–8. Epub 2017/03/17. https://doi.org/10.1002/hast.688.
56. Halpern SD. Shaping end-of-life care: behavioral economics and advance directives. Semin Respir Crit Care Med. 2012;33(4):393–400. https://doi.org/10.1055/s-0032-1322403.
57. Halpern SD, Loewenstein G, Volpp KG, Cooney E, Vranas K, Quill CM, et al. Default options in advance directives influence how patients set goals for end-of-life care. Health Aff. 2013;32(2):408–17. https://doi.org/10.1377/hlthaff.2012.0895.
58. Halpern SD, Ubel PA, Asch DA. Harnessing the power of default options to improve health care. N Engl J Med. 2007;357(13):1340–4. https://doi.org/10.1056/NEJMsb071595.
59. Hart J, Halpern SD. Default options in the ICU: widely used but insufficiently understood. Curr Opin Crit Care. 2014;20(6):662–7. Epub 2014/09/10. https://doi.org/10.1097/mcc.0000000000000146.
60. Anesi GL, Halpern SD. Choice architecture in code status discussions with terminally ill patients and their families. Intensive Care Med. 2016;42(6):1065–7. Epub 2016/03/10. https://doi.org/10.1007/s00134-016-4294-7.

Chapter 10
Sleep and Sleep Deprivation Among Families in the ICU

Stuti J. Jaiswal, Amy L. Bellinghausen, and Robert L. Owens

Overview of Sleep: Background and Definitions

Sleep is the transient state in which all people spend 25–33% of their lifetimes. Its role in human health and disease is still poorly understood. However, it is increasingly recognized that sleep and sleep disorders have major impact on cardiovascular and neurocognitive health. For example, reported chronic short sleep duration—adjusted for all known covariates—is an independent risk factor for incident coronary artery disease [1], pneumonia [2], and weight gain [3]. Acute sleep restriction is associated with decreased antibody response to vaccination, suggesting immune modulation with short sleep [4, 5]. Recent epidemiological, basic and animal research has begun to examine links between sleep duration and cancer [6]. Thus, sleep is likely to be important, but we have much to learn, especially regarding the effects of acute sleep deprivation. In general, most society guidelines recommend 7–9 h of sleep per night [7, 8].

Sleep Stages

Sleep is typically divided into different sleep stages, based upon electroencephalographic (EEG), electrooculographic, and electromyographic patterns. The major division of sleep stages is between rapid eye movement (REM) and non-rapid eye

S. J. Jaiswal
The Scripps Research Institute, La Jolla, CA, USA

A. L. Bellinghausen · R. L. Owens (✉)
Pulmonary, Critical Care and Sleep Medicine Division, University of California San Diego, La Jolla, CA, USA
e-mail: rowens@health.ucsd.edu

© The Author(s), under exclusive license to Springer Nature Switzerland AG 2025

A. J. Vance et al. (eds.), *Families in the Intensive Care Unit*,
https://doi.org/10.1007/978-3-031-83786-9_10

movement (NREM) sleep. REM sleep shows characteristic conjugate eye movements and is also referred to as “dreaming” sleep, as most recalled dreaming activity takes place during this phase of sleep. NREM sleep is further classified into phases called N1, N2, and N3 sleep, based upon the EEG appearance and the rhythms (e.g., alpha, delta) that predominate. Because N3 is classified by delta wave activity (high amplitude, relatively slow frequency), it is sometimes referred to as slow wave sleep. In lay literature, either N3 or REM sleep are considered “deep” or “quality” sleep; however, the data to support these statements are incomplete. Although many studies consider the impact of sleep duration on a variety of outcomes (as above), the difficulty in reliably measuring the various sleep stages has limited the amount of studies that look at the various sleep stages and outcomes. Thus, most of the literature and this review will focus on overall sleep duration rather than specific sleep stages. Additionally, most data is based on total sleep duration, though sleep fragmentation (i.e., duration of the sleep segments that sum to the total sleep duration) is likely also important.

Typically, the sleep phases change throughout the night in a cyclical pattern of N1, N2, N3, then REM, and repeat (see normal hypnogram, Fig. 10.1) with a period of approximately 120 min. However, the timing and amounts of sleep can vary considerably according to multiple factors, including age, medication use, and genetics. For example, the amount of N3 sleep decreases with age. Alternatively, many commonly prescribed medications impact sleep stages, such as selective serotonin reuptake inhibitors (SSRIs) which suppress REM sleep, as well as most of the medications used in the ICU [9].

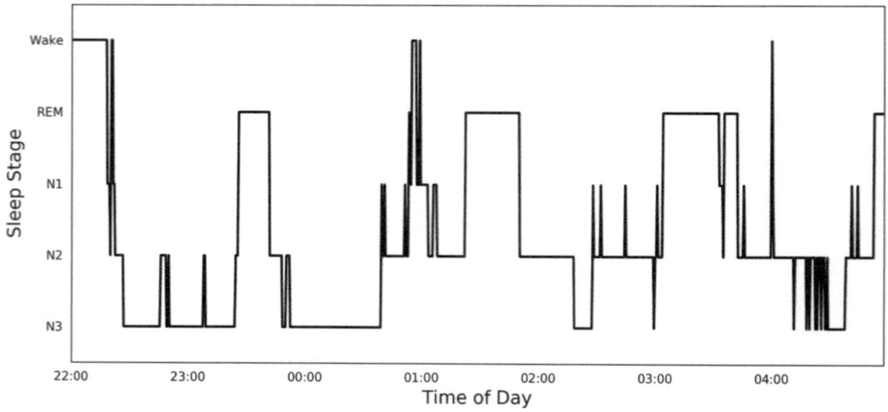

Fig. 10.1 An overnight hypnogram from a healthy subject that shows the pattern of the various sleep stages. The relative amounts of the sleep stages changes with age, medications, and other factors

Circadian Rhythm

One of the most important factors affecting the timing of sleep in general and its various phases is the endogenous circadian rhythm. The circadian rhythm typically has a period of close to 24 h, with most rhythms also aligned for sleep during the hours 10 p.m. to 6 a.m. (and sometimes in the early afternoon, see Fig. 10.2). The endogenous circadian rhythm is affected by a variety of external cues, with light the most powerful. There is also variability in both the period and alignment. For example, some individuals show either an advanced or delayed sleep phase, with marked preference for either early morning (so-called "morning larks") or late evening ("night owls"), respectively. However, when unable to accommodate to their preferred internal rhythm, symptoms of fatigue and sleepiness can result. The same mismatch between the internal circadian rhythm and the external environment commonly results in symptoms of "jet lag."

"I Can't Sleep": Lack of Opportunities for Sleep vs. Insomnia

Relevant to the ICU, family members of ICU patients often report difficulty sleeping. Broadly, this may be due either to lack of opportunities for sleep or insomnia, which have very different causes and treatments. Insomnia is defined as difficulty falling asleep, staying asleep, or non-restorative sleep *despite* an adequate opportunity for sleep. In the ICU, stress, anxiety, or other emotions could easily inhibit sleep in a family member even if the environment were conducive to sleep. However, the complaint of "I can't sleep" might more likely derive from the inability to find

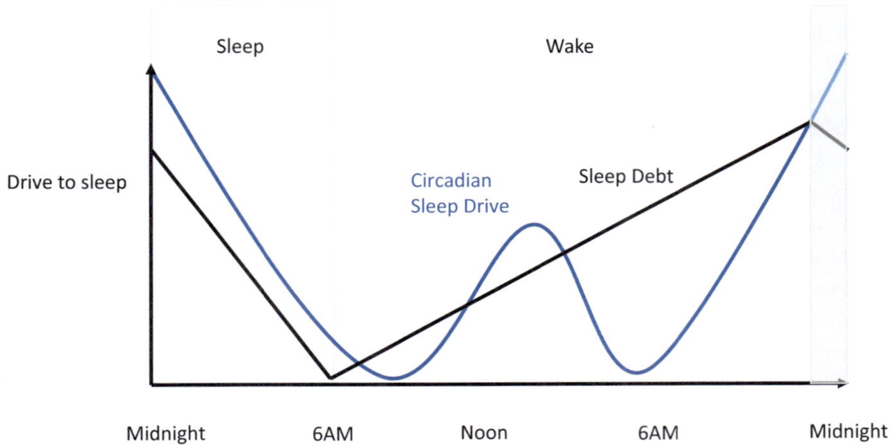

Fig. 10.2 The two stimuli for sleep are the endogenous circadian rhythm and sleep debt which accumulates during wake and recedes during sleep. Sleep during the night and with an early afternoon nap would mimic the endogenous circadian rhythm in most people

the right conditions for sleep in the ICU, and could be due to light, sound, frequent interruptions, or lack of a bed/chair in which to sleep. These are both considered below.

Lack of Opportunities for Sleep: "I Don't Have Enough (Time, Space, Quiet) to Get Some Sleep"

Sleep is notoriously bad in the ICU, for both patients and their family members due to multiple reasons, with most pointing to environmental factors and frequent care interactions [10, 11]. The primary rationale of the ICU is to group the sickest patients to allow for rapid response as needed. This comes into direct conflict with efforts to promote sleep. Patients themselves will have unique barriers to sleep, such as pain, dyspnea, and ventilator dyssynchrony. However, loud alarms from multiple different types of equipment (e.g., telemetry, ventilator alarms), frequent interactions with clinicians, and procedures will interfere with sleep for both patients *and their loved ones*. Multiple studies have found the ICU to be a very poor environment for sleep, with very high sound levels for example, frequently exceeding WHO recommended guidelines [12, 13]. Thus, the Society of Critical Care Medicine recommends promotion of the sleep environment by clustering routines, optimizing the environment for sleep, and promoting uninterrupted sleep times [14].

Efforts to improve the sleep environment in the ICU have been difficult. Multiple interventions, which require substantial staff education and changes in practice, may be required [15]. Even in the landmark study by Kamdar and colleagues that was designed to improve sleep quality and demonstrated an important reduction in ICU delirium, no improvement in subjectively reported patient sleep quality was found. While multimodal interventions are unlikely to be implemented easily, even more targeted interventions must be carefully considered. For example, "just" focusing on noise reduction can result in statistically significant changes in noise level, but these are small and unlikely to have clinical benefit [12]. Moreover, efforts to reduce noise levels may paradoxically increase difficulty sleeping since it is *changes* in sound level that actually lead to arousal from sleep [16, 17]. Consider the use of white noise machines to aid sleep, which work in part by increasing the average background noise level. Ear plugs and eye masks have been shown to modestly improve sleep (increasing sleep time by about 16 min per night) for healthy patients exposed to a simulated ICU environment [18]; however, comfort and acceptance of ear plugs in particular is low [19]. Finally, while efforts to reduce light during the circadian night are frequently recommended, light levels, when measured, have been low at night [20]. Instead, more light may be needed during the day to maintain a circadian rhythm, a finding seen in multiple studies [17, 20, 21].

Family members must encounter all these problems, and also frequently face additional challenges. First, some ICUs lack a physical space for family members to sleep, or that space is a communal waiting room which is not designed for sleep or privacy. Second, family members may have multiple other interruptions not related to the ICU environment such as updating other family members, work, and home obligations, etc. Third, family members may also travel from distance and deal with the effects of jet lag as well. Finally, stress and anxiety may cause insomnia, preventing sleep even when the ICU environment allows it. Indeed, family members themselves report anxiety, tension, and fearfulness as the three most common causes of sleep disturbance, much more commonly then environmental factors such as unfamiliar bed or too much noise [22]. Stress may not only be about the medical condition of their loved one, but family members can also face financial stress in the form of substantial nonmedical out-of-pocket expenses such as meals, lodging and parking, or from missed days at work [23].

How Well Do Family Members Sleep in the Hospital?

Emerging literature suggest that family members of critically ill patients are sleep deprived and that they have symptoms as a result, although the symptoms vary between individuals [24]. Subjectively, family members report poor sleep in and out of the hospital when a family member is critically ill [25, 26]. There are few studies that have objectively measured sleep times of family members in the ICU. In this regard, the work by Choi and colleagues, while based on a limited sample, is an important first step. Using actigraphy, they found that family members of ICU patients at the time of ICU admission averaged 328 ± 71 min (i.e., <5.5 h) of sleep per night [27]. Family members of ICU patients often report fatigue and difficultly sleeping [28]. Family members report inadequate rest, and nearly half report an inability to slow down or rest when *they themselves* are sick [29]. This follows a general pattern where family members prioritize presence in the ICU rather than their own health, missing doctor's appointments of their own, missing scheduled medications, skipping meals, etc.

Why Do Family Members Put Themselves Through These Conditions?

Multiple studies have shown that family members want to stay with patients for a variety of reasons. Primarily, most report a desire to safeguard and support their loved ones [30, 31]. But open visitation is also associated with improved family satisfaction [32, 33], reduced family anxiety [34], and has the practical benefit of improved communication with clinicians [35]. Recognizing these benefits, guidelines for family-centered care recommend open visitation and promote family presence [36]. However, increased family presence may worsen family, and potentially, patient sleep.

Could Family Presence Lead to Poor Patient Sleep?

Some families may visit loved ones according to their own schedule, such as late at night after work or during other designated rest times. While no evidence exists that such visits should be discouraged, families should be educated on the importance of uninterrupted rest time [37]. Conversely, families should understand that periods of wake and mobilization are equally important, and that sedation and sleep are not the same. For example, some family members may interpret the deeply sedated patient as sleeping comfortably, and discourage efforts to lighten sedation or perform interruptions of sedation, despite evidence that such efforts are beneficial [38]. Families may also defer opportunities for mobilization since their loved one is "sleeping," even though early mobilization may confer benefit [39]. Finally, some families may ask for pharmacological interventions, i.e., sleeping pills, to aid in sleep although risks usually outweigh any benefit [40].

Impact of Sleep Deprivation

There are very few studies carried out among ICU family members specifically. Thus, we extrapolate from the literature of acute sleep deprivation. One interesting study is by van Dongen and colleagues [41]. They exposed young healthy subjects to various degrees of sleep restriction/deprivation for up to 14 days. Each day, subjects rated their subjective sleepiness, and completed the psychomotor vigilance test (PVT), a test of alertness, daily. Subjects restricted to only 4 or 6 h per day felt tired, but their subjective sleepiness plateaued after a few days. In contrast, the objective PVT showed continued worsening every day. **Thus, one of the features of sleep deprivation is the inability for people to recognize how affected they are by sleep deprivation**. Relevant for families of ICU patients, families may not appreciate the degree of sleep deprivation they are experiencing or the impact of that sleep deprivation.

In general, the following domains impacted by acute sleep deprivation are likely to be important for family members, and their interaction with the health care team. Sleep deprivation can cause: increased number of lapses in attention; increased risk taking [42]; irritability; and decreased trust in others and increased aggressiveness [43]. One of the few studies to specifically test cognition in ICU family members found that most showed lapses in attention as measured by the psychomotor vigilance test [44]. Additionally, in this study, those subjects who were subjectively sleepy also experienced greater impairment in performing daily activities.

Taken together, lack of sleep may impact how families interact with clinicians, how they interpret information, and make decisions that affect their loved ones. Adequate sleep could be an important part of building a therapeutic bond between family and clinicians [45], and the atmosphere of the ICU is a factor identified as important in predicting family member dissatisfaction with intensive care [46]. For family members themselves, lack of sleep may impact decisions about their own care, such as ability to drive while drowsy [47]. Finally, family members and patients report feelings of dehumanization when sleeping schedules are not respected [48].

Management of Sleep Deprivation

In general, the treatment for sleep deprivation is adequate sleep, which could occur during the night or as naps throughout the day. Caffeine is also frequently used (by both providers and family members) to mitigate the impact of sleep deprivation. An important corollary is the avoidance of sedatives such as alcohol or sleeping pills (e.g., benzodiazepines) which cause increased sedation but are unlikely to be effective at promoting sleep unless the sleep environment is also improved.

Suggestions for Improving Family Sleep in the ICU

There are few data to suggest how best to improve family sleep. Until such data become available, the suggestions below are based on common sense. We emphasize that consideration of *both* patient and family member sleep might be useful, as has been suggested when assessing mental well-being of patient-caregiver dyads [49]. Finally, other efforts that are not sleep-specific—such as improved education and communication with families that generally reduces anxiety—have been advocated and may also be useful [50]:

1. *Improved physical space for sleeping*: This has been suggested as part of recent guidelines. Our own experience when physically relocating our ICU to new facilities (same type of patients, same providers, and same care policies in both ICUs) was an increase in nighttime visits by family members. While sleep and effects of sleep deprivation were not directly assessed, the average number of visitors in patient rooms at night increased from 50% of patients to 79% of patients [51]. In this regard, neonatal ICUs can lead the way, with sleeping areas for parents that allow closeness with their child and, at times, privacy [52]. The physical space for sleeping could be in the ICU room, a waiting area (ideally with bed provided), a dedicated sleeping room elsewhere in the hospital, or provided or subsidized accommodation near the hospital [53].
2. *Education for families about the importance of wake and sleep*: As above, information to educate and engage family members will be important. Interestingly, some patients and family members feel secure with abundant nighttime activity and alarms [10]. What many clinicians and some patients/family members interpret as barriers to sleep are interpreted as active monitoring by others. Thus, any intervention will need some element of education for patient and families to

provide reassurance. With appropriate education, family members may be the biggest advocates for uninterrupted rest time as well as periods of activity during the day. Furthermore, this information might also include education and resources about sleep after the ICU for both patients and family members. Sleeping pills should be discouraged for patients and family members.

3. *Active management of family member wake and sleep time*: Family member sleep could be encouraged both during the night and during rest ("nap") times during the day. Not only would such management improve family member sleep, but it may also improve patient sleep as well. For example, empowering family members to act as guardians of sleep time may also help reduce nighttime interruptions. During active periods during the day, family members might be encouraged to increase light levels in the room (which are frequently too low to entrain the circadian rhythm [17, 20]), and engage family members in conversations or simple cognitive activities (e.g., card playing) that might be useful in preventing or reducing delirium [54]. Similarly, if physically able and with appropriate guidance, they might participate in range-of-motion or other activities. This role for family members might provide a sense of usefulness for them, and foster teamwork with the clinical team (see Fig. 10.3). We note that family engagement is now considered in the design of clinical trials [55]. Importantly, such physical activity during the day could improve family member insomnia [56–58].
4. *Create protected sleep times at night and during the day for both patient and family*: We have previously advocated for a "Tuck In" time which would signal the start of the night time rest period for the patient [59]. For patients this might include management of pain and comfort, preparation of the room for sleep (lights down, TV off, setting of optimal desired temperature, etc.), and offering of ear plugs and eye masks. Importantly, the "Tuck In" could also be extended to

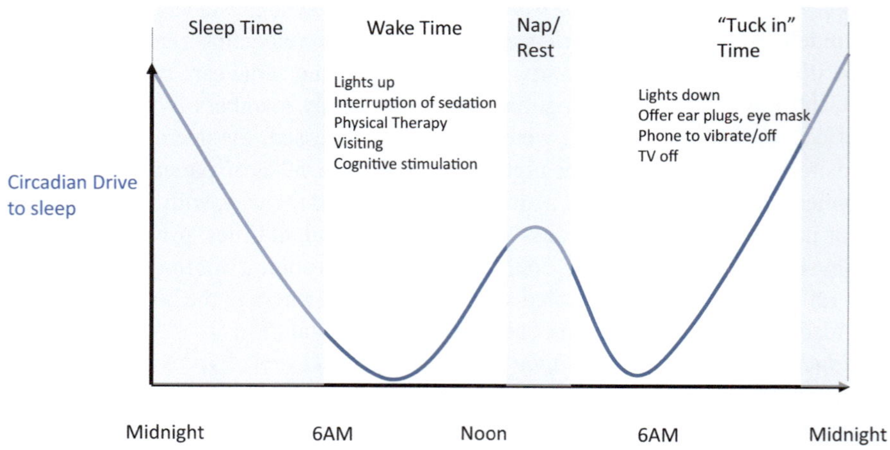

Fig. 10.3 Example protocol to optimize sleep in the hospital for both patients and family members. Activities during the day would ideally include family members. Bedtime Tuck-In would be aimed at patients and family members

family, as well, who could also be offered eye masks and ear plugs. Family members could also be encouraged to disengage from their mobile phone and other electronic devices.

Insomnia: "I Just Can't Seem to (Fall, Stay) Asleep"

A separate problem is insomnia—the inability to fall asleep despite an adequate opportunity to do so. Lack of an opportunity for sleep may occur mostly when families attempt to sleep in the ICU, but insomnia might occur outside of the ICU. Insomnia is one of the most common medical conditions, and some studies suggest that almost all Americans will have an episode of acute insomnia at some point during their lifetime. Insomnia can include difficulty falling asleep, staying asleep or waking up too early with inability to fall back asleep. This difficulty sleeping must also be paired with symptoms or distress from the poor sleep. Insomnia is endorsed frequently by ICU family members, and symptoms frequently correlate with stress or anxiety [22, 60, 61].

While insomnia may reflect stress or anxiety, it may persist and become the dominant symptom even after the initial stress/anxiety has resolved. For example, stress over a loved one's admission to the ICU may be the inciting event for prolonged insomnia even in family members of patients who recover well from critical illness. People with insomnia frequently have anxiety and frustration about their difficulty sleeping, and their responses to insomnia can further prolong or worsen sleep difficulties. People with difficulty falling asleep may perseverate on the problem by watching the clock or feel frustrated lying in bed awake. They may also compensate by staying in bed longer the next morning. All these behaviors will make it difficult to fall asleep the next night as well. Effective therapy focuses on eliminating the vicious cycle of these behaviors.

The cornerstone of therapy for insomnia is non-pharmacological. Education and cognitive behavioral therapy are the best initial treatment options. Education focuses on so-called sleep "hygiene"—the behaviors that help promote sleep, such as avoidance of naps (note that this is an effective strategy for sleep deprivation, but will worsen insomnia) and maintenance of a consistent sleep schedule. Avoidance of behaviors that promote frustration with sleep, such as avoidance of clock watching or staying in bed awake are recommended (i.e., stimulus control). For some, sleep restriction—the avoidance of too much time in bed—can also be very helpful. Medication would only be considered after an evaluation by a physician.

Sleep and Symptoms After the ICU

Both sleep deprivation and insomnia can occur after the ICU, depending on the course of illness for the patient. For those whose loved ones died in the ICU, the major post-ICU sleep abnormality may be insomnia in the setting of grief or subsequent depression. Conversely, those whose family members survive the ICU and return home may experience both insomnia and sleep deprivation as a result of the care they must provide to their loved ones. Multiple studies have shown high caregiver burden can be quite high and remain high after the ICU, particularly at the time of discharge [62–67]. The course of caregiver burden is variable [68], and results are generally few. As a starting point, in the study by Choi and colleagues, actigraphy was extended up to 2 months after the ICU [27]. We note that total sleep time at 2 months was highest in those whose family members died in the ICU, but their sleep tended to be more fragmented with more wake after sleep onset, a marker of insomnia. Conversely, those whose family members returned home got less sleep, which was less fragmented. Thus, sleep is likely to be poor in caregivers after ICU discharge for a variety of reasons and will fluctuate over time. (See Fig. 10.4 for conceptual examples.)

To improve sleep after the ICU, it will be important first to obtain sufficient history to understand why the family member "can't sleep." Education to family members about the signs and symptoms of insomnia, and basic sleep hygiene tips may be helpful. Persistent insomnia should prompt evaluation by a physician, and medication should be considered a last resort. If poor sleep is due to high caregiver burden, some caregiver relief will be needed.

Sleep and Relationship with PICS-F

Anxiety, depression, and post-traumatic stress disorder (PTSD) are now recognized complications for family members of ICU patients, and this constellation of symptoms has been termed post-ICU care syndrome-family (PICS-F) [69]. Poor sleep, then, may be a prominent symptom of PICS-F. Whether poor sleep in the hospital predisposes to PICS-F is not clear. Interestingly, some studies have shown that sleep deprivation after trauma reduces subsequent anxiety and development of PTSD [70–72]. It has been hypothesized that sleep deprivation slows or prevents new memory formation that could be used to reexperience the trauma. There are limited data that efforts to reduce PICS and PICS-F may improve sleep after the ICU. For example, participation in an ICU diary program improved sleep quality after discharge in cardiac ICU survivors and may have potential to improve post-ICU sleep in family members as well [73].

Regardless of any possible causal role, an emphasis on improving sleep and reducing insomnia may improve symptoms of anxiety or depression [74]. Alternatively, sleep symptoms in PTSD are often particularly refractory and may

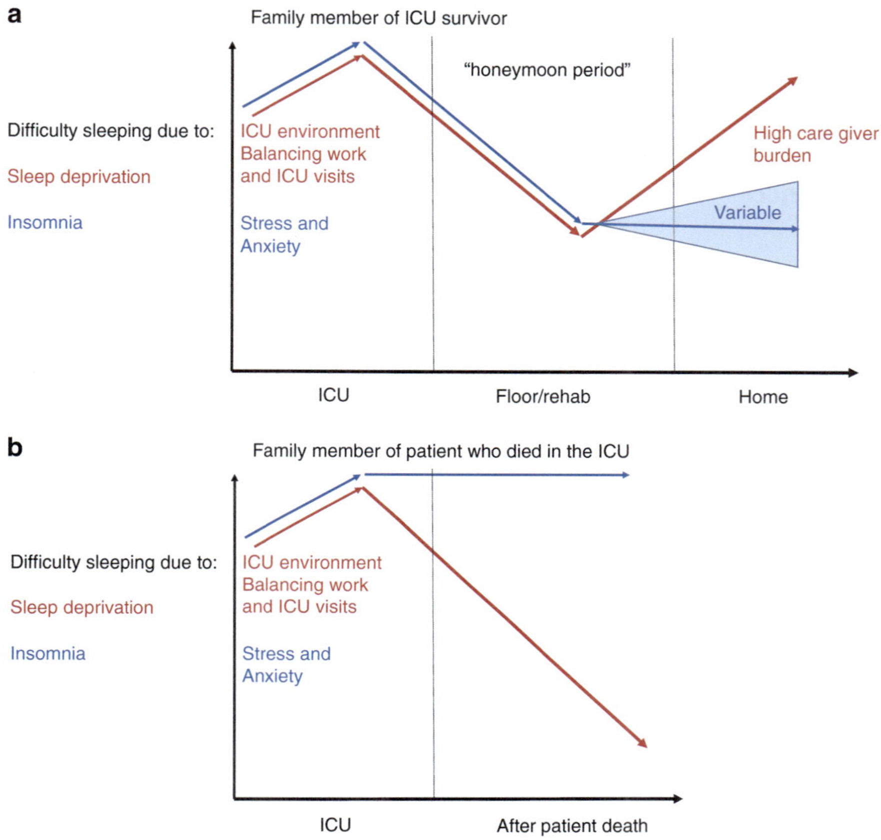

Fig. 10.4 Difficulty sleeping can be explained by lack of adequate sleep opportunity, or insomnia, or both. The relative contribution of each may also fluctuate during the hospital stay and based on the outcome of the ICU patient. In panel **a**, the patient survives to eventual home discharge. There may be a "honeymoon period" when caregivers sleep well, as patients improve yet remain cared for by others. This period may end when the patient returns home and caregiver burden increases, or as anxiety builds over the slow pace of recovery. In panel **b**, the patient does not survive to ICU discharge

need a focused approach [75]. Thus, a sleep history and a focus on sleep/difficulty sleeping will be important in family members after the ICU.

Summary

Difficulty sleeping is a problem not only for patients in the ICU, but also for their family members. Insufficient sleep causes symptoms in family members and may affect relationships with clinicians. An important first step is to differentiate between lack of opportunities for sleep vs. insomnia. Efforts to improve sleep for family members might also improve sleep for patients as well. Family members should be educated about symptoms of insomnia and first-step strategies to manage it.

References

1. Ayas NT, White DP, Manson JE, Stampfer MJ, Speizer FE, Malhotra A, et al. A prospective study of sleep duration and coronary heart disease in women. Arch Intern Med. 2003;163(2):205–9.
2. Patel SR, Malhotra A, Gao X, Hu FB, Neuman MI, Fawzi WW. A prospective study of sleep duration and pneumonia risk in women. Sleep. 2012;35(1):97–101.
3. Patel SR, Malhotra A, White DP, Gottlieb DJ, Hu FB. Association between reduced sleep and weight gain in women. Am J Epidemiol. 2006;164(10):947–54.
4. Spiegel K, Sheridan JF, Van Cauter E. Effect of sleep deprivation on response to immunization. JAMA. 2002;288(12):1471–2.
5. Prather AA, Hall M, Fury JM, Ross DC, Muldoon MF, Cohen S, et al. Sleep and antibody response to hepatitis B vaccination. Sleep. 2012;35(8):1063–9.
6. Owens RL, Gold KA, Gozal D, Peppard PE, Jun JC, Lippman SM, et al. Sleep and breathing and cancer? Cancer Prev Res (Phila). 2016;9(11):821–7.
7. Mukherjee S, Patel SR, Kales SN, Ayas NT, Strohl KP, Gozal D, et al. An official American Thoracic Society statement: the importance of healthy sleep. Recommendations and future priorities. Am J Respir Crit Care Med. 2015;191(12):1450–8.
8. Watson NF, Badr MS, Belenky G, Bliwise DL, Buxton OM, Buysse D, et al. Recommended amount of sleep for a healthy adult: a joint consensus statement of the American Academy of Sleep Medicine and Sleep Research Society. Sleep. 2015;38(6):843–4.
9. Weinhouse GL. Pharmacology I: effects on sleep of commonly used ICU medications. Crit Care Clin. 2008;24(3):477–91, vi.
10. Ding Q, Redeker NS, Pisani MA, Yaggi HK, Knauert MP. Factors influencing patients' sleep in the intensive care unit: perceptions of patients and clinical staff. Am J Crit Care. 2017;26(4):278–86.
11. Tronstad O, Flaws D, Lye I, Fraser JF, Patterson S. Doing time in an Australian ICU; the experience and environment from the perspective of patients and family members. Aust Crit Care. 2021;34(3):254–62.
12. Tainter CR, Levine AR, Quraishi SA, Butterly AD, Stahl DL, Eikermann M, et al. Noise levels in surgical ICUs are consistently above recommended standards. Crit Care Med. 2016;44(1):147–52.
13. Knauert M, Jeon S, Murphy TE, Yaggi HK, Pisani MA, Redeker NS. Comparing average levels and peak occurrence of overnight sound in the medical intensive care unit on A-weighted and C-weighted decibel scales. J Crit Care. 2016;36:1–7.
14. Barr J, Fraser GL, Puntillo K, Ely EW, Gelinas C, Dasta JF, et al. Clinical practice guidelines for the management of pain, agitation, and delirium in adult patients in the intensive care unit. Crit Care Med. 2013;41(1):263–306.
15. Kamdar BB, King LM, Collop NA, Sakamuri S, Colantuoni E, Neufeld KJ, et al. The effect of a quality improvement intervention on perceived sleep quality and cognition in a medical ICU. Crit Care Med. 2013;41:800.
16. Stanchina ML, Abu-Hijleh M, Chaudhry BK, Carlisle CC, Millman RP. The influence of white noise on sleep in subjects exposed to ICU noise. Sleep Med. 2005;6(5):423–8.
17. Jaiswal SJ, Garcia S, Owens RL. Sound and light levels are similarly disruptive in ICU and non-ICU wards. J Hosp Med. 2017;12(10):798–804.

18. Huang HW, Zheng BL, Jiang L, Lin ZT, Zhang GB, Shen L, et al. Effect of oral melatonin and wearing earplugs and eye masks on nocturnal sleep in healthy subjects in a simulated intensive care unit environment: which might be a more promising strategy for ICU sleep deprivation? Crit Care. 2015;19:124.
19. Hu RF, Jiang XY, Hegadoren KM, Zhang YH. Effects of earplugs and eye masks combined with relaxing music on sleep, melatonin and cortisol levels in ICU patients: a randomized controlled trial. Crit Care. 2015;19:115.
20. Fan EP, Abbott SM, Reid KJ, Zee PC, Maas MB. Abnormal environmental light exposure in the intensive care environment. J Crit Care. 2017;40:11–4.
21. Verceles AC, Liu X, Terrin ML, Scharf SM, Shanholtz C, Harris A, et al. Ambient light levels and critical care outcomes. J Crit Care. 2013;28(1):110.e1–8.
22. Day A, Haj-Bakri S, Lubchansky S, Mehta S. Sleep, anxiety and fatigue in family members of patients admitted to the intensive care unit: a questionnaire study. Crit Care. 2013;17(3):R91.
23. Clark ME, Cummings BM, Kuhlthau K, Frassica N, Noviski N. Impact of pediatric intensive care unit admission on family financial status and productivity: a pilot study. J Intensive Care Med. 2017;34:885066617723278.
24. Halm MA, Titler MG, Kleiber C, Johnson SK, Montgomery LA, Craft MJ, et al. Behavioral responses of family members during critical illness. Clin Nurs Res. 1993;2(4):414–37.
25. Saeid Y, Moradian ST, Ebadi A, Salaree MM. The family intensive care unit syndrome: a qualitative content analysis. Nurs Crit Care. 2021;27:401.
26. Dale CM, Carbone S, Istanboulian L, Fraser I, Cameron JI, Herridge MS, et al. Support needs and health-related quality of life of family caregivers of patients requiring prolonged mechanical ventilation and admission to a specialised weaning centre: a qualitative longitudinal interview study. Intensive Crit Care Nurs. 2020;58:102808.
27. Choi J, Tate JA, Donahoe MP, Ren D, Hoffman LA, Chasens ER. Sleep in family caregivers of ICU survivors for two months post-ICU discharge. Intensive Crit Care Nurs. 2016;37:11–8.
28. Celik S, Genc G, Kinetli Y, Asiliogli M, Sari M, Madenoglu Kivanc M. Sleep problems, anxiety, depression and fatigue on family members of adult intensive care unit patients. Int J Nurs Pract. 2016;22(5):512–22.
29. Choi J, Hoffman LA, Schulz R, Ren D, Donahoe MP, Given B, et al. Health risk behaviors in family caregivers during patients' stay in intensive care units: a pilot analysis. Am J Crit Care. 2013;22(1):41–5.
30. Burr G. The family and critical care nursing: a brief review of the literature. Aust Crit Care. 1997;10(4):124–7.
31. Elliott D, Davidson JE, Harvey MA, Bemis-Dougherty A, Hopkins RO, Iwashyna TJ, et al. Exploring the scope of post-intensive care syndrome therapy and care: engagement of non-critical care providers and survivors in a second stakeholders meeting. Crit Care Med. 2014;42(12):2518–26.
32. Roland P, Russell J, Richards KC, Sullivan SC. Visitation in critical care: processes and outcomes of a performance improvement initiative. J Nurs Care Qual. 2001;15(2):18–26.
33. Schnell D, Abadie S, Toullic P, Chaize M, Souppart V, Poncet MC, et al. Open visitation policies in the ICU: experience from relatives and clinicians. Intensive Care Med. 2013;39(10):1873–4.
34. Whitcomb JJ, Roy D, Blackman VS. Evidence-based practice in a military intensive care unit family visitation. Nurs Res. 2010;59(1 Suppl):S32–9.
35. Garrouste-Orgeas M, Philippart F, Timsit JF, Diaw F, Willems V, Tabah A, et al. Perceptions of a 24-hour visiting policy in the intensive care unit. Crit Care Med. 2008;36(1):30–5.
36. Davidson JE, Aslakson RA, Long AC, Puntillo KA, Kross EK, Hart J, et al. Guidelines for family-centered care in the neonatal, pediatric, and adult ICU. Crit Care Med. 2017;45(1):103–28.
37. Davidson JE, Savidan KA, Barker N, Ekno M, Warmuth D, Degen-De Cort A. Using evidence to overcome obstacles to family presence. Crit Care Nurs Q. 2014;37(4):407–21.
38. Kress JP, Pohlman AS, O'Connor MF, Hall JB. Daily interruption of sedative infusions in critically ill patients undergoing mechanical ventilation. N Engl J Med. 2000;342(20):1471–7.

39. Schweickert WD, Pohlman MC, Pohlman AS, Nigos C, Pawlik AJ, Esbrook CL, et al. Early physical and occupational therapy in mechanically ventilated, critically ill patients: a randomised controlled trial. Lancet. 2009;373(9678):1874–82.
40. Owens RL. Better sleep in the intensive care unit: blue pill or red pill or no pill? Anesthesiology. 2016;125(5):835–7.
41. Van Dongen HP, Maislin G, Mullington JM, Dinges DF. The cumulative cost of additional wakefulness: dose-response effects on neurobehavioral functions and sleep physiology from chronic sleep restriction and total sleep deprivation. Sleep. 2003;26(2):117–26.
42. Venkatraman V, Chuah YM, Huettel SA, Chee MW. Sleep deprivation elevates expectation of gains and attenuates response to losses following risky decisions. Sleep. 2007;30(5):603–9.
43. Anderson C, Dickinson DL. Bargaining and trust: the effects of 36-h total sleep deprivation on socially interactive decisions. J Sleep Res. 2010;19(1 Pt 1):54–63.
44. Verceles AC, Corwin DS, Afshar M, Friedman EB, McCurdy MT, Shanholtz C, et al. Half of the family members of critically ill patients experience excessive daytime sleepiness. Intensive Care Med. 2014;40(8):1124–31.
45. Huff NG, Nadig N, Ford DW, Cox CE. Therapeutic alliance between the caregivers of critical illness survivors and intensive care unit clinicians. Ann Am Thorac Soc. 2015;12(11):1646–53.
46. Hunziker S, McHugh W, Sarnoff-Lee B, Cannistraro S, Ngo L, Marcantonio E, et al. Predictors and correlates of dissatisfaction with intensive care. Crit Care Med. 2012;40(5):1554–61.
47. Jones CB, Dorrian J, Jay SM, Lamond N, Ferguson S, Dawson D. Self-awareness of impairment and the decision to drive after an extended period of wakefulness. Chronobiol Int. 2006;23(6):1253–63.
48. Basile MJ, Rubin E, Wilson ME, Polo J, Jacome SN, Brown SM, et al. Humanizing the ICU patient: a qualitative exploration of behaviors experienced by patients, caregivers, and ICU staff. Crit Care Explor. 2021;3(6):e0463.
49. Shaffer KM, Riklin E, Jacobs JM, Rosand J, Vranceanu AM. Mindfulness and coping are inversely related to psychiatric symptoms in patients and informal caregivers in the neuroscience ICU: implications for clinical care. Crit Care Med. 2016;44(11):2028–36.
50. Schmidt M, Azoulay E. Sleepless nights in the ICU: the awaken family. Crit Care. 2013;17(5):1003.
51. Huynh TDJ, Owens RL. Overnight ICU family presence in a model of family-centered care. Crit Care Med. 2018;46:412.
52. Edell-Gustafsson U, Angelhoff C, Johnsson E, Karlsson J, Morelius E. Hindering and buffering factors for parental sleep in neonatal care. A phenomenographic study. J Clin Nurs. 2015;24(5–6):717–27.
53. Tabah A, Ramanan M, Bailey RL, Chavan S, Baker S, Huckson S, et al. Family visitation policies, facilities, and support in Australia and New Zealand intensive care units: a multicentre, registry-linked survey. Aust Crit Care. 2021;35:375.
54. Jackson JC, Ely EW, Morey MC, Anderson VM, Denne LB, Clune J, et al. Cognitive and physical rehabilitation of intensive care unit survivors: results of the RETURN randomized controlled pilot investigation. Crit Care Med. 2012;40(4):1088–97.
55. Burns KEA, Devlin JW, Hill NS. Patient and family engagement in designing and implementing a weaning trial: a novel research paradigm in critical care. Chest. 2017;152:707.
56. Alessi C, Vitiello MV. Insomnia (primary) in older people: non-drug treatments. BMJ Clin Evid. 2015;2015:2302.
57. Hartescu I, Morgan K, Stevinson CD. Increased physical activity improves sleep and mood outcomes in inactive people with insomnia: a randomized controlled trial. J Sleep Res. 2015;24(5):526–34.
58. Kredlow MA, Capozzoli MC, Hearon BA, Calkins AW, Otto MW. The effects of physical activity on sleep: a meta-analytic review. J Behav Med. 2015;38(3):427–49.
59. Owens RL, Huynh TG, Netzer G. Sleep in the intensive care unit in a model of family-centered care. AACN Adv Crit Care. 2017;28(2):171–8.

60. Busse M, Stromgren K, Thorngate L, Thomas KA. Parents' responses to stress in the neonatal intensive care unit. Crit Care Nurse. 2013;33(4):52–9; quiz 60.
61. Lee SY, Kimble LP. Impaired sleep and well-being in mothers with low-birth-weight infants. J Obstet Gynecol Neonatal Nurs. 2009;38(6):676–85.
62. Davydow DS, Hough CL, Langa KM, Iwashyna TJ. Depressive symptoms in spouses of older patients with severe sepsis. Crit Care Med. 2012;40(8):2335–41.
63. van den Born-van Zanten SA, Dongelmans DA, Dettling-Ihnenfeldt D, Vink R, van der Schaaf M. Caregiver strain and posttraumatic stress symptoms of informal caregivers of intensive care unit survivors. Rehabil Psychol. 2016;61(2):173–8.
64. Cameron JI, Chu LM, Matte A, Tomlinson G, Chan L, Thomas C, et al. One-year outcomes in caregivers of critically ill patients. N Engl J Med. 2016;374(19):1831–41.
65. Comini L, Rocchi S, Bruletti G, Paneroni M, Bertolotti G, Vitacca M. Impact of clinical and quality of life outcomes of long-stay ICU survivors recovering from rehabilitation on caregivers' burden. Respir Care. 2016;61(4):405–15.
66. Gallop KH, Kerr CE, Nixon A, Verdian L, Barney JB, Beale RJ. A qualitative investigation of patients' and caregivers' experiences of severe sepsis*. Crit Care Med. 2015;43(2):296–307.
67. Cox CE, Docherty SL, Brandon DH, Whaley C, Attix DK, Clay AS, et al. Surviving critical illness: acute respiratory distress syndrome as experienced by patients and their caregivers. Crit Care Med. 2009;37(10):2702–8.
68. Van Pelt DC, Schulz R, Chelluri L, Pinsky MR. Patient-specific, time-varying predictors of post-ICU informal caregiver burden: the caregiver outcomes after ICU discharge project. Chest. 2010;137(1):88–94.
69. Needham DM, Davidson J, Cohen H, Hopkins RO, Weinert C, Wunsch H, et al. Improving long-term outcomes after discharge from intensive care unit: report from a stakeholders' conference. Crit Care Med. 2012;40(2):502–9.
70. Cohen S, Kaplan Z, Zohar J, Cohen H. Preventing sleep on the first resting phase following a traumatic event attenuates anxiety-related responses. Behav Brain Res. 2016;320:450.
71. Kuriyama K, Soshi T, Kim Y. Sleep deprivation facilitates extinction of implicit fear generalization and physiological response to fear. Biol Psychiatry. 2010;68(11):991–8.
72. Porcheret K, Holmes EA, Goodwin GM, Foster RG, Wulff K. Psychological effect of an analogue traumatic event reduced by sleep deprivation. Sleep. 2015;38(7):1017–25.
73. Wang S, Xin HN, Chung Lim Vico C, Liao JH, Li SL, Xie NM, et al. Effect of an ICU diary on psychiatric disorders, quality of life, and sleep quality among adult cardiac surgical ICU survivors: a randomized controlled trial. Crit Care. 2020;24(1):81.
74. Buysse DJ. Insomnia, depression and aging. Assessing sleep and mood interactions in older adults. Geriatrics. 2004;59(2):47–51; quiz 2.
75. Germain A, Buysse DJ, Nofzinger E. Sleep-specific mechanisms underlying posttraumatic stress disorder: integrative review and neurobiological hypotheses. Sleep Med Rev. 2008;12(3):185–95.

Chapter 11
Management of Family ICU Syndrome: Improving Family Outcomes in the ICU

Ji Won Shin, Truong-Giang Huynh, Samantha Gambles Farr, Suzette Jernigan, Steffanie A. Strathdee, Thomas Patterson, and Judy Elisa Davidson

Note: Standardized to use of term *clinician*, nurse used only when the intervention is specific to nursing. *Facilitated Sensemaking* (capitalized) is used in the sentence to reflect the name of the theoretical model. It is spelled in lower case when reflecting the process.

J. W. Shin (✉)
The Ohio State University College of Nursing, Columbus, OH, USA
e-mail: shin.527@osu.edu

T.-G. Huynh
Medical-Surgical ICU, University of California, San Diego Health, San Diego, CA, USA

S. G. Farr
Surgical Intensive Care, University of California, San Diego Health, San Diego, CA, USA
e-mail: sgambles@ucsd.edu

S. Jernigan
Burn ICU, Burn Special Care, University of California, San Diego Health, San Diego, CA, USA
e-mail: sjernigan@ucsd.edu

S. A. Strathdee
Harold Simon Professor of Global Health, Department of Medicine, University of California, San Diego, San Diego, CA, USA
e-mail: sstrathdee@ucsd.edu

T. Patterson
Department of Psychiatry, University of California, San Diego, San Diego, CA, USA
e-mail: tpatterson@ucsd.edu

J. E. Davidson
University of California, San Diego Health, San Diego, CA, USA
e-mail: jdavidson@ucsd.edu

© The Author(s), under exclusive license to Springer Nature Switzerland AG 2025
A. J. Vance et al. (eds.), *Families in the Intensive Care Unit*,
https://doi.org/10.1007/978-3-031-83786-9_11

Introduction

More than five million patients are admitted to an intensive care unit (ICU) in the United States each year [1]. This caregiving is often provided by direct family outcome members. Family, in the modern context, includes anyone the patient may have designated as family if they were able to do so, and is not restricted to direct lineage. From a review of the literature on family response to critical illness, it is estimated that 1/3 of families will suffer from anxiety, depression, and post-traumatic stress as a result of their exposure to the crisis of critical illness [2]. Stress disorders start in the ICU (Family ICU Syndrome) [3], but may last months to years following discharge or death of the patient (Post-Intensive Care Syndrome-Family) [4]. It is incumbent upon ICU clinicians to proactively provide family care in a manner that will minimize the risk of this trauma.

Without careful attention, the crisis of critical illness may also adversely affect social and physical endpoints in family members such as the intensity of caregiver burden, quality of life, ability to work, financial strain, marital strain, decompensation of preexisting health conditions, and the development of sleep disorders [5, 6]. Impaired or inadequate sleep may result in the inability to participate effectively in decision-making during the ICU stay [7]. In the event of patient death, families may also suffer complicated grief [4]. Although more research is needed, the prevailing wisdom is that the way we as clinicians, (a) communicate, and (b) involve families in care may affect these outcomes. Through an organized approach to family-centered care, communication and family engagement can be enhanced. Refer to Table 11.1 for constructs, definitions used throughout this chapter.

Table 11.1 Definitions of family constructs

Construct	Definition	Source
Family	Family is defined by the patient or, in the case of minors or those without decision-making capacity, by their surrogates. In this context, the family may be related or unrelated to the patient. They are individuals who provide support and with whom the patient has a significant relationship	Davidson JE, Aslakson RA, Long AC, Puntillo KA, Kross EK, Hart J, et al. Guidelines for Family-Centered Care in the Neonatal, Pediatric, and Adult ICU. Crit Care Med. 2017;45(1):103–28
Family-centered care	Family-centered care is an approach to healthcare that is respectful of and responsive to individual families' needs and values	Davidson JE, Aslakson RA, Long AC, Puntillo KA, Kross EK, Hart J, et al. Guidelines for Family-Centered Care in the Neonatal, Pediatric, and Adult ICU. Crit Care Med. 2017;45(1):103–28
Family ICU Syndrome	Morbidity and associated decision-making impairment experienced by many family members of patients with acute critical illness (in the ICU) and chronic critical illness (in the long-term acute care hospital)	Netzer G, Sullivan DR. Recognizing, naming, and measuring a family intensive care unit syndrome. Annals of the American Thoracic Society. 2014;11(3):435–41

(continued)

Table 11.1 (continued)

Construct	Definition	Source
Post-Intensive Care Syndrome Family	New or worsening problems with physical, cognitive, or mental health status arising after family exposure to critical illness and persisting past acute care hospitalization	Needham DM, Davidson J, Cohen H, Hopkins RO, Weinert C, Wunsch H, et al. Improving long-term outcomes after discharge from intensive care unit: report from a stakeholders' conference. Critical Care Medicine. 2012;40(2):502–9
Facilitated Sensemaking	Facilitated Sensemaking is a mid-range theory of family engagement with the goal of helping the family make sense of the situation their new role as caregivers in a structured manner ultimately decreasing negative outcomes resulting from exposure to critical illness	Davidson JE. Facilitated Sensemaking A Strategy and New Middle-Range Theory to Support Families of Intensive Care Unit Patients. Critical Care Nurse. 2010;30(6):28–39

Facilitated Sensemaking as a Framework for Family-Centered Care

Family members of intensive care patients are at high risk for anxiety, depression, and psychological distress that may extend well beyond their family members' ICU stay [3]. Often, the words spoken by family members seem rhetorical; 'I don't understand,' 'I can't deal with this,' and 'What am I going to do?' These seemingly rhetorical statements provide valuable insight into how we can help them through their crisis.

Facilitated Sensemaking [8] is a midrange theory of family engagement derived from two sources: Roy's Adaptation Model [9], and Wieck's business leadership Organizational Sensemaking model [10]. Roy's Adaptation Model states that in order to respond positively to change, an individual must adapt through two subsystems. The first system, which involves learning, emotion, perception, and judgment is named the Cognator system. The second, or Regulator system, involves neural, endocrine, and chemical channels. When people experience critical illness, they need to adapt to the situation, and the consequences of this exposure to crisis may result in a range of consequences, positive or negative, depending upon the nature of that process of adaptation [9]. Wieck's model emphasizes the role that leaders play in employee's perception of their roles and events occurring within the organization by providing feedback on employees' performance, expectations of roles, and an understanding or sense-making of events which may otherwise be misinterpreted. Leaders interpret the status of the organization, e.g., financial viability or successes in attaining targets, and 'message' this interpretation to staff to promote a positive image of the organization [8, 10].

In Facilitated Sensemaking, these same principles are applied to decoding the situation of critical illness for family members. Instead of leaving it up to family members to form an impression of what is happening from the cues in the environment, clinicians are encouraged to interpret the cues for family members to construct a reality-based narrative. Proactive communication is essential. We cannot assume that families will interpret what is happening around them accurately without interpretation from the healthcare team. For instance, simple things—such as the fact that family members are welcome to attend rounds—need to be articulated verbally.

Nursing interventions derived from the Facilitated Sensemaking theory initially help the family adapt to their loved one's illness or injury by assisting them to make sense of the immediate situation, helping them to do what is needed at the moment. The process is continuous and iterative. As the patient's condition changes, family interventions evolve. Family members' comfort with their new caregiving role and the ICU environment improves with communication and engagement in care. The questions 'What am I going to do' and 'How am I ever going to deal with this' are answered as family members eventually accept the new turn their life has taken, and the new roles which are theirs to assume. Fear and helplessness (antecedents to post-traumatic stress disorder (PTSD)) are replaced with knowledge, understanding, and purpose when family members are provided with the tools and knowledge to assist in the care of their loved one. When this process is used, it is welcomed by family members [11] and has been shown to decrease families' anxiety [12–15], depression [14], and PTSD-related symptoms [14, 15].

Physiologic Mechanisms of Facilitate Sensemaking (Fig. 11.1)

Reactivity to a traumatic situation is acute, transient, and self-limited for most of the population. Specific vulnerabilities such as genetics, prior trauma, female sex, trauma at developmental stages, injury, and hypocortisolism, create a greater vulnerability for the development of PTSD [16]. Facilitated Sensemaking provides the means to assuage the fear, horror, and helplessness experienced by loved ones of intensive care patients, potentially limiting the family's submersion into a vortex of nightmares, agitation, impulsivity, avoidance, and anger [8, 17]. A situation which may, at first, seem unsurmountable is broken down for the family into a scenario which makes sense, and in which they can engage in care to make a positive impact one day at a time.

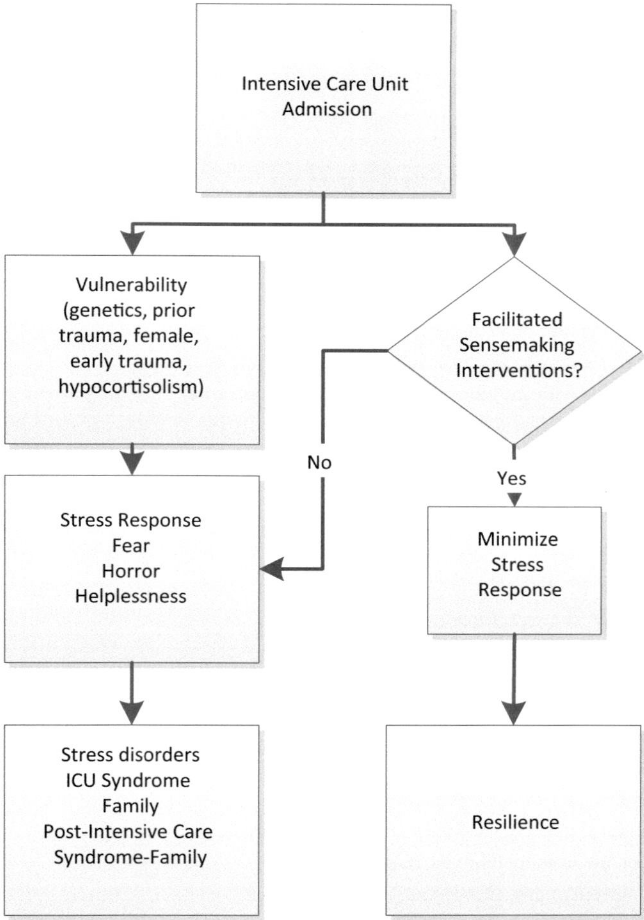

Fig. 11.1 Facilitated Sensemaking

Basic Bedside Strategies

Evidence-based guidelines on family-centered care were recently released by the Society of Critical Care Medicine (SCCM). The guidelines recommend many different clinical strategies to improve family-centered care with the goal of decreasing post-intensive care syndrome (PICS for patient/PICS-F for family) that can be used in the Facilitated Sensemaking process (Table 11.2). Here several strategies to translate recommendations into practice using Facilitated Sensemaking are described.

Table 11.2 Recommendations from Society of Critical Care Medicine guidelines

Presence
Open flexible family presence
Family presence on rounds
Family presence at resuscitation
Communication
Diaries White Board where family can write questions/suggestions
Communication tools that support patient-family communication while mechanical ventilation
Family education/leaflets
Shared decision-making/nurse involved in decision-making
Use validated decision-support tools for surrogate decision-making
Family conferences with structured approach to communication:
• Value input
• Acknowledge emotions
• Active listening
• Understand patient as person
• Elicit questions
• Messages of hope and non-abandonment
Consults as indicated
Spiritual support
Palliative care referrals
Ethics when value-laden conflict arises
Social workers to support family conference
Navigators (specially trained family liaisons)
Environmental/organizational considerations
Leaflet with helpful tips (e.g., visitation rules, time rounds usually occur)
Noise reduction/environmental hygiene/private rooms
Teach family sleep hygiene, provide family sleep surface
Develop policy for family-centered care
Staff education and training
Neonatal specific
Peer-to-peer support
Teach parents role and engage in care
Consider psychologist referral for cognitive behavioral therapy in mothers of preterm infants

There are four broad categories of interventions to be deployed within the Facilitated Sensemaking model intended to: develop caring relationships, enhance communication, encourage family presence and engagement, and support families in decision-making [18].

Caring Relationships

To build caring relationships, trust must first be established. Trust comes with demonstrating care through gentle touch, use of a caring voice, empathetic and active-listening, and inquiring about the patient and family as people. Families may exhibit a hypervigilant need to safeguard the patient until trust is formed. Though not studied scientifically, we posit that trust will develop sooner if the family witnesses care through presence, feels cared for, and is engaged as a team member. This could include the simple act of bringing a caregiver a cup of coffee or allowing the caregiver to provide observations or ask questions at the end of rounds. Following through on promises, such as answering questions or requests for pain medications in a timely manner, enhances trust. Many of the strategies listed below that enhance communication and engagement also help in forming the caring relationship.

Communication

Optimizing communication through actively promoting family presence and engagement coupled with structured frequent communication is recommended [19]. Effective communication between patients and family and physician correlates with health outcomes of both the patient and family, including decreased anxiety, depression, and symptoms of post-traumatic stress. Clear and open communication facilitates family decision-making process by reducing medical uncertainty. It is easy to make decisions when the medical prognosis is very good or very bad, but difficulty arises when the prognosis is uncertain [20].

One approach to improving communication is to practice family inclusion and engagement during interdisciplinary rounds. Members attending interdisciplinary rounds may include but are not limited to the intensivist, respiratory therapist, nurse, pharmacist, case manager, and family/surrogate decision-maker. In a concise review of the literature on family inclusion in rounds, families were more satisfied when included in rounds as compared to not being included, and when questioned over 95% would want to be included [21]. Family presence on rounds could serve to improve trust and relationship with the healthcare team. Further, when included, families have the opportunity to provide clinicians with important information regarding baseline status and previously failed or adverse reactions to treatments and medications [21]. Several observational studies specific to the ICU reported that family presence during rounds increased family knowledge, involvement in asking questions, and decision-making [19].

Once a trusting relationship has been established, communication on decoding the environment and reflective inquiry are important to reduce family stress. Families are generally unfamiliar with the ICU environment; one filled with lights, sounds, alarms, and different providers representing various disciplines coming in and out constantly. Decoding the environment includes explaining what the ICU monitors are, what the different numbers and alarms mean, and a basic explanation of each piece of equipment and how it relates to the treatment plan.

This means explaining to families the role each person on the care team plays because it is often not obvious, even from titles. Families also need to be cued into their new role as caregiver. The act of decoding the environment may need to be performed iteratively because stress may block learning and memory formation during the acute exposure to critical illness [18]. Families' enhanced understanding of what the patient is experiencing in the new ICU environment through effective patient-family communication may also facilitate sensemaking process. Such interventions that improve patient-family communication while mechanical ventilation may enable clear conversations on what the patient wants, needs, or how he/she feels, which directs families needed bedside activities, which may increase family engagement [22].

Families need to be assured that not all monitor alarms require immediate attention. This can decrease anxiety as well as mitigate forming an inappropriate impression of clinician inattention. In addition to decoding the environment, practicing reflective inquiry daily helps to identify false perceptions or myths regarding the situation. Reflective inquiry is another strategy of Facilitated Sensemaking in which clinicians can ask the family members open-ended questions such as, 'if you were going to tell the rest of your family the most important thing that happened in your (husband's, brother's, mother's daughter's) care today, what would it be?' [18]. In the case of the family labelled as difficult, were they upset because of the perception that the alarms were not tended to? In the reflective practice, the 'mythical realities' could be redirected towards a constructive truthful narrative.

Monitoring bedside conversations is important to assure the choice of words is healing not only to the patient, but to the listening family as well. Words can harm or heal. It has been demonstrated that the incidence of PICS-F is greater when clinicians are not perceived as caring [23]. Interteam conflict can erode family coping ability [24]. Even when patients appear not to be conscious enough to listen and retain information, many survivors report details of conversations that both helped them in the healing process and also those that scared them resulting in nightmares, hallucinations or flashbacks of a horrifying ICU experience [25]. Imagine the last time a colleague described a 'difficult' family member. Think back to the event and reflect upon whether the difficulty could have been iatrogenic. Did they overhear something that was said inappropriately? Did they distort information because of a lack of communication or insufficient information? Increased or improved communication may prevent or solve the tension between the family and the healthcare team and decrease the likelihood of a family member being labelled as 'difficult'. Clinicians need to be aware that in addition to decreased satisfaction, the likelihood of post-traumatic stress after they leave the ICU rises. According to the most recent *Diagnostic and Statistical Manual of Mental Disorders* (DSM-5), the threat or even perceived threat of actual or potential death to their family member may result in post-traumatic stress [26].

Engagement and Presence

Utilizing a tool designed to facilitate conversations during rounds such as the ABCDEF bundle can also improve patient and family outcomes [27]:

Assess, prevent, and manage pain
Both spontaneous awakening and breathing trials
Choice of analgesia and sedation
Delirium assessment
Early mobilization and exercise
Family engagement and empowerment

Use of this evidence-based bundle has demonstrated reductions in pain, delirium, agitation, and long-term consequences of critical illness. The **F** portion of the bundle implies that families support clinicians with attaining the ABCDE goals. They can be encouraged to report pain, report changes in mentation and cognition, coach the patient through breathing trials and attempts at mobilization, and keep the patient cognitively active to prevent delirium [28].

Family engagement in rounds empowers family members to help navigate decision-making and understand the severity of illness. It also influences clinicians' understanding of the family or patients' concept of illness to further individualize care [29]. Involving families in rounds can address current questions families have, facilitate communication, and clarify family role(s) during the ICU stay. This intervention also demonstrates respect for persons increasing the speed and quality with which a trusting relationship is formed. Structuring time out of each day to have open conversation between physician-patient and nurse-patient is also indicated. The time spent in proactive communication may decrease the need for after-hours phone calls later in the day.

A simple beside poster or whiteboard that is tailored toward 'persons' rather than 'patients' and their families also conveys messages of care. Some refer to these as 'All About Me' posters, in which clinicians and the family members can fill in information about what the patient likes or dislikes, their preferred name, spiritual beliefs, hobbies, what gives them meaning, favorite foods, music, etc. Family pictures and a picture of the patient at baseline health can be posted. Each clinician that enters the room can use the information to develop a better image of who the person is behind the patient, which in turn can be used to form a trusting and caring relationship. Care, stemming from the information provided, can be tailored to the individual to create a healing environment such as playing their favorite music in the background, sharing a prayer, or not feeding them their most disliked foods. This simple yet effective strategy involves families as partners in designing the ideal environment and care for their loved one.

The SCCM guidelines recommend that family presence in the ICU should be open and flexible with the intent to accommodate patient and family presence 24 h a day [19]. Family members now move past the concept of being visitors or visiting, to being present and engaged in the caring process. Family presence paired with empowerment can improve outcomes for both the patient and family [30, 31]. In a randomized controlled trial of mothers whose child was in a pediatric ICU, the mothers who were encouraged to visit and engage in care activities taught to them by the nurse reported significantly less stress and PTSD symptoms than those who were not [32, 33].

Encouraging family presence is necessary to facilitate sensemaking. How can families understand what is happening or what their role is if they are not present? In the process of Facilitated Sensemaking, family members are encouraged to be present, are welcomed by clinicians, and provided opportunities to perform simple bedside care, if desired [18]. An assessment is necessary to identify the family's preference for inclusion in care and determine which care activities would be most appropriate in this situation. Providing a comforting presence, assisting with care, participating in rounds and goal setting are some of the ways in which family members who to serve as a surrogate decision-makers can be empowered [18]. Following the assessment, family members are offered tailored interventions. Perhaps the family members are very stressed, anxious, and pacing around the room. The nurse can provide them with an invitation to perform a very basic task, such as holding or massaging the patient's hand or providing a hand massage with lotion. Activities can further progress to applying lip balm, reading, playing cards, letter recognition from word puzzles, passive range of motion, or simply praying together.

Once the patient is more awake and interactive, families can be encouraged to be their individualized coach [18]. The role of the coach is to motivate the patient to recovery. Encouraging the ICU patient to practice active range of motion exercises or mobilizing while intubated or on dialysis can be best accomplished by the familiar voice and encouragement of the family. Explain why mobilizing or exercising is good for the patient to the family, who can then in turn convey the message to their loved one in a manner they would best understand. Knowing that mobility can prevent delirium, and that they played a role in this important preventive health strategy is empowering for the family; giving them purpose in crisis which can be protective to their mental health.

Other coachable opportunities include encouraging the patient to brush their own teeth or hair, help bathe themselves, help them use a phone or laptop, or be as independent as possible. In addition to encouraging activities, the family member can also encourage the patient to sleep and rest. Sleep is vital to the patient's outcome as evidence demonstrates patient sleep in the ICU is very poor [30]. If present at night, families are in a great position to facilitate nighttime hours and a nighttime routine, turning the lights out at 10 p.m. and ensuring quiet hours [31]. In turn, family members can also sleep during those hours to promote their own health so they can better take care of their loved one during daytime hours [31].

Decision-Making

The role of surrogate decision-maker needs to be explained to the person within the family assuming this role and explained to the entire family unit to prevent role and family conflict. It is important for them to know that requesting whether the patient has an advanced directive, living will, durable power of attorney or other advanced planning document is routine part of practice and not because death is imminent. Usually, these explanations are done by the physician and reinforced by the nurse. The physician also assesses the preference for inclusion in decision-making. Due to the volume of time nurses spend with family members, they may advocate by providing the physician with their assessment of the family's desire for participation in decision-making as well as quantity of information desired. Decision-regret amongst family members can be avoided by reminding surrogates that their role is to inform the clinical team of what the patient would have wanted if they had been able to voice their own opinion. Therefore, the decisions are really that of the patient and not what the surrogate would do for themselves in a similar situation. Care is taken to help the family through disparate views on next steps to prevent family fragmentation. Detailed policy statements regarding how to engage families in decision-making have been published elsewhere [34, 35].

Provider Success with Practice and Training

Providers may need assistance to incorporate the interventions which solidify each of the four components of Facilitated Sensemaking as a whole. Whereas technical skills are often taught and tested, teaching and evaluating competency in family care, though recommended, is generally not, resulting in a wide range of skill when working with families. All components of Facilitated Sensemaking require interpersonal skills: development of caring relationships, encouraging family presence and engagement, encouraging participation in decision-making, and facilitating communication.

It is no longer acceptable to care for the patient without tending to the family [19]. Care of the patient encompasses not only the singular patient, but the family as well. In an environment which dictates proficiency, efficiency, and critical thought, it is easy for the clinician to become so entrenched in the tasks of the moment that they allow little room for the caring self to shine through. It is important that the family know that their clinician is not only competent but also that they care. Further, feeling-cared for is an important factor that can affect family health and well-being as well as their capacity to optimally engage in health-promoting self-care [36]. Clinicians need to take the time for empathic listening in order to be open to the family's suffering, hear their fears, and recognize their needs, preferences, and desires [18].

The clinician must also be aware of available resources which can be utilized if the medical goals of care conflict with the family's desires. A family conference can provide the setting for information exchange, role clarification, resolution of conflict, an opportunity for the family to express their wishes in a supportive environment, and if appropriate, revision of goals. When this is not effective, or when conflict exists despite standard communication efforts, an ethics consult may be indicated [19]. It has been recommended that, at a minimum, family conferences are organized when death is determined to be a potential outcome, there are significant changes in prognosis, multiple consults on the case with conflicting messages, and every 7 days [37].

The hurried pace of the ICU, frequent shift changes, and cramped quarters may interfere with the type of communication needed to provide the greatest family support. Though the clinician is knowledgeable of and familiar with the ICU environment, the family, most likely, is not. Part of clinician training may include developing lay language scripts to explain treatments, equipment, alarms, and/or manifestations of illness. The use of medical jargon should be avoided. Verbal explanations should supplement any visual aide provided. A combined approach of verbal, written, and video educational materials are recommended. Inquiring as to the family's understanding of the day's events or of what was said to them by other clinicians may provide clarification and avoid false impressions. Lastly, a review of how the family felt that the patient's or their needs were met or not met is an important factor in communication which clinicians should include in daily conversation [18]. With practice, clinicians will not only learn to incorporate the family into a collaborative approach to patient care, recognizing and valuing the family as their partner in care, and look forward to family presence.

Vulnerable Populations

Neonates

Patients in the Neonatal Intensive Care Unit (NICU) are infants whose births, and quite possibly, whose futures, have been complicated through complicated pregnancies, intrauterine accidents, premature births, syndromes, malformations, and the inability to adapt to life outside of their mothers' womb. Having hoped for, envisioned, or planned for a different beginning, parents are forced into the painful realization that the plans which they had for their children's births have changed [38].

Parents whose children begin their lives in an NICU must deal with an enormity of feelings and emotions. Tubes, machines, monitors, alarms, their infant's physical appearance, a new language, and not knowing what to expect may shock and overwhelm them [39, 40]. Fathers are uneasy, as they accompany the infant from the delivery room to the NICU, where mom is left behind. Both may feel that they are incapable of keeping their family together. They experience a strong desire to be close to and touch their newborn so that the infant knows that they are, but at the same time, fear that their infant would not like being touched or that they would cause harm [41]. Parents may feel that they may be judged that they decided to sustain the life of the baby whose termination was advised [42]. Some may feel that their faith is being tested, while others may feel that they are being abandoned and punished by God [43]. Some families, upon giving up hope, allow a sense of powerlessness to consume them [44]. Many wrestle between fear of their infants' death and concern over the long-term effects should the infant survive, knowing that it may be years until the full extent of neurological and sensory injuries are known [39, 45].

The vast extent of feelings and emotions experienced by the parents of infants in the NICU can result in long-term emotional struggles. Coping with grief, anxiety, helplessness, depression, and unmatched healthcare needs of their children, families may be left vulnerable to isolation and impaired relationships [43]. PTSD is an outcome for some parents, which is associated with severity of illness in the infant [40, 45, 46]. Severe PTSD in mothers has been associated with impaired maternal-infant relationships based on a pattern of control, inconsistency, and insensitivity in interactions with their infants. While patterns of control in maternal-infant relationships are associated with later behavioral problems, mothers' inconsistencies and insensitivities in interactions with their infants may also affect their infants' cognitive and social development [45]. The impact of how care is delivered in the early days of the infant's life can have a significant effect on the early and long-term experiences of parents and their infants [47]. Early interventions to support the formation of healthy maternal-infant dyads may help to reduce psychological distress in parents and developmental and behavioral problems in their infants [45].

Traditionally, parents have been left on the periphery while care is focused on the infant. Powerless, intimidated, and left to observe while others take care of the child that they long to hold, parents struggle to see themselves as parents and define their role [47–49]. But with the increasing integration of family-centered care practices, there is a greater recognition that parents are not visitors. Moved from the sidelines to the bedside, parents are introduced to the NICU environment and learn about the complexities of their infants' problems [38]. Parents express an increased connection to their infants and increased satisfaction with their parenting role when holding their infants skin to skin. Mothers' milk production increases, as does their bonding experience, sensitivity, and expression of affectionate behaviors toward their infants [38]. Benefits of skin to skin care for the infants include less episodes of apnea, better sleep regulation, regularity of heart rates, reduced bouts of infection, less advanced retinopathy, and less chronic lung disease [38, 50]. Exposure to mothers' voices and odors were also shown to have a positive influence on feeding progression as well as to contribute to their infants' cardiorespiratory stability and state regulation [47].

As they become increasingly comfortable with their infants, parents are instructed on feeding, bathing, dressing, diaper changes, and administering oral medications under the supervision of the clinician [47, 51]. Parents' increasing participation in their infants' care has demonstrated reduced lengths of stay, increased rates of weight gain, increased rates of breastfeeding at discharge, decreased hospital acquired infections, less maternal anxiety, and depression, and more positive interactions with their infants. Fathers who participate in their infants' care state that they were able to communicate with their infants, and that eye contact and their infants' reaction to their voices were especially important [41, 52].

Involvement in infant care is vital for both parents and infant. Protecting mothers from overwhelming stress improves the maternal-infant relationship. Lasting behavioral outcomes are associated with daily interactions between mothers and their NICU infants and the mother's ability to interact successfully with her infant. Positive parenting provides premature infants with the gift of resilience [40]. Family-centered care reconnects parent and child. Therefore, care of the family is essential for the well-being of the child and is an essential part of the scope of ICU clinicians, not an afterthought.

Pediatrics

> I can still recall the night which changed our lives forever. I was coming back with a friend in the car when I received an urgent call from one of my neighbors asking me where I am at the moment—she said that she saw smoke and my house was on fire. I started to panic and tried calling everyone's phone number to find out more about the situation. I finally got hold of my ex-husband to check on the kids who were left in the care of their aunt and boyfriend. I drove home without ever realizing how fast I was driving. I had 3 children—Fernando, 11 years old, Junior, 5-years-old, and Ezmi, 3-years-old who were being watched over by their aunt and her boyfriend. The children were asleep at the back room of the house when the fire from the space heater slowly engulfed the house. Their aunt's boyfriend tried to get the children, but he was only able to get Junior out who was passed out due to smoke inhalation. Ezmi was also unconscious, but Fernando died on the scene. When I got to UCSD Burn Unit, I was unsure what I was going to see. I wanted to be with my children, but I know that they need to be taken cared of because they were severely burned. I try to be strong for my children. Everyone was helping us—doctors, nurses, social worker, case manager and other staff to get through this challenging times. I stayed in the room on Ezmi more because she was awake, but I also go to see Junior when he was intubated. Physically and emotionally, I am drained throughout the hospitalization, but I do know that my faith help me move forward instead of putting blame on others for the accident. Junior and Ezmi are now at home playing like normal kids. We still do regular doctor's follow-up for Junior because of his trach. They cannot sleep without each other or someone else in the room at night. Both are in school doing well.—paraphrased from testimony with permission by Juanna Vasquez Nunez (Mother).

As is seen in other pediatric critical care admissions, anxiety, depression, and post-traumatic stress disorder for both parents and burn-injured children are significantly elevated and may remain abnormal for many years after discharge. Parents also suffer from guilt [53]. The burn event is always unexpected and coping with the trauma can be further complicated by the patient's pain, elevated anxiety, fear, uncertainty of outcome, need for multiple surgeries, the sight of wound care sessions, grueling rehabilitation therapy, disfigurement, and the extended period of time away from home.

In this case the immediate need was to provide burn care to the injured live children, but the staff were conflicted with how and when to approach the mother with news that her third child had not survived. All clinicians support the parents with understanding the sights, sounds, and expectations of the ICU environment.

However, clinicians also expect to fill in the social-emotional gap when parents are not present for their children or need to trade off time between children. Targeted support for these needs may be provided by a variety of resources.

Certified Child Life Specialists support the healthcare team with developmental, social, and emotional needs of hospitalized children and their families. It is the goal of the child life program to minimize the fear and anxiety often experienced in the healthcare setting by providing knowledgeable, compassionate, and developmentally appropriate support services (Personal communication: Kathryn Hamelin, Certified Child Life Specialist Manager, July 2017). In this case, the situation was further complicated by the death of the oldest child and competing priorities providing support for the two burn surviving children. Early activation of a child-life specialist, family navigator [19] or family ombudsman is essential for prompt attention to emotional and psychological of the parent/child needs during the critical care admission while clinicians are stabilizing the patient and providing direct care.

As ever greater number of children and youth survive serious burn injuries, more focus will be placed on preparing parents and siblings of survivors for caregiving after discharge. Providing care is the normal expectation of parents. However, the role of pediatric burn patient's parent/caregiver, and at times siblings, is often expanded to include unfamiliar nursing and physical and occupational therapy duties. Once discharged, parents provide wound care, change dressings, perform scar massage/hydration, and ensure that their child engages in a home exercise program: all responsibilities outside the normal and expected realm of parenting. Allowing them to be present during such care can offer them the opportunity to gradually learn the skills necessary for these tasks is indicated.

After initial stabilization, role modeling bedside behaviors and care will help parents to find their desired level of involvement. Because anxiety can be shared between humans [54] it is important for clinicians to remain calm at the bedside and provide parent's permission to take a break from the bedside when needed. A psychologist may also be necessary [19]. Given the high prevalence of persistent mental health issues, it is prudent upon transfer, discharge, or death, to include the possible necessity of a psychologist or psychiatrist referral with handoff communication and parent education. Additionally, early spiritual assessment can be helpful to identify the value structure of the family and activate the faith community, when indicated, to provide support [37].

In addition, clinicians can predict that hospitalized children will need parental presence, and parents will want to be present but will require help in learning how to participate in care and support their child. In the special case of burns, parents will need to overcome the dramatic change in appearance of their child as well as receive help to cope with witnessing their pain. With enough support, the parents, in turn, can be taught to provide the role of coach, encouraging their child to adhere to the treatment plan and endure the difficult treatments. Parental presence during rounds may be a way to support parents in learning how to participate in care; parental presence on rounds is recommended by the Society of Critical Care Medicine (SCCM) and endorsed by many other professional societies [19]. Although concerns have been raised by clinicians over the quality of teaching, the quantity of time parents may take during rounds with questions, and issues of privacy, in a review, it was found that families find information a higher priority than privacy and a full 95% would want to be present during rounds [21].

In pediatric burns and other similar situations, families may benefit from a navigator. Emerging evidence suggests that specially trained care coordinators or communication specialists called navigators may improve family satisfaction with physician communication, reduce cost of care, length of ICU and hospital stay, and decrease family psychological symptoms. The use of a family navigator is recommended [19], yet the cost of adding a member to the team may be prohibitive. Navigators are clinicians whose role is to step aside from patient care activities to provide family members with the information they need to make sense of the immediate situation, offer emotional support, and foster adaptive coping skills [19, 55]. Navigators may bridge the gap between the medical team and the family throughout the hospitalization, provide ongoing support, help parents understand the present and developing needs of their child, and provide anticipatory guidance throughout the hospitalization [56]. Once discharged, children are dependent upon their parents for care far beyond the care that their childhood once entailed. Support provided to parents in the acute care setting might help diminish distress and caregiving burden after hospital discharge.

Non-Native English Speakers

Communication is likely the single-most important aspect of family-centered care. It is well known that the timeliness, quality and quantity of communication drives both satisfaction and psychological outcomes [57]. Quality includes provision of information in the surrogate's preferred language. For example, accreditation standards in the United States require interpretation for patients and their surrogates so that they can understand the plan of care and thoughtfully consent to tests and treatments [58]. Nonetheless, communicating with non-English speaking families can remain challenging. Even though the technology exists to provide translation of the written word and interpretation of oral conversation through video and phone interpreters, time pressures promote the inappropriate tendency to take short cuts and use of family members, use of native speakers not tested for medical fluency, or not to communicate at all.

Use of family members as the interpreter is not acceptable for several reasons. First, the family may filter the discussion to the patient or surrogate so that only issues they feel should be discussed, are relayed. Secondly, the privacy of the patient is compromised when a family member who is not the surrogate is used to convey sensitive information like prognosis, tests, or diagnoses of sexually transmitted communicable diseases. And finally, culturally based gender issues might make it inappropriate for a man to discuss issues such as women's health concerns with a female family member who is not their wife. Minors should never be used for any reason as interpreters [19, 21]. Even when using professional interpreters, interpreters may add, omit, substitute, and editorialize words, which may cause misinterpretation of the meaning of conversation. It is recommended that healthcare providers need to maintain eye contact and speak to family members, not to the interpreters, when using interpreters in family meetings [59].

Appropriate, timely, transparent, high quality communication builds trust, decreasing risk of litigation even amidst negative patient outcomes [21, 60]. Despite standards to encourage compliance with interpretation and keen focus on interpretation during regulatory and accreditation on-site audits, wide variation occurs from organization to organization in available resources and the practice of holding clinicians accountable for appropriate use of interpreters. Leaders in the clinical environment can work to assure that the interpretation phone/video system is available in all conference rooms used for family conferences. Having a nurse or social worker present during family meetings to set up equipment and advocate for interpretation may increase compliance. Prescheduling daily interpretation sessions with non-English speaking surrogates, to provide updates for the plan of care and obtain consent for planned tests and procedures, is warranted.

Lesbian Gay Bisexual Transgender Queer or Questioning Intersex, Asexual (LGBTQIA) Population

The U.S. Department of Health and Human Services (HHS) Lesbian, Gay, Bisexual and Transgender (LGBT) Policy Coordination Committee worked diligently to improve the health and well-being of LGBT communities. Note that while recognizing that the initial ‘Q’ for queer or questioning, ‘I’ for intersex, and ‘A’ for asexual are now commonly added to the acronym LGBT, the titles of the regulatory standards at the time they were written, referred to only LGBT. With the signing of the Patient Protection and Affordable Care Act (PPACA) on March 23, 2010, under 42 CFR 482.608(a) this legislature guaranteed that all people, including LGBT people, have the right to be visited by their loved ones while in the hospital [61]. This provision also addressed who can make medical decisions on their behalf through advance directives. Under previous legislation, LGBTQIA patients and their families suffered prejudiced practices regarding family involvement. Historically, the definition of family consisted of only blood-related relatives.

The definition of ‘family’ used for this legislation was taken from the Institute for Patient- and Family-Centered Care [62] and is consistent with the definition published by the Society of Critical Care Medicine which was specifically vetted by members of the LBGTQIA population prior to adopting into practice (Table 11.1) [19]. In both definitions, family refers to two or more persons who are related in any way, biologically, legally, or emotionally. ***Family is defined by the patient***. The patient designates who should be considered family members, as able, for the purpose of visitation [63]. Family members and surrogates of the LGBTQIA patient are awarded the same rights as those of any other patient.

Of the LGBTQIA population, possibly the most vulnerable for medical and communication errors are individuals whose gender identity is different from the sex assigned to that person at birth (e.g., transgender, queer or questioning), also protected by PPACA legislation. Gender identity is an individual's internal sense of gender. Individuals may identify as male, female, neither or some combination of male and female and the patients' pronouns should be reflected in the medical records. Instead of assuming pronouns based on physical appearance, it is always best to ask the patient for the pronoun to use and document. Special attention is needed so that once assessed, clinicians accurately record gender in the medical record along with legal name change as indicated. Because some people have both a legal name and a different changed (but not legal) name, it is important to assess patients for both. For family members, there is only a need to know the legal name when it is related to matching the person to the name on legal papers such as a medical directive or Power of Attorney. It is a matter of respect to ask family about the use of pronoun when unsure, so that the proper pronoun can be used during conversation.

Clinically it is important that providers are cognizant of the birth gender of the patient, current gender identity, and the pronoun and name by which the patient wishes to be addressed. Solutions can be provided by vendors of the electronic health record software to assure this information is available in a readily retrievable manner once the social situation is assessed and recorded. The risk of making errors in documentation or communication is high if the patient transitioned to a new gender and name after becoming a patient to that healthcare organization. A full description of clinical considerations is beyond the scope of this chapter, but most importantly to the discussion of patient- and family-centered care, it can be psychologically damaging to repeatedly use the wrong pronoun or name when referring to a person; either to the patient themselves or when communicating with family. According to the general principal of respect for humans it is important to use the gender pronoun and name as directed by the patient, or when unable, their surrogate.

The Unbefriended Patient

The unbefriended patient is one who does not have a surrogate to act on their behalf as a healthcare proxy. Legislation from state to state varies regarding patients who are decisionally incapacitated and lack an identified healthcare surrogate. Historically, the largest proportion of unbefriended patients have been those suffering from mental illness, homeless, or baby boomers [64]. As the numbers of elderly people and therefore people with dementia rises, the number of unbefriended patients also rises [65].

Providers caring for critically ill patients often perform emergent, life-saving procedures as surrogate decision-makers until surrogates can be identified. However, if the patient remains unbefriended, a surrogate decision-maker may be appointed by court order [64]. In 2016, the American Geriatric Society (AGS) issued a policy statement issuing a call for action to create national (vs. state) standards regarding the unbefriended patient. At this writing, however, the issue is still handled at the state level and readers are encouraged to research the laws in the state in which they practice. The AGS policy statement also stated that healthcare teams, and not individual clinicians, should make the decisions for these patients according to best interest standards. Hospital ethics consultation is advised prior to court-ordered surrogate placement. Early Medical Social Worker (MSW) consultation is indicated to deploy due diligence to attempt to locate family [65]. It is incumbent upon providers of patients on a trajectory towards dementia or cognitive incapacitation to prevent them from becoming unbefriended by encouraging the appointment of a surrogate while still able to make medical decisions [65].

Approximately 16% of ICU patients are unbefriended [66] and 5.5% of ICU patients who die lack an advocate for decision-making [66]. This unbefriended population of patients within the ICU require special care considerations while hospitalized. In addition to legal issues, the healthcare team may fulfill the social role of family while the patient is hospitalized. The importance of acts of caring are heightened because without conscious recognition and attention to the human need for affiliation [36], the patient will not benefit from the healing power of presence and caring human touch. Healthcare providers need to play a large role in decision-making for unbefriended patients especially when they are dying in the ICU, which may cause burdens in both practical and ethical aspects. To what degree physicians need to be involved in the decision-making process is unclear. There is also concern over providers' ability to predict patient preferences and values accurately, which plays a crucial role in providing appropriate treatment for unfriended patients. Failure to avoid unnecessary and prolonged treatment may negatively impact the quality of death of the patients as well as moral distress in healthcare providers.

In response to the aforementioned concerns, end-of-life doulas have been discussed as a potential solution to reduce healthcare providers' burdens and improve the decision-making process for unbefriended ICU patients [67, 68]. End-of-life doulas are trained professional who serve as companions and advocates for those who are dying. The end-of-life doula 'movement' is recently evident in many countries including United States, Australia, Canada, and United Kingdom [69]. As non-medical members of the healthcare team, they provide a balancing, advocating voice on behalf of the patient. They may diffuse the moral burden in providers and help reduce inappropriate treatment and delays in care, so ultimately, ensure optimal, ethical care for unbefriended, dying ICU patients.

Additional Strategies to Support ICU Patients, Families, and Clinicians

Diaries have been used to support **ICU patients and their families** since the 1980s [70]. ICU diary programs vary throughout the world. A review of recent United States literature shows that diaries are typically comprised of a collaboration of authors including physicians, nurses, family, and visitors [71]. Entries are written to the patient rather than about the patient, offering messages of hope and caring. Some diaries include pictures of common ICU equipment and/or the view of the room as the patient might see it [72]. Clinical staff may provide more clinically focused entries in lay terms and are encouraged to write about issues that often stimulate nightmares or hallucinations such as restraint, endotracheal tubes, the magnetic resonance imaging machine, and urinary catheters, in addition to messages of hope and caring. Family and visitors offer more emotional messages [72]. Studies have shown that when patients survive the critical illness and are able to read their illness narrative, the diary helps fill in memory gaps or reconstruct delusional memories towards reality [73].

In addition to improving patient and family outcomes [74, 75], ICU diaries can influence family members and nurses. Families have reported that reading messages of care, empathy, and support humanized the clinical staff [76]. ICU diaries with multiple family member are more cohesiveness if all members share the same inner narrative. Opposing or family members in disagreement might not benefit from the jointly authored diary. When multiple family members contribute to a diary, a leader emerges in influencing the illness narrative which can shape the future perception of the ICU experience for the patient [77].

The use of diaries can be utilized as a starting point for conversations between family members and family to staff [77, 78]. The use of diaries allows staff to discern family frustrations and identify areas requiring additional education or resources [72]. Diaries provide an opportunity for clinicians to monitor the illness narrative for myths, distortions, and concerns so that communication can be course-corrected in real time.

Nurses and physicians report that writing in the ICU diary allowed them to connect to the person behind the patient and therefore strengthen the relationship between clinician and patient. Writing messages to preserve hope when a patient deteriorated is difficult but learning these skills foster professional development and exposure to written reflection; a skill that may need to be cultivated [62].

Joint ICU diary entries between staff and families have a potential to improve family communication and satisfaction [72]. Though families anecdotally and through qualitative research consistently report that diaries are helpful, family satisfaction scores may be slow to improve after starting a diary program or may not be the best measure of success [79].

Though ICU diary implementation practices vary throughout organizations, the underlying goal of improving patient and family outcomes related to PICS and PICS-F remains constant. Diaries may also be useful as a screening tool to refer patients to a post-ICU recovery clinic, where a trained professional can debrief the patient and family on their experience and screen for symptoms of PICS or PICS-F [79]. It has been suggested that use of a trained professional in ICU stay debriefing adds a deeper level of caring and empathy ultimately decreasing the likelihood of post-traumatic stress [80].

The SCCM family-centered care guidelines recommends the use of ICU diaries to improve psychological effects from critical illness exposure. The guidelines based their recommendation upon on the evidence supporting decreased patient and family stress disorders and improved communication with no evidence of harm [19]. Literature supports the use of ICU diaries in decreasing PICS and PICS-F however continued studies on the mechanism in which diaries have this effect needs to be addressed [78].

For **ICU clinicians**, there is an increasing emphasis on the psychological health for staff providing direct clinical care [81]. Cumulative stress may lead to second victim syndrome; being a victim of one's own work environment. This stress can result in burnout and/or compassion fatigue [82]. Clinicians have a moral and professional obligation to care for critically ill patients and their families in often challenging situations [83]. They provide emotional and psychological support to the family who have come to trust them; experiencing directly the raw emotions of agony, despair, grief, and suffering on a regular basis. This caregiving may take a toll on clinicians, especially when conflicts arise between their moral values about how the medical treatment of the patient is being managed, or when exposed to repeated traumatic events such as death or disfigurement. Family trust and ability to cope can be negatively affected when they sense or witness conflict within the team [24].

Stress debriefing has been shown to be an effective technique for stress management and helps in improving overall staff psychological well-being [84]. Through debriefings clinicians may be able to learn through the experience which may lead to post-traumatic growth rather than stress disorders [85]. Debriefings may be led by a chaplain, social worker, specially trained nurse, counselor, ethics consultant or palliative care expert and offered to all disciplines involved in the care of a critical ill patient whose case triggers an emotional response. During a debriefing, clinicians are welcome to share their thoughts about how it felt to be involved in patient's hospitalization; what went well and what went wrong. This form of psychological assistance helps staff to express emotions which they are unable to show, or kept to themselves, while taking care of critically ill patients and the family who rely on them for support.

Emotional grand rounds can also be conducted to focus on the emotional toll of providing care in challenging cases for clinicians. These interprofessional forums help clinicians to process their feelings and build recognition that they are not alone in their thoughts or feelings. Debriefings also promote the concept and culture that it is an acceptable practice to tend to self-care in the work environment [86]. Lastly, in the moment when the team experiences a patient death, one helpful practice is to perform a 'pause' for 45 s after the death for everyone involved to honor the person that has passed and reflect upon the efforts made to save that person's life or provide a peaceful death [87]. These forms of self-care are an essential component of family-centered care because it is only when we are emotionally healthy that we can provide the optimal care to those we serve [36].

Conclusion

In conclusion, family-centered care is a matter of public health with the potential to optimize the mental health and quality of life of millions of ICU family members in the United States every year. A well-rounded program of family-centered care may reduce PICS-F, but requires forethought, practice, education, and organizational support. Communication, caring, and engagement are key elements of any program of family-centered care. Facilitated Sensemaking is one tested method to organize care to deploy the evidence-based recommendations published by the Society of Critical Care Medicine and to better support ICU patients and their families.

References

1. Barrett ML, Smith MW, Elixhauser A, Honigman LS, Pines JM. Utilization of intensive care services, 2011. Healthcare cost and utilization project (HCUP) statistical briefs. Rockville, MD: Agency for Healthcare Research and Quality (US); 2006.
2. Davidson JE, Jones C, Bienvenu OJ. Family response to critical illness: postintensive care syndrome-family. Crit Care Med. 2012;40(2):618–24.
3. Netzer G, Sullivan DR. Recognizing, naming, and measuring a family intensive care unit syndrome. Ann Am Thorac Soc. 2014;11(3):435–41.
4. Needham DM, Davidson J, Cohen H, Hopkins RO, Weinert C, Wunsch H, et al. Improving long-term outcomes after discharge from intensive care unit: report from a stakeholders' conference. Crit Care Med. 2012;40:502–9.
5. Society of Critical Care Medicine. Critical care ethics: a practice guide. 2nd ed. Mount Prospect, IL: Society of Critical Care Medicine; 2009. 229 p.
6. Davidson JE, Netzer G. Family response to critical illness. In: Bienvenu OJ, Jones C, Hopkins RO, editors. Psychological and cognitive impact of critical illness. New York: Oxford University Press; 2017. p. 191–209.
7. Benner P. From novice to expert. Menlo Park: Addison-Wesley Publishing Company; 1984.
8. Davidson J. Facilitated sensemaking a strategy and new middle-range theory to support families of intensive care unit patients. Crit Care Nurse. 2010;30:28–39.
9. Roy C, Andrews HA. The Roy adaptation model. Prentice Hall; 1999.
10. Weick KE. Sensemaking in organizations. Sage; 1995.
11. Davidson JE, Daly BJ, Agan D, Brady NR, Higgins PA. Facilitated sensemaking: a feasibility study for the provision of a family support program in the intensive care unit. Crit Care Nurs Q. 2010;33(2):177–89.
12. Skoog M, Milner KA, Gatti-Petito J, Dintyala K. The impact of family engagement on anxiety levels in a cardiothoracic intensive care unit. Crit Care Nurse. 2016;36(2):84–9.
13. Shin JW, Happ MB, Tate JA. VidaTalk patient communication application "opened up" communication between nonvocal ICU patients and their family. Intensive Crit Care Nurs. 2021;66:103075.
14. Huang H, Dong H, Guan X, Zhang L, Zhou Q. The facilitated sensemaking model as a framework for nursing intervention on family members of mechanically ventilated patients in the intensive care unit. Worldviews Evid Based Nurs. 2022;19(6):467–76.
15. Shin JW, Tan A, Tate J, Balas M, Dabelko-Schoeny H, Happ MB. Preliminary efficacy of the vidatalk™ communication application on family psychological symptoms in the intensive care unit: A pilot study. Heart & Lung. 2025;70:14–22.

16. Gill J, Saligan L, Henderson W, Szanton S. PTSD know the warning signs. Nurse Pract. 2009;34:30–6.
17. Netzer G, Davidson J. Creating patient and family-focused care in the intensive care unit. In: Person-focused health care. Springer Publishing Company; 2016. p. 39–62.
18. Davidson JE, Zisook S. Implementing family-centered care through facilitated sensemaking. AACN Adv Crit Care. 2017;28(2):200–9.
19. Davidson JE, Aslakson RA, Long AC, Puntillo KA, Kross EK, Hart J, et al. Guidelines for family-centered care in the neonatal, pediatric, and adult ICU. Crit Care Med. 2017;45(1):103–28.
20. Ganz FD. Improving family intensive care unit experiences at the end of life: barriers and facilitators. Crit Care Nurse. 2019;39(3):52–8.
21. Davidson JE. Family presence on rounds in neonatal, pediatric, and adult intensive care units. Ann Am Thorac Soc. 2013;10(2):152–6.
22. Shin JW, Tate JA, Happ MB. The facilitated sensemaking model as a framework for family-patient communication during mechanical ventilation in the intensive care unit. Crit Care Nurs Clin. 2020;32(2):335–48.
23. Siegel MD, Hayes E, Vanderwerker LC, Loseth DB, Prigerson HG. Psychiatric illness in the next of kin of patients who die in the intensive care unit. Crit Care Med. 2008;36(6):1722–8.
24. Fassier T, Azoulay E. Conflicts and communication gaps in the intensive care unit. Curr Opin Crit Care. 2010;16(6):654–65.
25. Davidson JE, Harvey M, Schuller J, Black G. Post-intensive care syndrome: what it is and how to help prevent it. Am Nurse Today. 2013;8(5):32–7.
26. American Psychiatric Association. Diagnostic and statistical manual of mental disorders (DSM-5®). American Psychiatric Association Publishing; 2013.
27. Maley JH, Mikkelsen ME. Short-term gains with long-term consequences. Clin Chest Med. 2016;37(2):367–80.
28. Ely EW. The ABCDEF bundle: science and philosophy of how ICU liberation serves patients and families. Crit Care Med. 2017;45(2):321–30.
29. ICU Liberation Mount Prospect, Illinois: Society of Critical Care Medicine. 2015. http://www.sccm.org/Research/Quality/Pages/ICU-Liberation.aspx.
30. Elliott R, McKinley S, Cistulli P. The quality and duration of sleep in the intensive care setting: an integrative review. Int J Nurs Stud. 2011;48(3):384–400.
31. Owens RL, Huynh T-G, Netzer G. Sleep in the intensive care unit in a model of family-centered care. AACN Adv Crit Care. 2017;28(2):171–8.
32. Melnyk BM, Small L, Carno MA. The effectiveness of parent-focused interventions in improving coping/mental health outcomes of critically ill children and their parents: an evidence base to guide clinical practice. Pediatr Nurs. 2004;30(2):143–8.
33. Melnyk BM, Alpert-Gillis L, Feinstein NF, Crean HF, Johnson J, Fairbanks E, et al. Creating Opportunities for Parent Empowerment: program effects on the mental health/coping outcomes of critically ill young children and their mothers. Pediatrics. 2004;113(6):e597–607.
34. Kon AA, Shepard EK, Sederstrom NO, Swoboda SM, Marshall MF, Birriel B, Rincon F. Defining futile and potentially inappropriate interventions: a policy statement from the Society of Critical Care Medicine Ethics Committee. Crit Care Med. 2016;44(9):1769–74.
35. Kon AA, Davidson JE, Morrison W, Danis M, White DB. Shared decision-making in intensive care units. Executive summary of the American College of Critical Care Medicine and American Thoracic Society Policy Statement. Am J Respir Crit Care Med. 2016;193(12):1334–6.
36. Duffy JR. Quality caring in nursing and health systems: implications for clinicians, educators, and leaders. 2nd ed. New York: Springer; 2013. 312 p.
37. Davidson JE, Powers K, Hedayat KM, Tieszen M, Kon AA, Shepard E, et al. Clinical practice guidelines for support of the family in the patient-centered intensive care unit: American College of Critical Care Medicine Task Force 2004–2005. Crit Care Med. 2007;35(2):605–22.
38. Gooding J, Cooper L, Blaine A, Franck L, Howse J, Berns S. Family support and family centered care in the neonatal intensive care unit: origins, advances, impact. Semin Perinatol. 2011;35:20–8.

39. Pepper D, Rempel G, Austin W, Ceci C, Hendson L. More than information: a qualitative study of parents' perspectives on neonatal intensive care at the extremes of prematurity. Adv Neonatal Care. 2012;12:303–9.
40. Zimmerman K, Bauersachs C. Empowering NICU parents. Int J Childbirth Educ. 2012;27:50–3.
41. Martel M, Milette I, Bell L, St-Cyr Tribble D, Payot A. Establishment of the relationship between fathers and premature infants in neonatal units. Adv Neonatal Care. 2016;16:390–8.
42. Stafford C. A case study of Trisomy 13: balancing hope and reality. Adv Neonatal Care. 2015;15:285–9.
43. Brelsford G, Ramirez J, Veneman K, Doheny K. Sacred space religious and secular coping and family relationships in the neonatal intensive care unit. Adv Neonatal Care. 2016;16:315–22.
44. Amendolia B. Hope and parents of the critically ill newborn. Adv Neonatal Care. 2010;10:140–4.
45. Borghini A, Habersaat S, Forcada-Guex M, Nessi J, Pierrehumbert B, Ansermet F, Muller-Nix C. Effects of an early intervention on maternal post-traumatic stress symptoms and the quality of mother-infant interaction: the case of preterm birth. Infant Behav Dev. 2014;37:624–31.
46. Feeley N, Zelkowitz P, Cormier C, Charbonneau L, Lacroix A, Papageorgiou A. Posttraumatic stress among mothers of very low birthweight infants at 6 months after discharge from the neonatal intensive care unit. Appl Nurs Res. 2011;24:114–7.
47. Jiang S, Warre R, Qiu X, O'Brien K, Lee S. Parents as practitioners in preterm care. Early Hum Dev. 2014;90:781–5.
48. Bracht M, O'Leary L, Lee S, O'Brien K. Implementing family integrated care in the NICU: a parent education and support program. Adv Neonatal Care. 2013;13:115–26.
49. Galarza-Winton M, Dicky T, O'Leary L, Lee S, O'Brien K. Implementing family-integrated care in the NICU: educating nurses. Adv Neonatal Care. 2013;13:335–40.
50. O'Brien K, Bracht M, MacDonell K, McBride T, Robson K, O'Leary L, et al. A pilot cohort analytic study of Family Integrated Care in a Canadian neonatal intensive care unit. BMC Pregnancy Childbirth. 2013;13:1–8.
51. Lee S, O'Brien K. Parents as primary caregivers in the neonatal intensive care unit. Can Med Assoc J. 2014;186:845–7.
52. O'Brien K, Robson K, Bracht M, Cruz M, Lui K, Alvaro R, et al. Effectiveness of Family Integrated Care in neonatal intensive care units on infant and parent outcomes: a multicentre, multinational, cluster-randomised controlled trial. Lancet Child Adolesc Health. 2018;2(4):245–54.
53. Bakker A, Maertens KJ, Van Son MJ, Van Loey NE. Psychological consequences of pediatric burns from a child and family perspective: a review of the empirical literature. Clin Psychol Rev. 2013;33(3):361–71.
54. Eley TC, McAdams TA, Rijsdijk FV, Lichtenstein P, Narusyte J, Reiss D, et al. The intergenerational transmission of anxiety: a children-of-twins study. Am J Psychiatry. 2015;172(7):630–7.
55. Torke A, Worial L, Johns S, Sachs G, Callahan C, Bosslet G, et al. The family navigator: a pilot intervention to support intensive care unit family surrogates, vol. 25. Am Assoc Crit Care Nurses; 2016. p. 498–506.
56. Jacobs C, Dobbins C. From rough waters to smooth sialing: NICU population management model. Newborn Infant Nurs Rev. 2016;16:164–7.
57. Shaw DJ, Davidson JE, Smilde RI, Sondoozi T, Agan D. Multidisciplinary team training to enhance family communication in the ICU. Crit Care Med. 2013;42:265.
58. Joint Commission on Accreditation of Healthcare Organizations. Comprehensive accreditation manual for hospitals: the official handbook. CAMH: Joint Commission Resources; 2007.
59. Schenker Y, Smith AK, Arnold RM, Fernandez A. "Her husband doesn't speak much English": conducting a family meeting with an interpreter. J Palliat Med. 2012;15(4):494–8.
60. Lambert BL, Centomani NM, Smith KM, Helmchen LA, Bhaumik DK, Jalundhwala YJ, McDonald TB. The "Seven Pillars" response to patient safety incidents: effects on medical liability processes and outcomes. Health Serv Res. 2016;51(S3):2491–515.

61. PUBLIC LAW 111–148—MAR. 23, 2010 124 STAT. 119 Washington: Government Printing Office. 2010. https://www.gpo.gov/fdsys/pkg/PLAW-111publ148/pdf/PLAW-111publ148.pdf.
62. Ednell A-K, Siljegren S, Engström Å. The ICU patient diary—a nursing intervention that is complicated in its simplicity: a qualitative study. Intensive Crit Care Nurs. 2017;40:70–6.
63. Burwell S. Advancing LGBT Health and Well-being: 2016 cover letter announcing report of the HHS LGBT policy coordinating committee. Washington: HHS.gov; 2016. https://www.hhs.gov/programs/topic-sites/lgbt/reports/2016-cover-letter.html.
64. Pope TM. Legal briefing: adult orphans and the unbefriended: making medical decisions for unrepresented patients without surrogates. J Clin Ethics. 2015;26(2):180–8.
65. Farrell TW, Widera E, Rosenberg L, Rubin CD, Naik AD, Braun U, et al. AGS Position Statement: making medical treatment decisions for unbefriended older adults. J Am Geriatr Soc. 2016;65:14.
66. White DB, Curtis JR, Lo B, Luce JM. Decisions to limit life-sustaining treatment for critically ill patients who lack both decision-making capacity and surrogate decision-makers. Crit Care Med. 2006;34(8):2053–9.
67. Rawlings D, Tieman J, Miller-Lewis L, Swetenham K. What role do death doulas play in end-of-life care? A systematic review. Health Soc Care Community. 2019;27(3):e82–94.
68. Flaherty A, Meurer A. Unbefriended, uninvited: how end-of-life doulas can address ethical and procedural gaps for unrepresented patients and ensure equal access to the "good death". Clin Ethics. 2023;18(1):55–61.
69. Krawczyk M, Rush M. Describing the end-of-life doula role and practices of care: perspectives from four countries. Palliat Care Social Pract. 2020;14:2632352420973226.
70. Egerod I, Christensen D, Schwartz-Nielsen KH, Ågård AS. Constructing the illness narrative: a grounded theory exploring patients' and relatives' use of intensive care diaries. Crit Care Med. 2011;39(8):1922–8.
71. Hester M, Ingalls NK, Hatzfeld JJ. Perceptions of ICU diary utility and feasibility in a combat ICU. Mil Med. 2016;181(8):895–9.
72. Blair KTA, Eccleston SD, Binder HM, McCarthy MS. Improving the patient experience by implementing an ICU diary for those at risk of post-intensive care syndrome. J Patient Exp. 2017;4(1):4–9.
73. Aitken LM, Rattray J, Hull A, Kenardy JA, Le Brocque R, Ullman AJ. The use of diaries in psychological recovery from intensive care. Crit Care. 2013;17(6):253.
74. Garrouste-Orgeas M, Coquet I, Perier A, Timsit JF, Pochard F, Lancrin F, et al. Impact of an intensive care unit diary on psychological distress in patients and relatives. Crit Care Med. 2012;40(7):2033–40.
75. Jones C, Backman C, Griffiths RD. Intensive care diaries and relatives' symptoms of post-traumatic stress disorder after critical illness: a pilot study. Am J Crit Care. 2012;21(3):172–6.
76. Garrouste-Orgeas M, Perier A, Mouricou P, Gregoire C, Bruel C, Brochon S, et al. Writing in and reading ICU diaries: qualitative study of families' experience in the ICU. PLoS One. 2014;9(10):e110146.
77. Nielsen AH, Angel S. Relatives perception of writing diaries for critically ill. A phenomenological hermeneutical study. Nurs Crit Care. 2016;21(6):351–7.
78. Beg M, Scruth E, Liu V. Developing a framework for implementing intensive care unit diaries: a focused review of the literature. Aust Crit Care. 2016;29(4):224–34.
79. Huynh TG, Covalesky M, Sinclair S, Gunter H, Norton T, Chen A, Yi C. Measuring outcomes of an intensive care unit family diary program. AACN Adv Crit Care. 2017;28(2):179–90.
80. Knowles RE, Tarrier N. Evaluation of the effect of prospective patient diaries on emotional well-being in intensive care unit survivors: a randomized controlled trial. Crit Care Med. 2009;37(1):184–91.
81. Moss M, Good VS, Gozal D, Kleinpell R, Sessler CN. A Critical Care Societies collaborative statement: burnout syndrome in critical care health-care professionals. A call for action. Am J Respir Crit Care Med. 2016;194(1):106–13.

82. Sabo BM. Compassion fatigue and nursing work: can we accurately capture the consequences of caring work? Int J Nurs Pract. 2006;12(3):136–42.
83. American Nurse's Association. Code of ethics for nurses with interpretive statements. Silver Springs, MD: Nursebooks.org; 2015.
84. Hanna DR, Romana M. Debriefing after a crisis. Nurs Manag. 2007;38(8):38–42.
85. Mealer M, Jones J, Moss M. A qualitative study of resilience and posttraumatic stress disorder in United States ICU nurses. Intensive Care Med. 2012;38(9):1445–51.
86. Thompson A. How Schwartz rounds can be used to combat compassion fatigue: Alison Thompson reflects on an initiative that helps to maintain staff wellbeing and quality of patient care. Nurs Manag. 2013;20(4):16–20.
87. Bartels JB. The pause. Crit Care Nurse. 2014;34(1):74–5.

Chapter 12
End-of-Life Care for ICU Patients

Jennifer L. McAdam

Introduction

Intensive care units (ICUs) offer aggressive treatments with the goal of helping patients recover from life-threatening conditions. When these efforts are unsuccessful, the next measures rely on end-of-life care. Mortality rates in ICUs remain high, where on average one in five patients will die either in the unit or shortly thereafter [1]. In many of these cases, patients die after the decision is made to withdraw or withhold life-sustaining therapies [2, 3]. During this process, ICU families who participate in making these difficult decisions may suffer both physically and psychologically [4, 5]. They often face challenges they are not equipped to understand [6]. Families may experience confusion, frustrations, anger, or shock [7]. They are preparing for the loss of their loved one, often not knowing what to expect during this time [8]. This burden impacts families in many ways and may lead to negative sequelae [9]. An ICU patient's wife demonstrates this suffering,

> *The one thing I wish…I mean, the hope probably kept me from completely falling apart, but nobody ever really explained like when you go on a respirator, that could be the last time you talk to somebody. And when they said they were going to intubate him, the one thing I wish I knew—I mean, we always said we loved each other but [crying]…I didn't realize that I would never get to talk to him again…* [7, p. 18]

Providing family-centered care in the ICU is a recommended practice [10]. Optimizing the support given to families using evidence-based strategies may help improve family and patient outcomes. These approaches should be a high priority for the healthcare team. This chapter will cover the care of families of dying ICU patients. It will focus on the symptom burden experienced by families as they transition from intervention to end-of-life care and will offer practical interventions to

---

J. L. McAdam (✉)
College of Nursing, Samuel Merritt University, Oakland, CA, USA
e-mail: jmcadam@samuelmerritt.edu

© The Author(s), under exclusive license to Springer Nature Switzerland AG 2025
A. J. Vance et al. (eds.), *Families in the Intensive Care Unit*,
https://doi.org/10.1007/978-3-031-83786-9_12

help alleviate families' symptom burden. This chapter will also provide suggestions on how best to support families that are in conflict during end-of-life decision-making. In addition, it will discuss strategies that help families prepare for and cope during the transition where the patient is actively dying. Finally, issues affecting end-of-life care of families of underrepresented and LGBTQ+ populations will be discussed.

Family Symptom Burden

ICUs can be an extremely stressful environment for families. In a recent scoping review, researchers focusing on 22 studies of ICU families found that they had a high prevalence of symptoms such as anxiety, depression, traumatic stress, sleep disturbances, fatigue, fear, sadness, helplessness, and uncertainty [11]. This type of psychological distress during and after the ICU visit can affect families in multiple ways. First, these symptoms have been associated with long-term negative consequences such as PTSD, anxiety, prolonged grief, and major depression [12]. Occurring well past the ICU stay, this constellation of symptoms has been termed post-intensive care syndrome-family [13, 14]. Second, a high symptom burden may impact the way families' process information and deal with situations in the ICU. For example, high levels of stress and anxiety may affect the families' ability to participate in decision-making [15]. When they are stressed or anxious, they may over or under estimate the effectiveness of treatment options [16]. Or, they may have trouble concentrating and understanding information presented to them [17]. As a nurse noted in one study, "…[we know] when communication is not working such as when [the family's] eyes glaze over" [18, p. 692]. The consequences of a high symptom burden affect the well-being of the family, affects patient care, and may lead to frustration for the healthcare team.

Interventions to Help Alleviate Families' Symptom Burden (See Table 12.1)

The high symptom burden of ICU families is typically influenced by several components including the information needs of the family, decision-making stressors, and preexisting risk factors [15]. In order to better support ICU families, interventions targeting the multifactorial nature of their symptom burden are needed. The first component, information, has consistently been reported in the literature as one of the most important needs of ICU families [19]. Although formal education and structured family care conferences are recommended to provide information [10], other techniques can be effective. Families who are stressed and anxious may better process only the most critical information, requiring this information multiple times

Table 12.1 Multifactorial approach to help alleviate ICU family symptom burden

Informational needs	Decision-making	Pre-existing family symptoms
• Provide only the most critical information [20, 21] • Repeat critical information several times if needed [20, 21]	• Tailor the decision-making approach to the individual family case but active and shared decision-making are recommended [46]	• Routinely assess families for risk factors (i.e., female family members, spouses, poor coping skills, etc.) [36]
• Use multiple formats to deliver information (e.g., electronic tablets and written brochures) [14, 20, 21]	• Remain honest and unbiased [30, 32]	• Routinely assess families for symptom burden [36]
• Provide daily updates [21]	• Avoid personal opinions [30, 32]	• Use validated tools such as the Hospital Anxiety and Depression Scale [37] and the Impact of Event Scale Revised [38, 39] to assess common symptoms such as anxiety, depression, and traumatic stress
• Allow time to process information [20]	• Accept the families' decision [32]	
• Provide consistent information [21]		

Sources: Davidson et al. [14]; Seaman et al. [21]; Wholihan (2019) [30]; Berlin [32]; de Ridder et al. [36]; Zigmond et al. [37]; Creamer et al. [38]; Weiss [39]; Kerckhoffs et al. [46]

[20–23]. This will assist the family in focusing on the main issues and help to mitigate overload. In addition, they may need the information given in multiple formats such as verbal, written, or electronic [20, 21, 23]. One group of researchers found that providing written daily care summaries along with traditional communication approaches significantly reduced anxiety, depression, and acute stress in ICU families [20]. Utilizing multiple communication interventions may provide families more time to process information and decrease confusion and frustration [21, 22]. As stated by one family member, "[The doctors]…answered all of our questions, spent as much time as we needed…if we needed to talk with them when they came around, they would sit and answer all of our questions" [7, p. 17].

The second component in reducing families' symptom burden is related to decision-making stressors. Surrogate decision-makers often face uncertainty, experience empathetic suffering and tension, and have conflicting emotional needs [24, 25]. The negative outcomes associated with this state are that families may focus on small details rather than the big picture. They may seek more positive prognostic information. However, they may disbelieve this information and demand inappropriate treatments [26, 27].

By recognizing in advance, the strain this role may place on families, interventions can be initiated to help support them. The current recommendation to best support surrogate decision-makers includes tailoring the decision-making process (i.e., shared, active, or passive) to each individual case [28]. In a recent study, researchers reported that when physicians incorporated shared decision-making behaviors into the family care conference, it significantly improved family member trust [29]. Other supportive interventions cited by family decision-makers include that the healthcare team remain honest, unbiased, avoid personal opinions, and accept the decision of the family [30–32]. This improves families' relationships with the healthcare team and reduces families' decisional regret and psychological burden [33]. See Chap. XX for more detailed information on family decision-making.

Finally, the third component to consider is preexisting family risk factors. Researchers have reported female family members [5, 11, 34, 35], spouses [11, 34, 35], families of patients of a younger age [11, 34, 35], families of a race other than white [11, 34, 35], and poor family coping [15] tend to have a higher symptom burden. Although most of these are non-modifiable, it is recommended that families are routinely assessed for their risk factors and symptom burden while in the ICU [36]. Using validated tools such as the Hospital Anxiety and Depression Scale [37] and the Impact of Event Scale-Revised [38, 39] to recognize these high risk families, interventions can begin early in the ICU stay. Appropriate referrals such as counseling, palliative care, spiritual care, and ethics consultations can be given to help reduce potential negative consequences [34, 40, 41].

Supporting Families During Transitions in Care (See Table 12.2)

Transition from active treatment to end-of-life care in the ICU is complex for multiple reasons. Identification of patients who will not survive the ICU stay is difficult [42]. A lack of agreement often exists between different disciplines regarding the goals of end-of-life care [43, 44]. The families may be in denial and not ready to accept the outcome [26]. Having an understanding of the key transitional stages describing the end-of-life trajectory in the ICU is helpful in overcoming some of these challenges. These transitions as described by Coombs and colleagues [45] include the following:

- Admission to the ICU where there is still hope of recovery
- Transition from aggressive treatment to end-of-life care
- The actively dying patient

Table 12.2 Interventions to support families in each transition phase

Hope of recovery	Intervention to EOL	Actively dying patient
• Prepare families for what they may see, hear, and experience [21]	• Consider the length of the transition that patient is in the ICU (acute condition vs. chronic condition) [33]	• Use end-of-life protocols to help guide withdrawing and/or withholding of life-sustaining measures [64]
• Hold a family meeting early in the ICU stay (within 3–5 days) [21, 46]	• Give families time to adjust to this phase [8, 18, 19]	• Avoid the use of the term "withdrawal of care" [70]
• Use a family coordinator of care [47–50]	• Deal with family conflicts by using relationship building communication skills [56]	• When a decision is made to withhold or withdraw life-sustaining measures, there should be no delays, it should occur as soon as possible [64]
	• Use a family coordinator of care [47–50]	• Keep the patient in the ICU [72]
	• Incorporate palliative care principles early in the ICU stay [57]	• Maintain consistent staff caring for the patient and family [72]
	• Clarify information and help assist families recognize the deteriorating status of their loved one [8, 19]	• Do not abandon the patient and family [8]
	• Assess non-verbal cues and utilize these as indicators of family readiness [18]	• Display caring behaviors [7]
	• Consider the use of an ICU Diary [73]	• Prepare families for the dying process (what they may see, hear the timeframe) [8, 72]
		• Allow families to be present and participate in patient care [72]
		• Prepare the room for the dying process by creating a sacred space [72]

Sources: Erikson et al. [7]; Wiegand et al. [8]; Bloomer et al. [18]; Kentish-Barnes et al. [19]; Seaman et al. [21]; Jennerich et al. [33]; Kerckhoffs et al. [46]; Torke et al. [47]; Curtis et al. [48]; White et al. [49]; Parks Taylor et al. 50; Kayser et al. [56]; Aslakson et al. 57; Downar et al. [64]; DeForest (2019) [70]; Jensen et al. [72]; Galazzi et al. [73]

Supporting Families During the Transition Stage: Admission with Hope of Recovery

In the first transition, the use of full and intensive interventions predominate patient care. This is also the stage where families begin their adjustment to the ICU. In this stage, the healthcare team should prepare families on what they may see, hear, or experience while visiting their loved one in the ICU [21]. It is important to hold family meetings early in the ICU stay, within 3–5 days if possible [21, 46].

Additionally, ICUs should consider utilizing a variety of family support strategies. These could include the use of a dedicated family support coordinator [47–50] as well as having the bedside nurse provide the family daily updates [20]. In a randomized control trial, researchers who utilized a family support intervention found that families significantly rated the quality of communication higher and the patient ICU length of stay was significantly shorter in the intervention group versus the control group [49]. Since the ICU is stressful for families and the care can often seem fragmented [41], supporting families during this time can improve communication, satisfaction, and patient-centered care [51, 52].

Supporting Families During the Transition Stage: Intervention to End of Life

The second transition is typically initiated when the healthcare team notes a continued deterioration in the condition of the patient. This stage is usually the most problematic and challenging to navigate for both the healthcare team and families [8, 30, 53]. This transition, from intervention to end of life, occurs when the patient's condition is not improving and decisions need to be made on how to proceed. The duration of this transition period can affect how families perceive the dying process in the ICU. For example, when a patient dies suddenly, families may report feeling shocked and unable to prepare for the death or process their feelings [7]. Conversely, when the patient's hospital course is lengthy, this may benefit families as it may give them time to prepare for the death [54]. It is important to realize that families' experiences will differ depending on the time it takes to process the information. As one group of researchers noted, "time is a valuable commodity where we give families the opportunity to move from a position of hope for recovery to understanding the discussions and impact of end-of-life care" [45, p. 524].

During this transition from intervention to end of life, families often have interpersonal conflicts that need to be addressed and managed. Families struggle with not wanting to feel responsible for their loved ones death, the desire to continue to pursue recovery, and the need to preserve the family well-being [8, 55]. This can lead to confusion, anxiety, depression, and stress in families [55]. This in turn can lead to poor coping strategies within families and misunderstandings and miscommunication with the healthcare team [33, 53].

Several strategies can help families in conflict. One approach, discussed earlier, is the use of a dedicated family support coordinator [47–50]. This approach has been shown to help conflicted families by improving their satisfaction with ICU communication and care. Other strategies include updating families daily with factual information and gradually helping them face bad news assisted families in making difficult decisions [20, 49]. Nurses can be key in this area, by interpreting and clarifying the medical information for the family and by helping the family recognize the deteriorating status of the patient [8, 19]. As one nurse observed, "…they've just had really bad news, so there's got to be a bit of [emotional processing] with what they do, and I try and give it to them in small increments so they don't get a big waft of information all at once" [18, p. 694]. In addition, the healthcare team can assess the nonverbal cues (e.g., body positioning such as crossed arms, avoidance actions such as leaving the room) of families and use these indicators to balance when the most appropriate time should be for delivering information which may reduce conflict [18].

Another effective intervention for dealing with family conflict involves the development of communication skills that are relationship-building rather than task-related. Relationship-building communication skills consist of respecting families, supporting them emotionally, and expressing empathy. For comparison, task-oriented communication skills ensure families understand medical facts and their role as a decision-maker. In managing conflicts, the use of relationship-building communication has been found to be more effective in helping deal with family disagreements [56]. Other relationship building techniques such as the VALUE tool and NURSE mnemonic have been reported in the literature to be helpful in dealing with conflicted families making end-of-life decisions [30]. See Chap. XX for more details on the VALUE tool and the NURSE mnemonic.

Another strategy to support families during the transition from intervention to end of life is to incorporate palliative care principles early in the patient's ICU stay. This approach improves the quality of life of both patients and families who are experiencing a life-threatening illness. Palliative care includes such tenets as communication, symptom management, and early goal setting that is in line with the patients' wishes [57]. Incorporating palliative care into the ICU can occur by use of a consultative model, an integrative model—or a combination of both models. The consultant model focuses on increasing the involvement of individuals, outside of the ICU who have specialty training in palliative care [58]. The integrative model focuses on embedding palliative care principles and interventions (e.g., communication and symptom management) into the daily practice of the ICU team [58]. There are trade-offs to each model (see Table 12.3) [59] but the use of the consultative model appears to be used much more frequently in the acute care setting [60, 61].

When incorporating palliative care into the ICU it should be done early and it should be ongoing. This allows families the opportunity to develop relationships and build trust with the healthcare team. In a current randomized controlled trial, families that received three strategically designed family meetings that incorporated palliative care principles had significantly lower symptoms of prolonged grief than families who did not receive the intervention [62]. In addition, others found that the use of palliative care interventions significantly decreased families' symptom distress (e.g., depression and anxiety) along with increasing their satisfaction with ICU care [58].

Table 12.3 Pros and cons of the main models for integrating palliative care in the intensive care unit

Model	Consultation by palliative care service	Integration by critical care team in daily ICU practice
Advantages	• Expert input from interdisciplinary team of specialists • Expertise already exists, additional training unnecessary • Empirical evidence of benefit • Continuity of care before, during, and after ICU • Facilitation of transfer out of ICU for end-of-life care, if appropriate	• Availability of palliative care for all ICU patients and families • Palliative care service not required • Clearly acknowledges importance of palliative care as core element of intensive care • Systematization of ICU work processes promotes reliable performances of palliative care
Disadvantages	• Requires palliative care service with adequate staffing and other resources • Palliative care clinicians may be seen as "outsiders" in ICU • Consultants may lack familiarity with biomedical and nursing aspects of critical care • Activities of palliative care and ICU teams may overlap and/or conflict • Consultants must rapidly establish effective relationship with patients/families • Fragmentation of care may be compounded • ICU team may have less incentive to improve palliative care knowledge and skills	• Requires education of ICU clinicians in palliative care knowledge and skills • Depends on commitment of critical care clinicians and supportive ICU culture • Requires dedication of staff and other resources that my be lacking in ICU • Requires handoff to new team for post-ICU palliative care for patients who cannot benefit from or no longer need the ICU

ICU intensive care unit

© Used with Permission from Wolters Kluwer

Nelson, J.E., Bassett, R., Brasel, K.J., et al. (2010). Models for structuring a clinical initiative to enhance palliative care in the intensive care unit: a report from the IPAL-ICU Project (Improving Palliative Care in the ICU). *Crit Care Med*, 38(9):1765–72. https://www.ncbi.nlm.nih.gov/pubmed/20562699

Supporting Families During the Transition Stage: The Actively Dying Patient

In the final stage, when the patient is actively dying, making the patient comfort and ensuring that families are adequately supported becomes the goal [53]. Interventions during this transition focus mainly on palliation for the patient and grief and bereavement support for families. These interventions will be discussed in terms of end-of-life protocols, healthcare team factors, educational needs, and environmental elements.

End-of-Life Protocols

Protocols or guidelines surrounding both end-of-life care and treatment withdrawal are complex, used inconsistently, or may be lacking in many ICUs [63]. However, it is clear that having standardized protocols of these practices is helpful for all involved [64]. For example, Epker and colleagues, using a standardized protocol for end-of-life care, found that patients' achieved adequate comfort, were well sedated, and showed few signs of distress such as terminal restlessness, death rattle, or stridor [65]. Others have found similar benefits when using a standardized protocol on withdrawing mechanical ventilation [66] and providing end-of-life care [18].

In general, removal of life-sustaining measures and ventilator support should include the following:

- Ensure a do-not-resuscitate (DNR) order has been documented [67].
- Ensure that analgesics and sedatives are at the bedside, with the recommendation for both infusions and bolus doses as needed [64].
- Discontinue any treatments that do not provide comfort (i.e., lab draws, antibiotics, vasopressors, dialysis, IV fluids, neuromuscular blockade agents) [64].
- The typical order of withdrawal of life-sustaining measures is vasopressors and inotropes followed by mechanical ventilation [64].
- Consider two approaches for ventilator removal: terminal weaning or immediate extubation. The suggested method is immediate extubation, however, the strategy chosen should be individualized to reflect the patient situation and their values and preferences [64]. See Table 12.4 for description of both methods of ventilator removal along with the positives and negatives of both approaches [68, 69].

Finally, when the decision to withdraw life-sustaining measures is made, two key principles may be kept in mind. The first is avoiding the phrase "withdrawal of care" as it is factually inaccurate and can make families and patients feel abandoned [70]. Care continues regardless of the goals of care change from intervention to comfort. The second is that once the decision to remove life-sustaining measures is made, the plan of care should be implemented promptly, ensuring that delays are avoided at all possible. Delays can impact families in a negative way as discussed in a current systematic review where families of patients who died while they were still on vasopressors and remained intubated were more likely to experience complicated grief after the death [71].

Table 12.4 Two primary methods of mechanical ventilation removal

Immediate extubation	Terminal weaning
Description: • Abruptly removing the patient from the ventilator by extubation • Provide suctioning (if necessary) • Provide humidified air or oxygen to prevent airway drying	Description: • Gradual withdrawal of ventilator assistance by decreasing the amount of inspired oxygen, decreasing the ventilator rate and mode, and/or removal of positive end-expiratory pressure (PEEP) • Usual time for extubation can range from 30 to 60 min but in some cases may be over days
Positives: • Patient free of tubes • Dying process less likely to be prolonged	Positives: • Allows titration of medications for better symptom management • Maintains airway for suctioning (if necessary) • Patient has less potential to develop upper airway obstruction • Moral burden on family may decrease because method appears less active
Negatives: • Dyspnea • Potential for airway obstruction and gasps • Potential to be more stressful to patient/family • Time course to death is unpredictable but is typically shorter than terminal weaning	Negatives: • May prolong dying • Patient unable to communicate • Barrier of technology/machine between patient and family • Time course to death is unpredictable

Sources: Downar et al. [64]; Robert et al. [68, 69]

Healthcare Team Factors

When patients are actively dying, one important consideration for the healthcare team is ensuring that consistent staff are caring for the patient and their family [72]. In addition, the healthcare team needs to be present with the dying patient and their family. Do not abandon them during this stage [8]. Families have reported feelings of anger and disappointment when the healthcare team disappears [31]. Equally important to families is that physician(s) visit with them, even if they are no longer treating the patient, to assess how they are doing. Families have reported that these visits helped them answer questions, provided them with recommendations, and provided them with clarification of information [31]. Other benefits of this to families include a feeling of confidence, the opportunity to have all of their questions answered, the ability to build trust in the healthcare team, and a significant reduction in PTSD, prolonged grief, depression, and guilt [31, 55]. Finally, it is imperative that the healthcare team display caring behaviors. While this point may seem obvious, many ICU families still feel that the team is not always respectful and caring [7]. Families report small acts such as combing the patient's hair, calling them by their name, making sure the patient is clean, are very meaningful to them during the dying transition [72].

Educational Needs

An important educational need for families of actively dying patients is for them to know what to expect during the dying process and withdrawal of life-sustaining measures [8]. Education should include the expected duration, which can be anywhere from minutes to days. An important point to highlight to families is if the team feels death may be delayed or prolonged. Most families believe that once life-sustaining measures are discontinued the dying process will be quick. When it is not, families may become distraught and frustrated [31]. As stated by a family member in one study, "I was originally told he would only live 2–3 days, but [he] lived three weeks. I was not prepared…I was never warned of what could happen" [32, p. 1034]. Education should also include what to expect, such as the sounds the patient may make and changes in breathing patterns [72]. Assuring families that the patient will be comfortable is vital. Another potential helpful tool for families is a diary. In a systematic review, a group of authors found that ICU diaries helped reduce families symptom burden and may help families in the grief process [73]. Finally, when providing family education, it should take several forms (i.e., verbal, brochures, videos) depending on family needs, background, characteristics, and emotional state. Effective education occurs when it is delivered in a sensitive, empathetic, respectful, and patient-specific manner [20, 21, 23].

Environmental Elements

Several environmental and organizational elements should be considered during this transition. First, keep the dying patient in the ICU and only transfer them if it is absolutely necessary or requested by the family [72]. Second, allow families to have patient access at all times and allow them to be present when the patient is actively dying if they wish [72]. Third, prepare the ICU room for the dying process [74]. This is achieved by giving families privacy, providing comfortable chairs, providing beverages and snacks, and removing all unnecessary equipment [74]. It is important to create this space to both encourage and allow families to say goodbye. Finally, ICUs should consider allowing families to participate in care, if they desire, by providing a bed bath, massage, oral care, and even postmortem care [74].

The End-of-Life Care Needs of Underrepresented Populations

End of life in the ICU is challenging, but can be more so for underrepresented populations. Families from an ethnic minority group are at higher risk of conflict and stress due to differences in their cultural background [74]. In these populations, common issues that occur revolve around communication and information sharing, religious beliefs, cultural norms and values, care practices, and attitudes toward illness and treatments as well as attitudes toward death and dying [74–76]. The potential for miscommunication increases when there are multiple cultures and languages involved [77]. When this happens, the use of specific religious leaders, community leaders, or professional interpreters have been shown to be helpful [74]. Attitudes and beliefs toward illness, treatments, death and dying, and decisions to withdraw or withhold life-sustaining treatments vary depending on the patient and families' cultural backgrounds and religious preferences [74]. Conflict can be reduced by treating these as clinical procedures that deserve the same preparation and expectation of quality as other procedures [78].

Differences in cultural norms and values as well as care practices between the ethnic minority and ethnic majority are daily challenges in the ICU. In a study from Norway, nurses discussed challenges they experienced when caring for patients and families that immigrated to their country. These challenges included language and interpreter issues, differences in religious and cultural values, and the burden of family involvement [79]. As one nurse stated, "There have been challenges related to that…Neighboring patients are often affected by the fact that there are so many visitors and they are there for a long time" [79, p. 7]. In another study, Van Keer and colleagues discussed end-of-life decision-making conflicts that ICU professionals in a Belgium ICU experienced when caring for immigrants from Southern Europe, Turkey, North Africa, and Central Africa. The main issues the healthcare professionals had were difficulty establishing trust of the family and difficulty in getting the family to make and agree upon a decision. They also noted that many of the families wanted the patients to receive maximal curative therapy until death even if the provider disagreed. In addition, most families did not want to talk about the patient's end of life and thought it was inappropriate, making these conversations frustrating for the providers [74]. Both of these studies highlight the challenges but there are steps healthcare professionals can incorporate that will help deliver culturally sensitive care. First, they can facilitate cultural and religious rituals such as prayer or blessings [80]; they can involve religious leaders [81], they can ensure that an interpreter is used to translate key information [81], and finally they can manage differences in cultural values and beliefs by acknowledging these differences occur, avoid stereotyping individuals, and negotiating compromises [81].

The End-of-Life Care Needs of the LGBTQ+ Community

There is documentation that socially excluded populations such as lesbian, gay, bisexual, transgender, and queer or questioning (LGBTQ+) communities may receive poorer access to end-of-life care than their heterosexual counterparts [82]. Members of this population often hide their identities due to fear of stigmatization [82, 83]. This can lead to feelings of isolation and may prevent or delay them from seeking appropriate healthcare resources [84]. Members of this population have stated that although healthcare providers' attitudes towards them were vital to their care [83], discrimination is still common in healthcare settings [83, 85]. Below is a discussion of the key issues that LGBTQ+ partners often face at the end of life, along with strategies that may better support this population.

Research has shown that families of LGBTQ+ individuals experience a lower quality of end-of-life care [86]. When facing the patient's end of life, LGBTQ+ partners may struggle with living openly for fear of discrimination [83]. This fear could prevent them from accessing supportive end-of-life resources such as palliative care or hospice care because of stigmatization [82]. This anticipated discrimination leads to feelings of caregiver burden, isolation, and vulnerability [82, 87]. One strategy that may promote inclusion is representing LGBTQ+ language and imagery in promotional materials for these services. This may decrease the invisibility felt by this population and may improve perception that these resources are inclusive [85]. Other concerns for LGBTQ+ partners are being excluded from participating in decision-making or being denied access to the patient at the time of death [87–89]. A strategy that may alleviate this concern is to encourage advanced care planning [83, 90]. This will provide a legal framework for the partner to be involved with the patient's care and will prevent any confusion on the patient's choice of surrogate [90].

Other issues cited by LGBTQ+ partners are feelings of social isolation and the need to silently mourn their loved one [91]. Strategies that may help mitigate these emotions can be as simple as asking them about their needs, their well-being, and whether they feel they have enough support [87, 88]. In addition, offering support groups that are specific for the needs of LGBTQ+ people could be beneficial [88]. Another area of concern for LGBTQ+ partners is around religion and spirituality. This is an area often ignored even though many in this population can be deeply rooted in faith [85, 87]. Healthcare workers need to consider the role of religion and spirituality in this population to better deliver holistic end-of-life care [92]. Finally, heterosexual assumptions about identity and family structure are also commonplace [85, 87]. A key way to improve this is to promote inclusive language. Asking the patient who they would like to be involved with their care or using straightforward questions such as "who are the most important people in your life?" or, "what is your preferred name?" can help start conversations between patients, families, and providers and create an open, nonjudgmental environment [85, 90]. As stated by one LGBTQ patient,

I don't think your sexuality should be an issue at all within the healthcare setting, because humanity is so diverse. Whatever your personal thoughts, you're in a profession to treat people… [88, p. 32]

Conclusion

Supporting the ICU family is important for healthcare professionals in providing family-centered care. Recognizing and alleviating the symptom burden in families both during and after the ICU stay can help reduce negative outcomes. Supporting families through ICU transitions from the hope of recovery, to patient decline, to the actively dying patient is essential. Finally, it is necessary to understand the barriers of providing quality end-of-life care and the importance of overcoming those barriers in providing effective care to all ICU families.

References

1. Angus DC, Barnato AE, Linde-Zwirble WT, et al. Use of intensive care at the end of life in the United States: an epidemiologic study. Crit Care Med. 2004;32(3):638–43.
2. Mark NM, Rayner SG, Lee NJ, Curtis JR. Global variability in withholding and withdrawal of life-sustaining treatment in the intensive care unit: a systematic review. Intensive Care Med. 2015;41(9):1572–85.
3. Sprung CL, Ricou B, Hartog CS, et al. Changes in end-of-life practices in European intensive care units from 1999 to 2016. JAMA. 2019;322(17):1692–704.
4. Pattison NA, White C, Lone NI. Bereavement in critical care: a narrative review and practice exploration of current provision of support services and future challenges. J Intensive Care Soc. 2021;22(4):349–56.
5. Kentish-Barnes N, Chaize M, Seegers V, et al. Complicated grief after death of a relative in the intensive care unit. Eur Respir J. 2015;45(5):1341–52.
6. Scheunemann LP, Ernecoff NC, Buddadhumaruk P, et al. Clinician-family communication about patients' values and preferences in intensive care units. JAMA Intern Med. 2019;179(5):676–84.
7. Erikson AE, Puntillo KA, McAdam JL. Bereavement experiences of families in the cardiac intensive care unit. Am J Crit Care. 2022;31(1):13–23.
8. Wiegand DL, Cheon J, Netzer G. Seeing the patient and family through: nurses and physicians experiences with withdrawal of life-sustaining therapy in the ICU. Am J Hosp Palliat Care. 2019;36(1):13–23.
9. Shear MK. Clinical practice. Complicated grief. N Engl J Med. 2015;372(2):153–60.
10. Davidson JE, Aslakson RA, Long AC, et al. Guidelines for family-centered care in the neonatal, pediatric, and adult ICU. Crit Care Med. 2017;45(1):103–28.
11. Abdul Halain A, Tang LY, Chong MC, Ibrahim NA, Abdullah KL. Psychological distress among the family members of intensive care unit (ICU) patients: a scoping review. J Clin Nurs. 2022;31(5–6):497–507.
12. Wen FH, Prigerson HG, Chou WC, et al. How symptoms of prolonged grief disorder, posttraumatic stress disorder, and depression relate to each other for grieving ICU families during the first two years of bereavement. Crit Care. 2022;26(1):336.

13. Zante B, Camenisch SA, Schefold JC. Interventions in post-intensive care syndrome-family: a systematic literature review. Crit Care Med. 2020;48(9):e835–40.
14. Davidson JE, Jones C, Bienvenu OJ. Family response to critical illness: postintensive care syndrome-family. Crit Care Med. 2012;40(2):618–24.
15. Butler JM, Hirshberg EL, Hopkins RO, et al. Preliminary identification of coping profiles relevant to surrogate decision making in the ICU. PLoS One. 2016;11(11):e0166542.
16. Hengen KM, Alpers GW. Stress makes the difference: social stress and social anxiety in decision-making under uncertainty. Front Psychol. 2021;12:578293.
17. Hallion LS, Steinman SA, Kusmierski SN. Difficulty concentrating in generalized anxiety disorder: an evaluation of incremental utility and relationship to worry. J Anxiety Disord. 2018;53:39–45.
18. Bloomer MJ, Endacott R, Ranse K, Coombs MA. Navigating communication with families during withdrawal of life-sustaining treatment in intensive care: a qualitative descriptive study in Australia and New Zealand. J Clin Nurs. 2017;26(5–6):690–7.
19. Kentish-Barnes N, Jensen HI, Curtis JR. The legacy of the interprofessional family meeting. Intensive Care Med. 2022;48:933.
20. Greenberg JA, Basapur S, Quinn TV, et al. Daily written care summaries for families of critically ill patients: a randomized controlled trial. Crit Care Med. 2022;50(9):1296–305.
21. Seaman JB, Arnold RM, Scheunemann LP, White DB. An integrated framework for effective and efficient communication with families in the adult intensive care unit. Ann Am Thorac Soc. 2017;14(6):1015–20.
22. Bennett F, O'Conner-Von S. Communication interventions to improve goal-concordant care of seriously ill patients: an integrative review. J Hosp Palliat Nurs. 2020;22(1):40–8.
23. Kennedy NR, Steinberg A, Arnold RM, et al. Perspectives on telephone and video communication in the intensive care unit during COVID-19. Ann Am Thorac Soc. 2021;18(5):838–47.
24. Schenker Y, Crowley-Matoka M, Dohan D, Tiver GA, Arnold RM, White DB. I don't want to be the one saying 'we should just let him die': intrapersonal tensions experienced by surrogate decision makers in the ICU. J Gen Intern Med. 2012;27(12):1657–65.
25. Nunez ER, Schenker Y, Joel ID, et al. Acutely bereaved surrogates' stories about the decision to limit life support in the ICU. Crit Care Med. 2015;43(11):2387–93.
26. Beckstrand RL, Mallory C, Macintosh JLB, Luthy KE. Critical care nurses' qualitative reports of experiences with family behaviors as obstacles in end-of-life care. Dimens Crit Care Nurs. 2018;37(5):251–8.
27. White DB, Carson S, Anderson W, et al. A multicenter study of the causes and consequences of optimistic expectations about prognosis by surrogate decision-makers in ICUs. Crit Care Med. 2019;47(9):1184–93.
28. Michalsen A, Long AC, DeKeyser Ganz F, et al. Interprofessional shared decision-making in the ICU: a systematic review and recommendations from an expert panel. Crit Care Med. 2019;47(9):1258–66.
29. Lincoln TE, Buddadhumaruk P, Arnold RM, et al. Association between shared decision-making during family meetings and surrogates' trust in their ICU physician. Chest. 2022;163:1214.
30. Wholihan D. Psychological issues of patient transition from intensive care to palliative care. Crit Care Nurs Clin North Am. 2019;31(4):547–56.
31. Morris SE, Manan MN, Block SD. Insights from bereaved family members about end-of-life care and bereavement. J Palliat Med. 2020;23(8):1030–7.
32. Berlin A. Goals of care and end of life in the ICU. Surg Clin North Am. 2017;97(6):1275–90.
33. Jennerich AL, Hobler MR, Sharma RK, Engelberg RA, Curtis JR. Unplanned admission to the ICU: a qualitative study examining family member experiences. Chest. 2020;158(4):1482–9.
34. Amass T, Van Scoy LJ, Hua M, et al. Stress-related disorders of family members of patients admitted to the intensive care unit with COVID-19. JAMA Intern Med. 2022;182(6):624–33.
35. McAdam JL, Dracup KA, White DB, Fontaine DK, Puntillo KA. Symptom experiences of family members of intensive care unit patients at high risk for dying. Crit Care Med. 2010;38(4):1078–85.

36. de Ridder C, Zegers M, Jagernath D, Brunnekreef G, van den Boogaard M. Psychological symptoms in relatives of critically ill patients: a longitudinal cohort study. Crit Care Explor. 2021;3(7):e0470.
37. Zigmond AS, Snaith RP. The hospital anxiety and depression scale. Acta Psychiatr Scand. 1983;67(6):361–70.
38. Creamer M, Bell R, Failla S. Psychometric properties of the Impact of Event Scale—Revised. Behav Res Ther. 2003;41(12):1489–96.
39. Weiss D. Assessing psychological trauma and PTSD. 2nd ed. New York: The Guilford Press; 2004.
40. Rhoads S, Trikalinos T, Levy M, Amass T. Intensive care based interventions to reduce family member stress disorders: a systematic review of the literature. J Crit Care Med. 2022;8(3):145–55.
41. Rhoads S, Amass T. Communication at the end-of-life in the intensive care unit: a review of evidence-based best practices. R I Med J (2013). 2019;102(10):30–3.
42. Keuning BE, Kaufmann T, Wiersema R, et al. Mortality prediction models in the adult critically ill: a scoping review. Acta Anaesthesiol Scand. 2020;64(4):424–42.
43. Pecanac K, King B. Nurse-family communication during and after family meetings in the intensive care unit. J Nurs Scholarsh. 2019;51(2):129–37.
44. Mehter HM, McCannon JB, Clark JA, Wiener RS. Physician approaches to conflict with families surrounding end-of-life decision-making in the intensive care unit. A qualitative study. Ann Am Thorac Soc. 2018;15(2):241–9.
45. Coombs MA, Addington-Hall J, Long-Sutehall T. Challenges in transition from intervention to end of life care in intensive care: a qualitative study. Int J Nurs Stud. 2012;49(5):519–27.
46. Kerckhoffs MC, Senekal J, van Dijk D, et al. Framework to support the process of decision-making on life-sustaining treatments in the ICU: results of a Delphi study. Crit Care Med. 2020;48(5):645–53.
47. Torke AM, Wocial LD, Johns SA, et al. The family navigator: a pilot intervention to support intensive care unit family surrogates. Am J Crit Care. 2016;25(6):498–507.
48. Curtis JR, Treece PD, Nielsen EL, et al. Randomized trial of communication facilitators to reduce family distress and intensity of end-of-life care. Am J Respir Crit Care Med. 2016;193(2):154–62.
49. White DB, Angus DC, Shields AM, et al. A randomized trial of a family-support intervention in intensive care units. N Engl J Med. 2018;378(25):2365–75.
50. Parks Taylor S, Short RT, Asher AM, Muthukkumar R, Sanka P. Family Engagement Navigators: a novel program to facilitate family-centered care in the intensive care unit during Covid-19. NEJM Catal. 2020;2020:1–10.
51. Coventry A, Ford R, Rosenberg J, McInnes E. A qualitative meta-synthesis investigating the experiences of the patient's family when treatment is withdrawn in the intensive care unit. J Adv Nurs. 2020;76(9):2222–34.
52. Guerra-Martin MD, Gonzalez-Fernandez P. Satisfaction of patients and family caregivers in adult intensive care units: literature review. Enferm Intensiva (Engl Ed). 2021;32(4):207–19.
53. Stokes H, Vanderspank-Wright B, Fothergill Bourbonnais F, Wright DK. Meaningful experiences and end-of-life care in the intensive care unit: a qualitative study. Intensive Crit Care Nurs. 2019;53:1–7.
54. Bandini JI. Beyond the hour of death: family experiences of grief and bereavement following an end-of-life hospitalization in the intensive care unit. Health (London). 2020;26:1363459320946474.
55. Chen C, Michaels J, Meeker MA. Family outcomes and perceptions of end-of-life care in the intensive care unit: a mixed-methods review. J Palliat Care. 2020;35(3):143–53.
56. Kayser JB, Kaplan LJ. Conflict management in the ICU. Crit Care Med. 2020;48(9):1349–57.
57. Aslakson RA, Cox CE, Baggs JG, Curtis JR. Palliative and end-of-life care: prioritizing compassion within the ICU and beyond. Crit Care Med. 2021;49(10):1626–37.

58. Metaxa V, Anagnostou D, Vlachos S, et al. Palliative care interventions in intensive care unit patients. Intensive Care Med. 2021;47(12):1415–25.
59. Nelson JE, Bassett R, Boss RD, et al. Models for structuring a clinical initiative to enhance palliative care in the intensive care unit: a report from the IPAL-ICU Project (Improving Palliative Care in the ICU). Crit Care Med. 2010;38(9):1765–72.
60. Cobert J, Cook AC, Lin JA, O'Riordan DL, Pantilat SZ. Trends in palliative care consultations in critically ill patient populations, 2013–2019. J Pain Symptom Manag. 2022;63(2):e176–81.
61. Ma J, Chi S, Buettner B, et al. Early palliative care consultation in the medical ICU: a cluster randomized crossover trial. Crit Care Med. 2019;47(12):1707–15.
62. Kentish-Barnes N, Chevret S, Valade S, et al. A three-step support strategy for relatives of patients dying in the intensive care unit: a cluster randomised trial. Lancet. 2022;399(10325):656–64.
63. Efstathiou N, Vanderspank-Wright B, Vandyk A, et al. Terminal withdrawal of mechanical ventilation in adult intensive care units: a systematic review and narrative synthesis of perceptions, experiences and practices. Palliat Med. 2020;34(9):1140–64.
64. Downar J, Delaney JW, Hawryluck L, Kenny L. Guidelines for the withdrawal of life-sustaining measures. Intensive Care Med. 2016;42(6):1003–17.
65. Epker JL, Bakker J, Lingsma HF, Kompanje EJ. An observational study on a protocol for withdrawal of life-sustaining measures on two non-academic intensive care units in The Netherlands: few signs of distress, no suffering? J Pain Symptom Manag. 2015;50(5):676–84.
66. Campbell ML, Yarandi HN, Mendez M. A two-group trial of a terminal ventilator withdrawal algorithm: pilot testing. J Palliat Med. 2015;18(9):781–5.
67. Canadian Critical Care Society Ethics Committee, Bandrauk N, Downar J, Paunovic B. Withholding and withdrawing life-sustaining treatment: the Canadian Critical Care Society position paper. Can J Anaesth. 2018;65(1):105–22.
68. Robert R, Le Gouge A, Kentish-Barnes N, et al. Sedation practice and discomfort during withdrawal of mechanical ventilation in critically ill patients at end-of-life: a post-hoc analysis of a multicenter study. Intensive Care Med. 2020;46(6):1194–203.
69. Robert R, Le Gouge A, Kentish-Barnes N, et al. Terminal weaning or immediate extubation for withdrawing mechanical ventilation in critically ill patients (the ARREVE observational study). Intensive Care Med. 2017;43(12):1793–807.
70. DeForest A. Better words for better deaths. N Engl J Med. 2019;380(3):211–3.
71. Sanderson EAM, Humphreys S, Walker F, et al. Risk factors for complicated grief among family members bereaved in intensive care unit settings: a systematic review. PLoS One. 2022;17(3):e0264971.
72. Jensen HI, Halvorsen K, Jerpseth H, Fridh I, Lind R. Practice recommendations for end-of-life care in the intensive care unit. Crit Care Nurse. 2020;40(3):14–22.
73. Galazzi A, Adamini I, Bazzano G, et al. Intensive care unit diaries to help bereaved family members in their grieving process: a systematic review. Intensive Crit Care Nurs. 2022;68:103121.
74. Van Keer RL, Deschepper R, Huyghens L, Bilsen J. Withholding/withdrawing life-sustaining treatment in a multiethnic critical care setting: an ethnographic study. J Palliat Med. 2021;24(3):338–46.
75. Chuang E, Fiter RJ, Sanon OC, et al. Race and ethnicity and satisfaction with communication in the intensive care unit. Am J Hosp Palliat Care. 2020;37(10):823–9.
76. Nugent SM, Golden SE, Chapa J, Tuepker A, Slatore CG, Vranas KC. "You're socially distant and trying not to be emotionally distant." Physicians' perspectives of communication and therapeutic relationships in the ICU during the COVID-19 pandemic: a qualitative study. Crit Care Explor. 2023;5(2):e0854.
77. Nayfeh A, Yarnell CJ, Dale C, et al. Evaluating satisfaction with the quality and provision of end-of-life care for patients from diverse ethnocultural backgrounds. BMC Palliat Care. 2021;20(1):145.
78. Curtis JR, Vincent JL. Ethics and end-of-life care for adults in the intensive care unit. Lancet. 2010;376(9749):1347–53.

79. Alkhaled T, Rohde G, Lie B, Johannessen B. Beyond challenges and enrichment: a qualitative account of cross-cultural experiences of nursing patients with an ethnic minority background in Norway. BMC Nurs. 2022;21(1):322.
80. Brooks LA, Manias E, Bloomer MJ. How do intensive care clinicians ensure culturally sensitive care for family members at the end of life? A retrospective descriptive study. Intensive Crit Care Nurs. 2022;73:103303.
81. Hunt J, Bristowe K, Chidyamatare S, Harding R. 'So isolation comes in, discrimination and you find many people dying quietly without any family support': accessing palliative care for key populations—an in-depth qualitative study. Palliat Med. 2019;33(6):685–92.
82. Sprik P, Gentile D. Cultural humility: a way to reduce LGBTQ health disparities at the end of life. Am J Hosp Palliat Care. 2020;37(6):404–8.
83. Rosa WE, Roberts KE, Braybrook D, et al. Palliative and end-of-life care needs, experiences, and preferences of LGBTQ+ individuals with serious illness: a systematic mixed-methods review. Palliat Med. 2023;37(4):460–74.
84. Lintott L, Beringer R, Do A, Daudt H. A rapid review of end-of-life needs in the LGBTQ+ community and recommendations for clinicians. Palliat Med. 2022;36(4):609–24.
85. Braybrook D, Bristowe K, Timmins L, et al. Communication about sexual orientation and gender between clinicians, LGBT+ people facing serious illness and their significant others: a qualitative interview study of experiences, preferences and recommendations. BMJ Qual Saf. 2023;32(2):109–20.
86. Kemery SA. Family perceptions of quality of end of life in LGBTQ+ individuals: a comparative study. Palliat Care Soc Pract. 2021;15:2632352421997153.
87. Bristowe K, Marshall S, Harding R. The bereavement experiences of lesbian, gay, bisexual and/or trans* people who have lost a partner: a systematic review, thematic synthesis and modelling of the literature. Palliat Med. 2016;30(8):730–44.
88. Bristowe K, Hodson M, Wee B, et al. Recommendations to reduce inequalities for LGBT people facing advanced illness: ACCESSCare national qualitative interview study. Palliat Med. 2018;32(1):23–35.
89. Bristowe K, Timmins L, Braybrook D, et al. LGBT+ partner bereavement and appraisal of the Acceptance-Disclosure Model of LGBT+ bereavement: a qualitative interview study. Palliat Med. 2023;37(2):221–34.
90. Rosa WE, Shook A, Acquaviva KD. LGBTQ+ inclusive palliative care in the context of COVID-19: pragmatic recommendations for clinicians. J Pain Symptom Manag. 2020;60(2):e44–7.
91. Lucas JJ, Bouchoucha SL, Afrouz R, Reed K, Brennan-Olsen SL. LGBTQ+ loss and grief in a cis-heteronormative pandemic: a qualitative evidence synthesis of the COVID-19 literature. Qual Health Res. 2022;32(14):2102–17.
92. Ferrell BR, Handzo G, Picchi T, Puchalski C, Rosa WE. The urgency of spiritual care: COVID-19 and the critical need for whole-person palliation. J Pain Symptom Manag. 2020;60(3):e7–11.

Chapter 13
Family Support and ICU Survivorship: Lessons Learned from the Pediatric Critical Care Experience

Bree Andrews, Nilu Rahman, and Neethi Pinto

Introduction

After the establishment of the first pediatric intensive care unit (PICU) in 1955, the field of pediatric critical care has achieved remarkable progress. Advances in pediatric medicine and technology have fueled tremendous growth of this subspecialty [1]. The centralization of care into PICUs with dedicated pediatric intensivists and development of fellowship training programs was accompanied by a decreased likelihood of mortality [1–3]. Notably, PICU mortality decreased from 11% in the 1980s to 4.8% in the mid-2000s [4]. The mortality rate among critically ill children has continued to decrease to a historic low during the last decade [4, 5]. This progress remains one of the most significant accomplishments in contemporary pediatrics.

However, the risk of mortality in the PICU is not equivalent among all patients who experience critical illness. For example, adult patients between the ages of 20 and 29 years who are admitted to the PICU (typically, patients with complex medical problems who continue to be cared for primarily by pediatricians and/or pediatric subspecialists) exhibit increased baseline morbidity, greater severity of illness, and a twofold higher risk of mortality when compared with younger PICU patients between the ages of 15–18 years [6]. This difference in mortality by age group is

B. Andrews
Section of Neonatology, The University of Chicago Comer Children's Hospital, Department of Pediatrics, The University of Chicago, Chicago, IL, USA

N. Rahman
Child Life Department, Johns Hopkins Children's Center, Baltimore, MD, USA

N. Pinto (✉)
Division of Critical Care Medicine, Department of Anesthesiology and Critical Care Medicine, Children's Hospital of Philadelphia, Philadelphia, PA, USA
e-mail: pintonp@chop.edu

© The Author(s), under exclusive license to Springer Nature Switzerland AG 2025

A. J. Vance et al. (eds.), *Families in the Intensive Care Unit*,
https://doi.org/10.1007/978-3-031-83786-9_13

consistent with overall trends in the adult intensive care unit (ICU) compared to the PICU, where overall mortality rates are 10–29% and 2–3%, respectively [7–9].

The landscape of pediatric critical care is changing, focusing on what happens to children after they leave the PICU environment. As more children survive, attention to improving outcomes and function *after* discharge has become more relevant. Today, children are increasingly using PICU resources, representing 12–15% of pediatric hospital encounters and 85% of children being admitted to ICUs in children's hospitals [10, 11]. While PICU mortality has decreased to 1.8% in 2019 [10], children survive with increased rates of moderate or severe disability compared to earlier rates of disability among PICU survivors [4, 8]. Better survival brings with it the conundrum that these survivors face increasing medical burdens placing them at high risk for sequelae and even readmission to the PICU.

With these increases in morbidity, it is not surprising that the majority (72% of nearly 53,000 patients admitted in 2008) of PICU patients have chronic conditions and most (53%) of these are complex. Similarly, between 2001 and 2019, 57% of 275,656 children admitted to the PICU had underlying morbidities and 23.5% of these patients had preexisting technology dependence [10]. These trends are concerning because children with complex chronic conditions are at increased risk of mortality compared to all other children admitted to the PICU [12]. Even among children surviving critical illness, an ongoing risk of poor long-term outcomes exists, with twice as many children experiencing morbidity and mortality up to 3 years after hospital discharge [13]. Thus, although in-hospital ICU mortality may be markedly improved compared to historic data, survivors of contemporary pediatric critical illness increasingly experience ongoing morbidity, chronicity of disease, and increased risk of mortality paralleling the natural history of their adult counterparts after discharge [14].

Adults and children who experience critical illness may experience similar sequelae from their disease as well as from requisite invasive life-saving therapies such as prolonged mechanical ventilation, central venous and arterial catheters, sedation, neuromuscular blockade, and use of vasoactive substances. Understanding the overlap of the pediatric and adult experiences during and after critical illness may be informative to both fields. Here, we focus on lessons from both the PICU and neonatal intensive care unit (NICU) that may have important implications for adult ICUs (Table 13.1).

Table 13.1 Parallels between pediatric and adult experiences

Pediatric	Adult
Decreasing mortality	Decreasing mortality
Increased disease chronicity	Multiple co-morbidities
Increased morbidity after critical illness	PICS[a]
Neuroplasticity and vulnerability	Resiliency
Parent/guardian as decision maker	Patient, spouse, child as decision maker
Loss of some parental control during illness	Power of attorney during and after illness
Re-adjusting with less support after illness	New caretaker/lack of independence after illness
School transition	Workplace transition
Impact on family	PICS-F[b]

[a]Post-Intensive Care Syndrome
[b]Post-Intensive Care Syndrome-Family

At the Onset of Critical Illness: A Focus on Recovery

Studies indicate that clinicians in the NICU and the medical intensive care unit (MICU) are unable to relably predict outcomes [15, 16]. Similarly, in the PICU, prognostication may be affected by level of confidence, experience, clinical skills, and patients' severity of illness or disease [17, 18]. With limited prognostic ability, it may be difficult to determine whether care is futile or to assess potential for recovery in certain clinical scenarios [15]. As a result, the typical initial approach to the critically ill pediatric patient is characteristically intense with an armamentarium of invasive measures undertaken. While this may raise concerns regarding resource utilization and ethics of provision of care unlikely to benefit the patient, the majority of care and resource consumption in the NICU and PICU settings is not futile [15, 19, 20]. This low percentage of care unlikely to benefit the patient may be secondary to the unique recovery potential associated with pediatric patients as well as advances in medicine and technology. In particular, children may be more resilient than adults with regard to physiologic recovery due to their typically fewer preexisting co-morbidities at the time of onset of critical illness, evidence of neuroplasticity and greater overall regenerative potential, and a dynamic developmental trajectory.

The Impact of Baseline Health

Although children typically have fewer co-morbidities than adults, an increasing percentage of children admitted to the PICU are chronically ill (Killien), and children with complex chronic conditions are at increased risk of readmission to the PICU within 11 year of discharge [21]. These include children with asthma, congenital heart disease, chronic lung disease, diabetes, cerebral palsy, and/or medical complexity, including technology dependence. Children who are readmitted to the ICU are at increased risk of mortality and longer lengths of stay with its attendant morbidity [22].

In contrast, children, who were previously healthy, had less severe disease at the onset of critical illness, or noncomplex chronic conditions exhibit better long-term outcomes [12, 13]. With this knowledge, concerted strategies such as multidisciplinary inpatient rounds and/or conferences and follow-up clinics with a focus on preventive health, parent, and caregiver education, and coordination of care to reduce both the short-term impact of co-morbidities and improve long-term control of complex chronic conditions may have important, lasting implications for children who experience critical illness.

A similar focus on preservation and restoration of baseline health for adult survivors of critical illness warrants attention because adults are even more likely to have complex co-morbidities both prior to and as an aftermath of critical illness.

Neuroplasticity and Resiliency

The concept of neuroplasticity, the ability of the central nervous system to adapt neural circuitry in response to environmental stimuli, may also explain the generally positive outcome trajectories of critically ill children [23]. For example, children who experience brain injury may exhibit near complete recovery of function, faring better than their adult counterparts due to the effects of neuroplasticity [24]. Similarly, children with congenital heart disease who require prolonged hospitalization (exposure to sedatives, neuromuscular blockade, etc.) do not necessarily exhibit increased neurocognitive delay when compared to healthy children [25]. However, there may be a spectrum of neural adaptability that ranges from neuroplasticity to early vulnerability predisposing some children to an increased risk of incomplete recovery. This "recovery continuum," the balance between early plasticity and early vulnerability, is subject to a multitude of influences including:

1. The nature, extent, and site of insult.
2. Age and developmental stage at the time of injury.
3. Environmental influences.
4. Rehabilitative interventions [23].

Just as neuroplasticity and neurodevelopment may influence the trajectory of outcomes after pediatric critical illness, the related concept of resiliency may be an important factor in survivorship in adult critical care [26, 27]. Resiliency refers to a psychological trait reflecting adjustment and adaptability to stress [28]. However, behavior that is adaptive to a stressful event may be unconventional, maladaptive, or self-detrimental. There may be a spectrum of adaptability, an "adaptability continuum," ranging from resiliency to maladaptation that parallels the recovery continuum for neuroplasticity and vulnerability. Similar to the aforementioned influences on the recovery continuum for children, adaptability may be influenced by:

1. *The nature and severity of critical illness.*
2. *Age, baseline adaptability, and cognitive loss or dementia (in lieu of developmental stage).*
3. *Environmental influences (supports, social networks, etc.).*
4. *Rehabilitative interventions* (including strategies for coping).

Understanding how to foster resiliency and adaptability may mitigate the overall impact of critical illness for adult survivors.

During Critical Illness: Family-Centered Care as Normative

In 2001, the Institute of Medicine (IOM) issued recommendations for patient-centered care, defined as care that is "respectful of and responsive to individual patient preferences, needs, and values" [29]. Subsequently, in 2007, the American College of Critical Care Medicine (ACCM) issued guidelines for patient and family-centered care in ICUs [30]. The 2012 American Academy of Pediatrics (AAP) Policy Statement on Patient- and Family-Centered Care and the Pediatrician's role similarly delineates the core principles of patient and family-centered care as care that is "based on the understanding that the family is the child's primary source of strength and support and that the child's and family's perspectives are important in clinical decision-making" [31]. The AAP recommendations for how all pediatricians (including pediatric intensivists and neonatologists) may integrate this patient- and family-centered care approach in hospitals include the development of collaborative relationships with patients and families, ensuring family presence during hospitalization, rounds, and procedures, facilitating family support and peer-to-peer support, attending to environmental issues that facilitate family presence, incorporating patients and families into decision-making, and ensuring appropriate transitions of care.

In 2013, the ACCM proposed new family-centered care recommendations [32]. The new recommendations called attention to:

1. Family presence in the ICU
2. Family support
3. Operational and environmental issues
4. Communication with family members
5. Use of specific consultations and ICU team members

PICUs and NICUs have embraced many of these recommendations from both the AAP and the ACCM with various components of family-centered care having been routinely adapted and becoming standard practice in the United States.

1. Family Presence in the ICU

   (a) Open Visitation

   In alignment with the aforementioned AAP Policy Statement, family visitation has shifted from historically restrictive policies to open visiting policies 24 h a day/7 days a week. In renovated or new PICUs, patient rooms often incorporate parent sleep spaces, fostering an environment conducive to unrestricted visitation, proximity of the child and family, and continual family presence [33]. Similarly, in prior decades, sibling visitation was either restricted or not permitted at all. Siblings likely experienced significant disruption of their routines due to absence of their parents and a lack of understanding of their affected sibling's illness. However, today, sibling visitation in the PICU is not only routinely expected but also commonly facilitated with the support of child life specialists who prepare siblings, facilitate questions, debrief after visits, anticipate the sibling's questions and reactions for the parent, educate health care providers regarding developmental stages, and utilize age-appropriate resources [34].

   Family satisfaction and knowledge has been shown to improve with open visitation in the adult ICU setting [32]. The model provided by child life specialists for critically ill children has important implications for critically ill adults; children may benefit from the opportunity to visit a critically ill parent or relative with appropriate assistance from child life specialists. Adults may benefit from active preparation by designated staff prior to and debriefing after visiting a critically ill relative or friend. (*See* Use of Specific Consultations and ICU Team Members)

   (b) Partnership in Rounds

   Family presence on rounds allows for bidirectional education. Parents and guardians are able to relay information about and advocate for their child while health care professionals are able to educate families about their child's condition, potentially reducing misunderstanding and miscommunication. Family-centered rounds also provide families and health care professionals with increased opportunities to interact, build trust, and develop relationships [34]. Overall, families report improved satisfaction when given the option to participate in rounds [32].

   Family-centered rounds may also pose some challenges [35]. Families may not understand terminology or topics discussed on rounds and may experience increased anxiety as a result of this lack of understanding. Further explanation and discussion on rounds may not be practical given the need to attend to other critical patients. Family understanding and participation is dynamic; families may understand less, feel less comfortable asking questions, not want bad news shared during rounds or need more information after rounds on the day of admission compared to subsequent days.[36]

   Additionally, parental presence may pose a challenge to open communication about sensitive topics such as noncompliance, medical abuse or neglect, and medical errors that warrant discussion among the health care team. Open visitation policies may also contribute to privacy concerns or interruption of rounds due to an unrestricted flow of visitors. Teaching on rounds may be negatively affected due to concerns for exposure of gaps in trainees' knowledge with resultant undermining of trainees' credibility with families [34].

Meert et al. note that an understanding of the true impact of family-centered rounds in the PICU is limited, as studies of family-centered rounds typically have selection bias since parents self-select whether or not to be present on rounds and partnership in rounds tends to occur predominantly in Western societies [34]. Keeping this selection bias in mind, parents report increased satisfaction, more contact with physicians, and better knowledge of test results. Nurses also report increased satisfaction with not being the intermediary between physicians and families. Physicians themselves report increased trust. Residents may benefit from exposure to family perspectives. However, there may be adverse consequences for trainees in a training environment; residents report decreased teaching opportunities on rounds when families are present and express preferences for being asked questions in a conference room rather than in front of family members [34].

Overall, the pediatric experience with family-centered rounds is generally favorable and adaptation of family-centered rounds to the adult setting should take into account the potential for perceived barriers regarding increased duration of rounds, increased family anxiety, difficulty discussing sensitive topics, concerns for privacy, and impact on trainee learning environment.

(c) Presence During Procedures

The option for family presence during invasive procedures, including cardiopulmonary resuscitation (CPR), was first recommended by the American Heart Association in 2000 [37]. Health care providers holding views supporting family presence suggest that family presence may facilitate understanding and grief due to direct observation of all measures taken. Opponents contend that family presence may exacerbate misunderstanding, generate interference, heighten anxiety and psychological trauma for the family, increase performance anxiety among health care providers, and result in medicolegal issues [32, 34]. Families themselves typically are supportive of family presence. In fact, parents believe their presence may directly help their child or help decrease their own anxiety about the procedure [34, 38, 39]. During an era where parental observation of invasive procedures was not standard practice, Powers *et al* demonstrated decreased parental procedure-related anxiety for their critically ill child when parents were allowed to be present for invasive procedures, including endotracheal intubation, central line placement, and chest tube placement [38]. Now, familial presence during invasive procedures in the PICU is more widely practiced; the spectrum of invasive procedures for which families may be present varies within and among individual institutions but may include endotracheal intubation, central line placement, arterial line placement, cardiopulmonary resuscitation, extracorporeal membrane oxygenation, and extracorporeal cardiopulmonary resuscitation. Similarly, there is variability with regard to families' preferences and decisions to remain present for any of these procedures.

In 2006, consensus recommendations regarding family presence during pediatric procedures recommended that specific definitions of family members and applicable procedures be identified [40]. Similarly, family preparation with presence of a facilitator, establishment of policies in the event of disagreements or obstruction to care, and attention to staff education and safety are key components of family presence during procedures that must be addressed at the institutional level to ensure that the needs of families and staff are met [32, 34]. Simulation training on how to support family during CPR has been shown to increase staff comfort with parental presence during procedures [41]. The American Academy of Pediatrics continues to reiterate the importance of patient and family-centered care, and the fundamental responsibility of the pediatrician to facilitate provision of patient and family-centered care, particularly for hospitalized children [31].

Adaptation of family presence during procedures in adult ICUs should be deliberately planned to ensure that clear definitions of family members and which procedures are appropriate for family presence exist. Attention to patient and staff safety must be paramount; policies and procedures including designation of a family facilitator who may help a grieving family or contend with disagreements or obstruction to care is essential prior to implementation of policies endorsing family presence during procedures.

2. Family Support

NICU care is fraught with concerns about parenting engagement and adjustment, as NICU care is often prolonged and in many cases prognosis is uncertain. Parents may not understand their exact role in the NICU as they observe an entire health care team attend to their child, and they may be uncertain of how to best engage with their new baby at the bedside [42]. This role uncertainty may lead to a gap between NICU parenting experiences and parenting expectations, which is particularly concerning because long-term maternal psychological outcomes (e.g., depression, anxiety, and PTSD) are negatively associated with the different parenting experiences and expectations [43]. Communication and education are key components for families to successfully navigate and make sense of the indeterminacies and chaotic circumstances created by a premature or complex birth and subsequent NICU hospitalization, which may extend over weeks to months for many neonates [44].

Conversely, the role of being a caregiver and assisting with care in the PICU is a natural extension of the expectations and responsibilities that parents and guardians hold prior to the child's critical illness. This is because children are inherently dependent on adult family members in order to meet their basic needs of food, clothing, shelter, health, and education (Fig. 13.1a). Thus, the challenge for families in the PICU is not in accepting the burden of the role, but in relinquishing some of this care to a myriad of new and relatively unknown health care

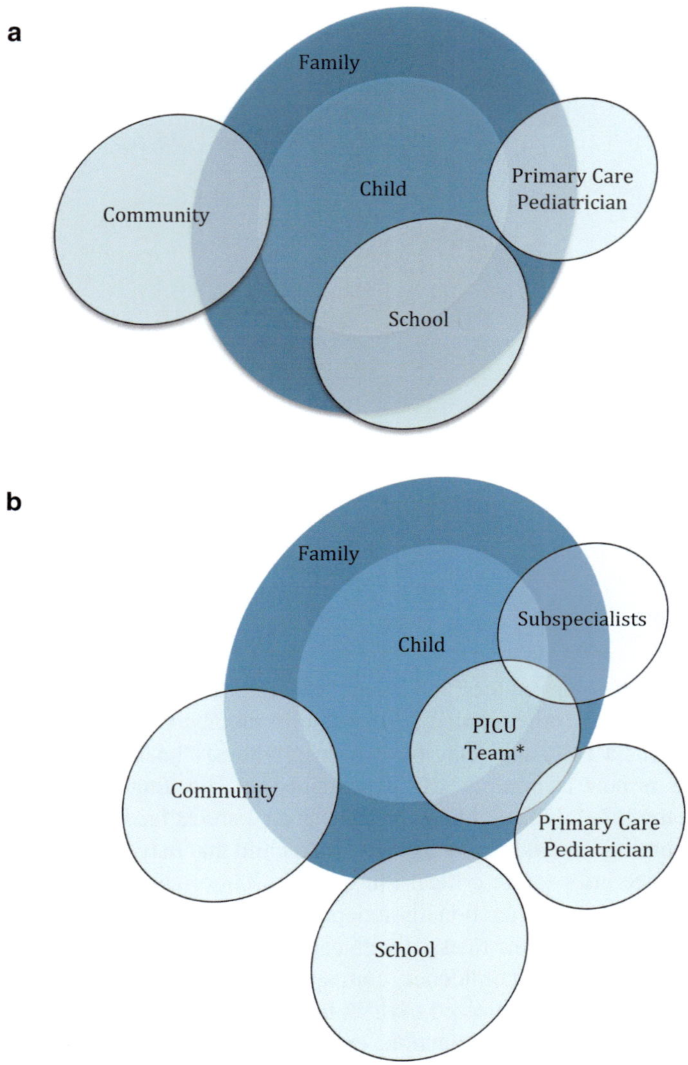

Fig. 13.1 (**a**) Prior to critical illness. (**b**) During critical illness. (**c**) After critical illness***PICU Team including:** Physicians**,** nurses, pharmacists**,** nutritionists, respiratory therapists, occupational therapists, physical therapists, speech therapists, case managers, social workers, child life specialists, family advocates, chaplain, other

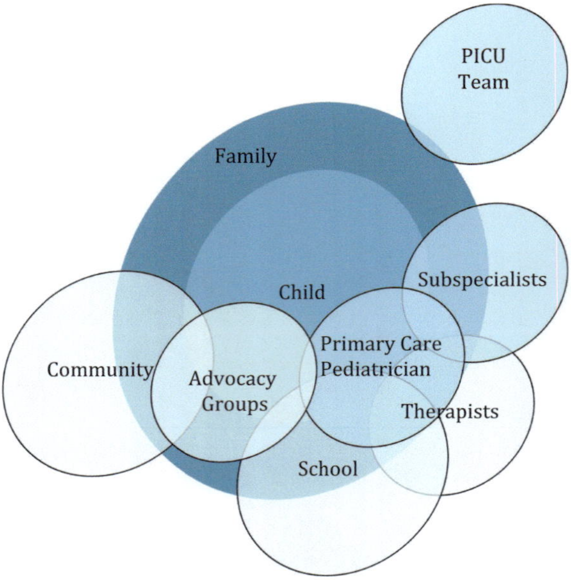

Fig. 13.1 (continued)

providers who comprise the PICU team [45] (Fig. 13.1b). As the child recovers from acute illness, other challenges for family members include learning complex care for a child that may have been previously healthy but due to their condition is now technologically dependent (e.g., needing a tracheostomy or gastrostomy tube). Indeed, in this circumstance, parents face enormous difficulties reassuming increased responsibility for a child that may have achieved some independence prior to the critical illness (e.g., school-aged children or adolescents) but no longer is functionally independent.

Teaching families how to assist with care of the critically ill neonate or child is pivotal to improving confidence, competence, and stress during and after the ICU stay [32]. Two randomized trials in the NICU population provide evidence for the improvement in satisfaction, enhanced active participation by parents, and possible reduction in readmissions with teaching families to participate in care while in the NICU [46, 47]. In addition to education, families also may benefit from professional, spiritual, and peer-to-peer support that is either organized or occurs informally in the context of shared, common spaces such as family lounges. In particular, evidence from observational studies in the NICU suggests that families report increased satisfaction and value peer-to-peer support [32]. Similarly, two randomized trials provide evidence for improved outcomes (including decreased anxiety, trauma, and depression) for mothers who received psychological interventions such as psychologist support, psychoeducation, cognitive behavioral therapy, and educational materials after the birth of a preterm infant [32].

Parents may also benefit from care coordination for follow-up appointments or assistance with determining their eligibility for early intervention or support from local school districts [44]. Additionally, families may need help navigating insurance barriers, obtaining durable medical equipment, and obtaining medication in a timely manner, etc. [44].

*In adult ICUs, there are direct parallels. The role of caregiving for an adult patient who is now dependent may be new for a friend or family member. Just as in the NICU and PICU, family presence on rounds and family support may facilitate an understanding of these transitions. Family education during hospitalization and gradual transition of bedside care from nurses to relatives may decrease stress after discharge by equipping family members with confidence and competence in their skills at providing care and managing levels of expectation regarding post-discharge outcomes. The importance of education and peer-to-peer support for both pediatric and adult ICU patients and their families is reflected by global resource development through organizations such as the Society of Critical Care Medicine's THRIVE initiative (*www.myicucare.org/thrive*) and ICUsteps (icusteps.org) Psychological support may also improve outcomes for adult patients with evidence of decreased post-traumatic stress disorder in adult patients who receive early psychological support* [32].

3. Operational and Environmental Issues

   Important to family presence and support is attention to the physical and social needs of parents during their child's PICU or NICU admission. For example, private rooms rather than open bays or curtained spaces, provision of parent beds or sleep spaces, self-care facilities, meal vouchers, and transportation have been reported to reduce parent stress and allow for increased family presence in the PICU and NICU [32–34].

   Other environmental areas that require ongoing attention from health care providers include the need to recognize the importance of noise reduction, normalization of sleep-wake and day-night cycles with regard to lighting, and minimization of sleep interruptions while providing necessary care due to the impact on child and parent stress, delirium, and outcomes.

   These same operational and environmental issues are likely to benefit the families of adult ICU patients. Increased family presence is more feasible when basic needs such as food, temporary lodging, parking, or transportation are addressed.

4. Communication with Family Members

   Also central to the effectiveness of family presence and family support is the role of communication between the health care team and the family. Although family presence during rounds facilitates the opportunity for daily communication, bidirectional time constraints may present challenges in providing parents and the health care team adequate daily opportunities to interact in person. For example, due to other responsibilities such as care for siblings or other family members, work constraints, transportation issues, and lack of financial resources, parents may not be able to be routinely present in the ICU particularly if the ICU stay is prolonged. Language barriers and routine use of interpreters to provide updates in the family's preferred language is also an important aspect of effective communication [48]. The health care team may need to attend to other critically ill patients, causing interruptions or limitations in the duration of a particular family discussion. Thus, in addition to daily face-to-face conversations about the child's status and plan, telephone conferences may be an important means of improving communication.

Effective communication beyond these relatively brief interactions is further facilitated by family conferences with discussion of a child's medical condition, prognosis, and treatment options. Clinicians' use of the VALUE mnemonic (Value family statements, Acknowledge family emotions, Listen to family, Understand the patient as a person, and Elicit family questions) may facilitate communication in these settings [49]. Mutual understanding between families and the health care team may benefit from these extended conversations. Moreover, family conferences that are multidisciplinary provide an opportunity to address family questions in a concerted, unified manner. In these conferences, consultative services may directly provide information to the family in the presence of the primary ICU team, harmonizing transfer of medical information. Considerations regarding the timing of the meeting (within the first 72 h of admission and/or on a weekly basis for prolonged stay patients) and the setting (private space separate from the child's room) are important as are acknowledgments of the families' concerns and need for empathy [34]. The family conference represents an opportunity for discussion of family preferences and values. With regard to end-of-life decision-making, clinicians and staff note that family conferences allow for improved communication among clinicians, information transfer between clinicians and family, and support of families [50]. Studies also suggest that families may benefit from family meetings after a child's death or discharge with decreased levels of depression and posttraumatic stress [51].

Parent functioning, coping, and adjustment to medical complexity and uncertainty also may be affected by the consistency of communication, clinical continuity (e.g., primary nursing), and the availability of tools for enhanced education for families.[44, 52–55] Empathetic support from the health care team toward parents is important for increasing parental well-being, engagement, and satisfaction [31, 56–59]; parents may benefit from mental health screening and supports [44]. Parents may utilize a diverse array of coping mechanisms and support options while in the ICU setting (e.g. acceptance, emotional support, active coping, positive reframing, religion, planning, social networks, and families with current or prior NICU experience) [44, 60]. These alternative support options need to be considered when developing parental support resources. For example, parents in the NICU have shown a preference for support programming that focuses on education about infant development [61] or meeting with other NICU parents [60].

The improved communication facilitated by family conferences has direct applicability to the adult ICU patient. In many MICUs, these conferences occur but are typically at the discretion of the primary attending. Incorporation of family conferences as a routine element of patient care will likely benefit patients and multiple family members who would gain the opportunity to obtain informa-

tion directly from health care providers. Additionally, educational information and the provision of resources such as ICU informational guides and diaries have been demonstrated to both improve patient and family understanding and satisfaction as well as reduce anxiety, depression, and stress [62, 63].

5. Use of Specific Consultations and ICU Team Members

   The role of the multidisciplinary team is also pivotal for improving communication; The PICU team and rounds may incorporate nurses, physicians (intensivists, primary care pediatricians, and other medical and surgical subspecialists), pharmacists, nutritionists, respiratory therapists, physical/occupational therapists, social workers, case managers, chaplains or spiritual advisors, family advocates or navigators, and child life specialists. In particular circumstances, this team may also include consultations to Palliative Care, Ethics, or Psychology. When families are able to participate in rounds or multidisciplinary conferences, their ability to interact with this vast team of care providers and their understanding of the multiple aspects of their child's recovery has the potential to increase exponentially.

   Child life specialists, in particular, are a fundamental part of this vast multidisciplinary team in the PICU. They actively use a multifaceted family-centered care approach to proactively identify the needs of a patient and family and collaborate with the medical team on how to best support those needs. They are able to address needs related to visitation, presence during invasive and noninvasive procedures, and operational and environmental issues while also directly focusing on reducing the stress and anxiety associated with the ICU setting. They normalize the hospital environment for the patient through play. Child life specialists in the PICU also serve an important role with legacy building and facilitating end-of-life conversations and interventions with the patient and family.

   Operationalizing a model similar to that of the child life specialists in the adult ICU may be particularly helpful to families. Children may benefit from increased preparation and opportunity to visit a critically ill parent or relative with the assistance of child life specialists and provision of developmentally appropriate educational resources. Similarly, spouses, siblings, relatives, and friends of critically ill adults may also benefit from a designated family advocate or team member who is equipped to prepare them for visits, facilitate questions, debrief after visits, and anticipate questions and reactions. These advocates or team members ideally would be able to educate health care providers and provide appropriate resources.

After Critical Illness: Embracing Multidisciplinary Follow-Up Care and Advocacy

After discharge, two modalities have been shown to improve patient outcomes as well as child and parental functioning. First, a multidisciplinary primary care clinic with pediatric or neonatal, nutrition, developmental, social work, and nursing expertise is an efficient and effective way to coordinate complex services in the first months and years after discharge. Second, systems of advocacy across the discipline of intensive care medicine with a focus on attainment of public and private benefits for patients can impact overall outcomes.

Multidisciplinary Follow-Up Clinics

The aforementioned concept of multidisciplinary rounding has been well embraced and includes a wide complement of professionals. However, follow-up care after admission to the PICU or NICU is not typically multidisciplinary and is often fragmented due to the complex logistics of coordinating various subspecialty and therapy providers. Ideally, a multidisciplinary follow-up clinic in which intensivists worked collaboratively with the other providers who (re)assume care in order to transition care for a patient would be implemented widely. The knowledge of the care the patient requires, and the new medical problems he/she may encounter is perhaps best understood by the ICU team. However, the provision of ongoing care is best undertaken by ambulatory providers. For example, collaboration between neonatologists and developmental and behavioral pediatricians may facilitate screening of former premature infants for developmental delays and appropriate institution of early therapy and resource implementation with resultant positive impact on the child's dynamic outcome trajectory [64].

Coordination of complex care and multiple (new) follow-up appointments and evaluations by subspecialists and therapists are often burdensome. For families, transportation, coordination of schedules, and missed school and work cause enormous challenges. Moreover, in the United States, transfer of relevant, summative health information after critical illness is often fragmented and incomplete. In neonatology, multidisciplinary clinics have been effective and efficient mechanisms to ensure appropriate medical care and support for parents traversing these difficulties after critical illness. Currently, in the United States and many other countries, if an institution offers high-level NICU services such as mechanical ventilation, extracorporal membrane oxygen, central lines, total parenteral nutrition, and pediatric surgical services, then the institution is expected to provide ongoing assessment and support for developmental delays and impairments until age 3 years in accordance with state and national public health guidelines for regional centers [65]. The extent to which hospitals offer these services varies, but this type of coordination of ongoing care has led to some of the most robust outcome evaluations, including behavioral, cognitive, academic, and emotional benefits, for a subset of intensive care patients across the globe [66–71]. Currently, clinical standards and best practices for multidisciplinary PICU follow-up programs have yet to be established but in a recent survey of 60 centers in the United States, Canada, Australia, and the United Kingdom, most respondents (>80%) endorsed the benefits of follow-up clinics [72]. However, only 1/3 of these programs had established programs [72].

This paradigm of follow-up clinics has gained widespread adaptation in neonatology; incorporating this model into pediatric and adult ICU post-discharge care as a standard of care would likely translate into improved outcomes for ICU survivors.

Advocacy

Transitions of care after NICU and PICU discharge to the primary care pediatrician and a multitude of specialists represent an important underdeveloped and understudied aspect of family support. In addition to providing ongoing medical care for survivors of critical illness, these primary and subspecialty health care providers often coordinate their patients' complex care and interface with important systems external to the health care setting to advocate for their patients (Fig. 13.1c).

For example, pediatricians often undertake an advocacy role with regard to the development of individualized education plans (IEPs) for qualifying children in accordance with the requirements of the 1975 Individuals with Disabilities Education Act. Pediatricians also provide referrals to Early Intervention programs for children between the ages of 0 and 3 years who have disabilities and developmental delays. Pediatricians also advocate for "504 plans" for children with disabilities per Section 504 of the Rehabilitation Act of 1973 that requires provision of a free and appropriate public education in the least restrictive environment to children with disabilities (including children with medical conditions that result in functional limitations such as attention-deficit hyperactivity disorder, asthma, and diabetes) [73]. Pediatricians can advocate for special education, speech therapy, or occupational therapy under the purview of this legislation. Similar interactions are often required for governmental and private agency social services and concurrent therapies (physical therapy, mental health counseling, etc.) Either parents or pediatric health care providers may be more effective in advocating for such services by partnering with legal services or disability advocates such as the Council of Parent Attorneys and Advocates and the National Disability Rights Network [73].

Neonatology follow-up clinics demonstrate the importance of a such an advocacy role in order to improve child functioning for intensive care graduates. One key arena for child and family functioning is through legal advocacy especially around public health benefits. Medical Legal Partnerships (MLPs) provide one way for lawyers to partner with physicians in clinical care to improve the social determinants of health [74]. In a recent study of the impact of preventative legal advocacy to assist the medical team in providing an action plan for parents, physicians, and lawyers to help children, the use of a written document with action items and information about issues including Early Intervention, Supplemental Food and Housing programs, Special Education and Social Security was 80% effective in surmounting barriers to attainment of these services for families [75]. Additionally, only 24% of families required legal representation after 1 year. While direct legal service is a model well known within

MLPs, widespread adaptation of such a preventative legal approach may lead to more care for patients.

Health care providers embracing the advocacy role and partnership with legal advocates have been an effective means of garnering resources for infants and children who survive critical illness with disabilities; adults who require additional assistance, therapies, nursing care, or assistance in the workplace may similarly benefit from such partnerships between their health care providers and advocacy organizations.

Lessons Learned from the COVID-19 Pandemic and Respiratory Surges in PICUs

Restrictions to Family-Centered Care Policies

In response to the COVID-19 pandemic, hospitals placed restrictions on some of these family-centered care policies in the PICU, specifically regarding open visitation and family presence during rounds or procedures. For example, families were restricted completely in Canada [76] and to 1–2 visitors in the United States [77] with potential exceptions at the end-of-life, traumatic diagnoses, parent mental health concerns, medical complexity, breastfeeding, and language barriers [78]. However, when we did not understand how SARS-CoV-2 was transmitted, the development of uniform standards for visitation policies was not possible, leading to variability in practice.

Downstream and Unintended Consequences of Restrictions

The variability in visitation resulted in incredibly different experiences for children and their families [79]. For example, in an Austrian NICU which promoted parental visitation throughout the pandemic, restricting to one parent per day, total daily visiting time and physical contact time with the neonate increased, and infant pain and stress scores decreased [80]. However, in institutions with more restrictive visitation policies, the outcomes were concerning. These restrictions, albeit deemed necessary for effective quarantine for health care workers and families, may have caused additional stress and anxiety for both children and their families, limited social support, impeded communication, family-centered care, and shared decision-making with the health care team, and negatively affected sibling adjustment and family functioning [78, 81–83].

Even when families were permitted to visit, they experienced restrictions with regard to leaving the PICU or hospital, resulting in challenges with availability and use of bathrooms, sleeping surfaces, obtaining meals, etc. [78]. During invasive procedures or resuscitative efforts, families, who may not have elected to be present in the pre-COVID-19 era, may have been unable to leave [78]. Additionally, cohorting potentially infected patients on "COVID" floors may also have increased stress, fear, and anxiety for families [81].

Limited In-Person Social Support

Prior to COVID-19, international differences already existed in family visitation policies with North America and Oceania allowing two family members 24 h per day as a normative practice, whereas this was generally not allowed in Africa and rarely allowed in Central and South America [84]. Telephone or video conferencing in lieu of visitation during the pandemic magnified, rather than offset, these same international differences [84]. Additionally, at the onset of the pandemic, variability also occurred within countries, resulting in families within a country having unequal access to their critically ill children [78]. The absence of family members may have important consequences for children's anxiety, sedation requirements, delirium, length of stay, early mobility, and outcomes [84]. Also, with regard to restrictions at end-of-life, in particular, the focus on infection containment may have precluded the cultural or religious beliefs of patients and families [84]. Restrictions to the number of visitors also posed challenges for family members who were present at the bedside; their social support was limited to virtual contact with friends and family, at best.

Reduced Communication

Among family members who were able to visit, there were likely reductions in the interactions with health care providers due to less time spent in the patient room, lack of family presence on rounds for COVID+ patients (especially prior to vaccine availability), virtual consultation, and limited nonverbal communication and reassurance due to use of personal protective equipment [81]. The overall impact of reduced interaction likely resulted in decreased communication and feelings of support for families [81].

Family Functioning

Visitation policies that were restricted to one visitor who was not permitted to leave the hospital had implications for other family members (including siblings) with disruption of normal routines, possible worsening of fear and anxiety with the inability to see the sick child, employment absences, etc. In the PICU at Johns Hopkins Children's Center (JHCC), and likely across many other medical centers in North America, multiple measures were taken to bridge these gaps in family support. Most rooms in the JHCC PICU, including the COVID-19 biodome, were equipped with an iPad that had telecommunication accessibility and a Bluetooth speaker to allow video visits with the patient and caregiver at the hospital and their family at home. The child life department created child-and-family-centered

COVID-19 educational resources and activity books that could be sent via email to the family at home and were readily available on the COVID-19 portal on the JHCC website. The child life specialists conducted video visits with siblings and family members at home to provide additional psychosocial support and facilitate these video visits with the patient at the bedside. In the event of a death when siblings and additional family members could not visit, the child life specialist would facilitate a video visit to give the siblings and family an opportunity to be involved in end-of-life support and to say goodbye. In collaboration with JHCC's Hospital Epidemiology and Infection Control department, child life specialists were able to still create certain memory art with the patient as keepsakes for the family to take home. Despite these interventions, patients, siblings, and family were greatly impacted by the restrictions, though necessary to maintain infection control, during the COVID-19 pandemic.

Thinking Outside the Box

With restrictions on bedside communication, telephone communication became more common in countries in North America, Europe, Oceania, and Asia but was less frequent in Africa, Central, and South America [84]. Similarly, video conferencing became more commonly used in North America and Oceania but was not widely used elsewhere [84]. Hospitals had to creatively adapt to the restrictions to family physical presence by utilizing these alternate methods of communication between health care providers and families as well as encouraging families to use both asynchronous and synchronous modes of communication such as journaling, telephone, text, and social media for support [85]. However, families with limited or no access to the Internet or devices with video capability would not have had reliable access to their children [82].

The COVID-19 pandemic and related visitor restrictions posed threats to family-centered care by leaving families feeling like they had inadequate in-person support, reduced communication and agency, and increased difficulty maintaining intact family function. Wherever possible, use of additional psychosocial virtual or in-person support using social workers, psychologists, and child life specialists and free Internet to facilitate communication with outside social support networks may be important to fostering support, communication, and family functioning that was impeded by pandemic-related restrictions and practices [84].

Summary

Patients who require intensive care across the age continuum may share similar challenges and opportunities at the onset, middle, and conclusions of their admission (Table 13.2). At the onset of critical illness, the neonatal and pediatric intensive

Table 13.2 Fundamentals of neonatal and pediatric intensive care unit management

	Onset of illness	During critical illness	After critical illness
Opportunities	Focus on Recovery Minority of care is futile	Family-centered care Shared decision-making	Advocacy (schools, services, etc.)
Challenges	Prognostication Uncertainty	Privacy concerns Perceived work burden Impact on teaching Legal implications	Transition to primary care Multidisciplinary follow-up clinics

care approach is grounded in an unwavering focus of recovery; attention to minimizing the impact of co-morbidities and disease chronicity and anticipation of neuroplasticity rather than early vulnerability facilitates this recovery focus. During neonatal and pediatric critical illness, family-centered care has become widely accepted. Experiences with families of infants and children suggest that thoughtfully constructed policies that foster open visitation, family partnership in rounds, family presence during procedures, family support, and communication are important and effective. In implementing such programs, one must carefully consider health care provider concerns and educational issues. Such measures may mitigate family stress, improve expectations, and smooth transitions after discharge from the ICU. The COVID-19 pandemic and restrictions to visitation and family-centered care reinforced how open visitation and family presence foster open communication and improved outcomes for children. After critical illness, experiences from both neonatology and pediatric critical care medicine suggest the need for post-ICU coordination of complex care in multidisciplinary follow-up clinics and a vital role for health care provider advocacy and partnership with legal and disability advocates to maximize resources and optimize long-term health for young survivors.

A focus on resiliency potential with an understanding that there may be potential limitations secondary to underlying disease and co-morbidities and widespread adaptation of family-centered care practices will likely have similar positive effects for critically ill adults. Adult survivors would benefit from advocacy efforts to garner services that may affect their long-term health and ability to transition out of the hospital to home. Goals for both adults and children are a return to productive lives in the community. Thus, the parallels between the neonatal, pediatric, and adult intensive care unit experiences are strong; sharing our collective experiences and operationalizing effective components of family-centered care will facilitate important advances for all ICU survivors.

In conclusion, health care teams must focus on resiliency at the onset of illness, the provision of family-centered care during illness, and an ongoing responsibility to transition care and advocate for patients after ICU discharge in order to optimize outcomes for critically ill patients across the lifespan.

References

1. Epstein D, Brill JE. A history of pediatric critical care medicine. Pediatr Res. 2005;58(5):987–96.
2. Pollack MM, Cuerdon TT, Patel KM, Ruttimann UE, Getson PR, Levetown M. Impact of quality-of-care factors on pediatric intensive care unit mortality. JAMA. 1994;272(12):941–6.
3. Pollack MM, Patel KM, Ruttimann E. Pediatric critical care training programs have a positive effect on pediatric intensive care mortality. Crit Care Med. 1997;25(10):1637–42.
4. Namachivayam P, Shann F, Shekerdemian L, Taylor A, van Sloten I, Delzoppo C, Daffey C, Butt W. Three decades of pediatric intensive care: who was admitted, what happened in intensive care, and what happened afterward. Pediatr Crit Care Med. 2010;11(5):549–55.
5. Aspesberro F, Mangione-Smith R, Zimmerman JJ. Health-related quality of life following pediatric critical illness. Intensive Care Med. 2015;41(7):1235–46.
6. Edwards JD, Houtrow AJ, Vasilevskis EE, Dudley RA, Okumura MJ. Multi-institutional profile of adults admitted to pediatric intensive care units. JAMA Pediatr. 2013;167(5):436–43.
7. Namachivayam SP, Butt W. Outcomes after pediatric critical illness: important to be accurate. Pediatr Crit Care Med. 2016;17(6):576–7.
8. Pollack MM, Holubkov R, Funai T, Clark A, Berger JT, Meert K, Newth CJ, Shanley T, Moler F, Carcillo J, et al. Pediatric intensive care outcomes: development of new morbidities during pediatric critical care. Pediatr Crit Care Med. 2014;15(9):821–7.
9. Critical Care Statistics (http://www.sccm.org/Communications/Pages/CriticalCareStats.aspx).
10. Killien EY, Keller MR, Watson RS, Hartman ME. Epidemiology of intensive care admissions for children in the US from 2001 to 2019. JAMA Pediatr. 2023;177(5):506–15.
11. Heneghan JA, Rogerson C, Goodman DM, Hall M, Kohne JG, Kane JM. Epidemiology of pediatric critical care admissions in 43 United States children's hospitals, 2014–2019. Pediatr Crit Care Med. 2022;23(7):484–92.
12. Edwards JD, Houtrow AJ, Vasilevskis EE, Rehm RS, Markovitz BP, Graham RJ, Dudley RA. Chronic conditions among children admitted to U.S. pediatric intensive care units: their prevalence and impact on risk for mortality and prolonged length of stay*. Crit Care Med. 2012;40(7):2196–203.
13. Pinto NP, Rhinesmith EW, Kim TY, Ladner PH, Pollack MM. Long-term function after pediatric critical illness: results from the survivor outcomes study. Pediatr Crit Care Med. 2017;18(3):e122–30.
14. Wunsch H, Guerra C, Barnato AE, Angus DC, Li G, Linde-Zwirble WT. Three-year outcomes for Medicare beneficiaries who survive intensive care. JAMA. 2010;303(9):849–56.
15. Meadow W, Cohen-Cutler S, Spelke B, Kim A, Plesac M, Weis K, Lagatta J. The prediction and cost of futility in the NICU. Acta Paediatr. 2012;101(4):397–402.
16. Meadow W, Pohlman A, Frain L, Ren Y, Kress JP, Teuteberg W, Hall J. Power and limitations of daily prognostications of death in the medical intensive care unit. Crit Care Med. 2011;39(3):474–9.
17. Marcin JP, Pretzlaff RK, Pollack MM, Patel KM, Ruttimann UE. Certainty and mortality prediction in critically ill children. J Med Ethics. 2004;30(3):304–7.
18. Marcin JP, Pollack MM, Patel KM, Sprague BM, Ruttimann UE. Prognostication and certainty in the pediatric intensive care unit. Pediatrics. 1999;104(4 Pt 1):868–73.
19. Sachdeva RC, Jefferson LS, Coss-Bu J, Brody BA. Resource consumption and the extent of futile care among patients in a pediatric intensive care unit setting. J Pediatr. 1996;128(6):742–7.
20. Goh AY, Mok Q. Identifying futility in a paediatric critical care setting: a prospective observational study. Arch Dis Child. 2001;84(3):265–8.
21. Keim G, Hsu JY, Pinto NP, McSherry ML, Gula AL, Christie JD, Yehya N. Readmission rates after acute respiratory distress syndrome in children. JAMA Netw Open. 2023;6(9):e2330774.
22. Edwards JD, Lucas AR, Boscardin WJ, Dudley RA. Repeated critical illness and unplanned readmissions within 1 year to PICUs. Crit Care Med. 2017;45(8):1276–84.
23. Anderson V, Spencer-Smith M, Wood A. Do children really recover better? Neurobehavioural plasticity after early brain insult. Brain. 2011;134(Pt 8):2197–221.

24. Mundkur N. Neuroplasticity in children. Indian J Pediatr. 2005;72(10):855–7.
25. Sterken C, Lemiere J, Van den Berghe G, Mesotten D. Neurocognitive development after pediatric heart surgery. Pediatrics. 2016;137(6)
26. Maley JH, Brewster I, Mayoral I, Siruckova R, Adams S, McGraw KA, Piech AA, Detsky M, Mikkelsen ME. Resilience in survivors of critical illness in the context of the survivors' experience and recovery. Ann Am Thorac Soc. 2016;13(8):1351–60.
27. Charney DS. Psychobiological mechanisms of resilience and vulnerability: implications for successful adaptation to extreme stress. Am J Psychiatry. 2004;161(2):195–216.
28. Connor KM. Assessment of resilience in the aftermath of trauma. J Clin Psychiatry. 2006;67(Suppl. 2):46–9.
29. Institute of Medicine (US) Committee on Quality of Health Care in America. Crossing the quality chasm: a new health system for the 21st century. Washington (DC): National Academies Press (US); 2001.
30. Davidson JE, Powers K, Hedayat KM, Tieszen M, Kon AA, Shepard E, Spuhler V, Todres ID, Levy M, Barr J, et al. Clinical practice guidelines for support of the family in the patient-centered intensive care unit: American College of Critical Care Medicine Task Force 2004–2005. Crit Care Med. 2007;35(2):605–22.
31. Committee On Hospital C, Institute For P, Family-Centered C. Patient- and family-centered care and the pediatrician's role. Pediatrics. 2012;129(2):394–404.
32. Davidson JE, Aslakson RA, Long AC, Puntillo KA, Kross EK, Hart J, Cox CE, Wunsch H, Wickline MA, Nunnally ME, et al. Guidelines for family-centered care in the neonatal, pediatric, and adult ICU. Crit Care Med. 2017;45(1):103–28.
33. Smith AB, Hefley GC, Anand KJ. Parent bed spaces in the PICU: effect on parental stress. Pediatr Nurs. 2007;33(3):215–21.
34. Meert KL, Clark J, Eggly S. Family-centered care in the pediatric intensive care unit. Pediatr Clin N Am. 2013;60(3):761–72.
35. Stickney CA, Ziniel SI, Brett MS, Truog RD. Family participation during intensive care unit rounds: goals and expectations of parents and health care providers in a tertiary pediatric intensive care unit. J Pediatr. 2014;165(6):1245–51. e1241
36. Aronson PL, Yau J, Helfaer MA, Morrison W. Impact of family presence during pediatric intensive care unit rounds on the family and medical team. Pediatrics. 2009;124(4):1119–25.
37. American Heart Association in Collaboration with the International Liaison Committee on Resuscitation. Guidelines 2000 for cardiopulmonary resuscitation and emergency cardiovascular care. Part 2: Ethical aspects of CPR and ECC. Circulation. 2000;102(Suppl. 8):I12–21.
38. Powers KS, Rubenstein JS. Family presence during invasive procedures in the pediatric intensive care unit: a prospective study. Arch Pediatr Adolesc Med. 1999;153(9):955–8.
39. Robinson SM, Mackenzie-Ross S, Campbell Hewson GL, Egleston CV, Prevost AT. Psychological effect of witnessed resuscitation on bereaved relatives. Lancet. 1998;352(9128):614–7.
40. Henderson DP, Knapp JF. Report of the National Consensus Conference on Family presence during pediatric cardiopulmonary resuscitation and procedures. J Emerg Nurs. 2006;32(1):23–9.
41. Pye S, Kane J, Jones A. Parental presence during pediatric resuscitation: the use of simulation training for cardiac intensive care nurses. J Spec Pediatr Nurs. 2010;15(2):172–5.
42. Fegran L, Helseth S, Fagermoen MS. A comparison of mothers' and fathers' experiences of the attachment process in a neonatal intensive care unit. J Clin Nurs. 2008;17(6):810–6.
43. Rodrigues SM, Shin SS, Pinto MD, Bounds DT, Terry J, Burton CW. Parenting expectations, NICU experiences, and maternal psychological outcomes: an exploratory mixed-methods study. Adv Neonatal Care. 2024;24(2):195–207.
44. Gorsky KG, Butala S, House M, Moon C, Calvetti S, Khando T, Kipke M, Lakshmanan A. Uncertainty and the NICU experience: a qualitative evaluation of family and provider perspectives. Children. 2023;10(11):1745.
45. Board R, Ryan-Wenger N. Long-term effects of pediatric intensive care unit hospitalization on families with young children. Heart Lung. 2002;31(1):53–66.

46. Franck LS, Oulton K, Nderitu S, Lim M, Fang S, Kaiser A. Parent involvement in pain management for NICU infants: a randomized controlled trial. Pediatrics. 2011;128(3):510–8.
47. Bastani F, Abadi TA, Haghani H. Effect of Family-centered care on improving parental satisfaction and reducing readmission among premature infants: a randomized controlled trial. J Clin Diagn Res. 2015;9(1):SC04–8.
48. Zurca AD, Fisher KR, Flor RJ, Gonzalez-Marques CD, Wang J, Cheng YI, October TW. Communication with limited English-proficient families in the PICU. Hosp Pediatr. 2017;7(1):9–15.
49. Curtis JR, White DB. Practical guidance for evidence-based ICU family conferences. Chest. 2008;134(4):835–43.
50. Michelson KN, Emanuel L, Carter A, Brinkman P, Clayman ML, Frader J. Pediatric intensive care unit family conferences: one mode of communication for discussing end-of-life care decisions. Pediatr Crit Care Med. 2011;12(6):e336–43.
51. Colville GA, Cream PR, Kerry SM. Do parents benefit from the offer of a follow-up appointment after their child's admission to intensive care? An exploratory randomised controlled trial. Intensive Crit Care Nurs. 2010;26(3):146–53.
52. Jackson K, Ternestedt BM, Schollin J. From alienation to familiarity: experiences of mothers and fathers of preterm infants. J Adv Nurs. 2003;43(2):120–9.
53. Garfield CF, Lee Y, Kim HN. Paternal and maternal concerns for their very low-birth-weight infants transitioning from the NICU to home. J Perinat Neonatal Nurs. 2014;28(4):305–12.
54. Horwitz SM, Storfer-Isser A, Kerker BD, Lilo E, Leibovitz A, St John N, Shaw RJ. A model for the development of mothers' perceived vulnerability of preterm infants. J Dev Behav Pediatr. 2015;36(5):371–80.
55. Stefana A, Lavelli M. Parental engagement and early interactions with preterm infants during the stay in the neonatal intensive care unit: protocol of a mixed-method and longitudinal study. BMJ Open. 2017;7(2):e013824.
56. Enke C, Oliva YHA, Miedaner F, Roth B, Woopen C. Communicating with parents in neonatal intensive care units: the impact on parental stress. Patient Educ Couns. 2017;100(4):710–9.
57. Boss RD, Donohue PK, Larson SM, Arnold RM, Roter DL. Family conferences in the neonatal ICU: observation of communication dynamics and contributions. Pediatr Crit Care Med. 2016;17(3):223–30.
58. Rossman B, Greene MM, Meier PP. The role of peer support in the development of maternal identity for "NICU moms". J Obstet Gynecol Neonatal Nurs. 2015;44(1):3–16.
59. Labrie NHM, van Veenendaal NR, Ludolph RA, Ket JCF, van der Schoor SRD, van Kempen A. Effects of parent-provider communication during infant hospitalization in the NICU on parents: a systematic review with meta-synthesis and narrative synthesis. Patient Educ Couns. 2021;104(7):1526–52.
60. Huenink E, Porterfield S. Parent support programs and coping mechanisms in NICU parents. Adv Neonatal Care. 2017;17(2):E10–8.
61. Varni JW, Seid M, Rode CA. The PedsQL: measurement model for the pediatric quality of life inventory. Med Care. 1999;37(2):126–39.
62. Azoulay E, Pochard F, Chevret S, Jourdain M, Bornstain C, Wernet A, Cattaneo I, Annane D, Brun F, Bollaert PE, et al. Impact of a family information leaflet on effectiveness of information provided to family members of intensive care unit patients: a multicenter, prospective, randomized, controlled trial. Am J Respir Crit Care Med. 2002;165(4):438–42.
63. Jones C, Backman C, Capuzzo M, Egerod I, Flaatten H, Granja C, Rylander C, Griffiths RD, Group R. Intensive care diaries reduce new onset post traumatic stress disorder following critical illness: a randomised, controlled trial. Crit Care. 2010;14(5):R168.
64. Andrews B, Myers P, Osterhout P, Pellerite M, Zimmerman A, Msall M. NICU follow-up care: the development and advocacy perspectives. NeoReviews. 2014;15(8):e336–43.
65. Bockli K, Andrews B, Pellerite M, Meadow W. Trends and challenges in United States neonatal intensive care units follow-up clinics. J Perinatol. 2014;34(1):71–4.
66. Marlow N, Wolke D, Bracewell MA, Samara M, Group EPS. Neurologic and developmental disability at six years of age after extremely preterm birth. N Engl J Med. 2005;352(1):9–19.

67. Doyle LW, Anderson PJ, Battin M, Bowen JR, Brown N, Callanan C, Campbell C, Chandler S, Cheong J, Darlow B, et al. Long term follow up of high risk children: who, why and how? BMC Pediatr. 2014;14:279.
68. Wilson-Costello D, Friedman H, Minich N, Fanaroff AA, Hack M. Improved survival rates with increased neurodevelopmental disability for extremely low birth weight infants in the 1990s. Pediatrics. 2005;115(4):997–1003.
69. Saigal S. Follow-up of very low birthweight babies to adolescence. In: Seminars in neonatology: 2000, vol. 5. Elsevier; 2000. p. 107–18.
70. Litt JS, Edwards EM, Lainwala S, Mercier C, Montgomery A, O'Reilly D, Rhein L, Woythaler M, Hartman T. Optimizing high-risk infant follow-up in nonresearch-based paradigms: the New England follow-up network. Pediatr Qual Safety. 2020;5(3):e287.
71. Broyles RS, Tyson JE, Heyne ET, Heyne RJ, Hickman JF, Swint M, Adams SS, West LA, Pomeroy N, Hicks PJ. Comprehensive follow-up care and life-threatening illnesses among high-risk infants: a randomized controlled trial. JAMA. 2000;284(16):2070–6.
72. Williams CN, Hall TA, Francoeur C, Kurz J, Rasmussen L, Hartman ME, O'meara AI, Ferguson NM, Fink EL, Walker T. Continuing care for critically ill children beyond hospital discharge: current state of follow-up. Hosp Pediatr. 2022;12(4):359–93.
73. Lipkin PH, Okamoto J, Council on Children with D, Council on School H. The individuals with disabilities education act (IDEA) for children with special educational needs. Pediatrics. 2015;136(6):e1650–62.
74. Raju TN, Pemberton VL, Saigal S, Blaisdell CJ, Moxey-Mims M, Buist S. Adults born preterm conference S, discussants: long-term healthcare outcomes of preterm birth: an executive summary of a conference sponsored by the National Institutes of Health. J Pediatr. 2017;181:309–18. e301
75. Redd L, Belcher R, Dotts B, Andrews B. A silver lining for neonatal intensive care (NICU) graduates: coordinated services from 0–6 years. Int Public Health J. 2018;10(3)
76. Fiest KM, Krewulak KD, Hiploylee C, Bagshaw SM, Burns KE, Cook DJ, Fowler RA, Kredentser MS, Niven DJ, Olafson K. An environmental scan of visitation policies in Canadian intensive care units during the first wave of the COVID-19 pandemic. Can J Anaesth. 2021;68(10):1474.
77. Vance AJ, Duy J, Laventhal N, Iwashyna TJ, Costa DK. Visitor guidelines in US Children's hospitals during COVID-19. Hosp Pediatr. 2021;11(6):e83–9.
78. Foster JR, Lee LA, Seabrook JA, Ryan M, Betts LJ, Burgess SA, Slumkoski C, Walls M, Garros D. Family presence in Canadian PICUs during the COVID-19 pandemic: a mixed-methods environmental scan of policy and practice. Can Med Assoc Open Access J. 2022;10(3):E622–32.
79. Kostenzer J, von Rosenstiel-Pulver C, Hoffmann J, Walsh A, Mader S, Zimmermann LJI. Parents' experiences regarding neonatal care during the COVID-19 pandemic: country-specific findings of a multinational survey. BMJ Open. 2022;12(4):e056856.
80. Giordano V, Fuiko R, Witting A, Unterasinger L, Steinbauer P, Bajer J, Farr A, Hoehl S, Deindl P, Olischar M, et al. The impact of pandemic restrictive visiting policies on infant wellbeing in a NICU. Pediatr Res. 2023;94(3):1098–103.
81. Balistreri KA, Lim PS, Tager JB, Davies WH, Karst JS, Scanlon MC, Rothschild CB. "It has added another layer of stress": COVID-19's impact in the PICU. Hosp Pediatr. 2021;11(10):e226–34.
82. Lessa ARD, Bitercourt VN, Crestani F, Andrade GRH, Costa CAD, Garcia PCR. Impact of the COVID-19 pandemic on patient-and family-centered care and on the mental health of health care workers, patients, and families. Front Pediatr. 2022;10:880686.
83. Vance AJ, Malin KJ, Miller J, Shuman CJ, Moore TA, Benjamin A. Parents' pandemic NICU experience in the United States: a qualitative study. BMC Pediatr. 2021;21(1):558.
84. Camporesi A, Zanin A, Kanaris C, Gemma M, Lanziotti VS. Impact of COVID-19 pandemic on pediatric intensive care unit (PICU) visiting policies: a worldwide survey. J Pediatr Intensive Care. 2021;
85. Tedesco B, Borgese G, Cracco U, Casarotto P, Zanin A. Challenges to delivering family-centred care during the coronavirus pandemic: voices of Italian paediatric intensive care unit nurses. Nurs Crit Care. 2021;26:10.

Chapter 14
Child Life in the Adult ICU: Including the Youngest Members of the Family

Jaime E. Bruce and Kathleen McCue

Child Life in the Adult ICU: Including the Youngest Members of the Family

Communication issues, decision-making challenges, negative psychosocial sequelae, and traumatic grief are all components of Family Intensive Care Unit Syndrome. In order to document both the depth and intensity of this syndrome and to plan for possible ways to ameliorate its devastating impact, it is necessary to consider the needs and reactions of children as well as adults in the family of the intensive care patient. Child life, as an applied psychosocial service, has been available to pediatric patients and their family members on a small scale since the early 1900s. However, it was only in the 1950s and 1960s that the impact of health care encounters on children's developmental, social, and emotional needs became well-documented in books and articles. In 1982, an organization called Child Life Council came into existence, and individuals who worked to provide for those needs unified under the title of child life specialists. This organization is now The Association of Child Life Professionals, and it is the only group that establishes standards, educational requirements, and certification for professionals in the field of child life.

This chapter first briefly describes the profession of child life, including philosophy, mission, training, credentials, and the profession's role within the pediatric

J. E. Bruce (✉)
Department of Medicine, Health and Society, Vanderbilt University, Nashville, TN, USA

Department of Child Life and Volunteer Services, Monroe Carell Jr. Children's Hospital at Vanderbilt, Nashville, TN, USA
e-mail: jaime.e.bruce@vanderbilt.edu

K. McCue
The Gathering Place, Cleveland, OH, USA

© The Author(s), under exclusive license to Springer Nature Switzerland AG 2025

A. J. Vance et al. (eds.), *Families in the Intensive Care Unit*,
https://doi.org/10.1007/978-3-031-83786-9_14

environment. The more recent movement of child life into the adult medical world will be documented, with special emphasis on child life services when families of adult patients are experiencing highly challenging medical events, such as trauma, complex and debilitating illness or injury, or end-of-life. Child life currently provides a wide range of services to these families, especially to the children in the family who are impacted by an adult's critical medical status. Finally, specific descriptions of the role and function of a child life specialist in an adult intensive care unit will be provided, along with tools to assist other professionals in meeting the needs of the expanded family, including any infants, children, and adolescents who are impacted by the hospitalization of an adult in the challenging environment of an intensive care unit.

Philosophy and Standards for Child Life

The Association of Child Life Professionals (ACLP) is constantly working to clarify and modernize the mission and vision of the profession. The current Mission Statement [1] is: *We, as child life professionals, help infants, children, youth, and families cope with the stress and uncertainty of illness, injury, and treatment. We provide evidence-based, developmentally appropriate interventions including therapeutic play, preparation, and education to reduce fear, anxiety and pain.* In a portion of the Vision Statement [1], the settings in which child life specialists may provide their services are expanded to state: *The philosophy and practice of child life will be applicable to any health care setting and transferable to other community settings or situations in which the potential for infants, children, and youth to cope, learn, and master is placed at risk.*

A significant level of training and skill is necessary to provide the services needed for at-risk populations in any of these settings. In order to ensure that a minimal level of skill has been acquired by the incoming child life specialist, educational and credentialing standards have also been set by ACLP. This skill level is measured by the requirements established by the Child Life Certification Commission, the ACLP, and a private testing agency. At this point in time, a bachelor's degree in any field of study, the completion of academic courses covering specific curricula, plus a full semester clinical internship are the basic requirements. To achieve certification, it is also necessary to pass a comprehensive written certifying examination. When those standards are met, the individual is eligible to hold the title of Certified Child Life Specialist (CCLS). However, the majority of child life specialists have continued their education to achieve a master's degree or higher. At this point in time, there is no state or national licensure in the United States for a professional in child life.

Much of the early child life programming focused on addressing and minimizing the negative emotional and developmental consequences of an inpatient hospital stay for a child. However, during the late 1900s, child life programming expanded to include emergency services, all aspects of a child's surgical experience, outpatient and specialty clinics, pediatric hospice and palliative care, and others. Even private pediatric medical offices and dental offices found value in the utilization of child life services for their stressed or challenged patients and families. Children today must face a wide array of difficult and potentially traumatic life events, and often parents and other responsible adults are not sure of the best ways to help and support the children for whom they are responsible. Child life specialists can, as a result of their training and experience, guide both children and adults to positive coping and successful outcomes.

As a result of the demonstrated success of child life professionals in the pediatric arena, the American Academy of Pediatrics has developed a policy statement on child life services. The most recent revision of the statement may be found in Pediatrics [2]. It includes strong recommendations for the inclusion of child life services across many different settings and concludes: *Child life services should be delivered as part of an integrated patient- and family-centered model of care and included as a quality indicator in the delivery of services for children and families in health care settings.*

Only in the last two decades has child life begun to consistently contribute to efforts to empirically document the value of various services and interventions. These services, skills, and competencies will be briefly reviewed later in this section. However, as early as 1988, a comprehensive study evaluated several dimensions of the impact of child life programming.

The evaluation by Wolfer et al. [3] of a model child life program indicated less emotional distress, better overall coping during hospitalization, a clearer understanding of procedures, and a more positive physical recovery for children enrolled in the study sample. Other, more recent studies [4–9], have found that child life interventions in specialty areas are correlated to lessening of children's fears and producing higher parent satisfaction ratings of the total care experience.

Child Life professionals are included in the larger Family-Centered Care movement. Family-Centered Care is an approach to health care that values partnership with patients and families in all aspects of care. Child life has been instrumental in supporting the inclusion of "emotional safety" as a major component of Family-Centered Care. Concern for the well-being of the entire family includes but is not limited to the promotion and understanding of emotional safety as it pertains to gender, race, culture, and spirituality.

Child Life Competencies

The Association of Child Life Professionals denote the following five areas of competency in which the certified child life specialist should be proficient: (A) care of infants, children, youth, and families; (B) professional responsibility; (C) education and supervision; (D) research fundamentals; and (E) administration.

For the purposes of this chapter, special attention will be paid to the two competencies that most frequently are connected to child life work with children of adult patients. This includes competency A (care of infants, children, youth, and families) which speaks to the clinical services of the child life specialist and competency B (professional responsibility) which reflects the interdisciplinary functions of child life.

Care of Infants, Children, Youth, and Families

The primary clinical role of the child life specialist in the health care setting is the direct care of patients and families. The child life professional utilizes knowledge based on theories of human development, family systems and play to address the psychosocial and developmental needs of patients of all ages and family members. Through formal and informal assessment techniques, child life is tasked with creating a plan of care that incorporates developmentally supportive interventions geared toward preparing the patient and family for the health care experience.

Specialists are trained in communicating information about medical diagnoses and procedures in accurate but minimally threatening language that is manageable for children and adolescents.

Through a practice known as psychological preparation, child life specialists are able to describe medical procedures to patients and family members of varying ages, backgrounds, and levels of health care experience. They have a basic knowledge of medical terminology, typical treatment plans, and clinical procedures that allow preparation techniques to best meet the needs of each member of the family. Sequential photographs of procedures may be utilized to illustrate what the patient and family will experience. The specialist will employ his or her knowledge of varying developmental levels and cognitive abilities to identify the appropriate combination of tools to assist each individual in the family in gaining an understanding of the experience.Throughout preparation activities, the specialist will be observing both verbal and nonverbal cues to ascertain points of distress. When distress is noted, the specialist adapts the teaching to the individual's level of tolerance. A key component of psychological preparation is instruction on coping strategies that will help the child or adult through stressful health care situations. Positive coping strategies such as stress reduction techniques, relaxation exercises, and distraction will promote a sense of control and feeling of being a participant in the care plan.

Professional Responsibility

The child life specialist is an integral part of the interdisciplinary team with a unique skill set and knowledge base. In this role, the specialist is charged with the responsibility to practice within "the scope of professional and personal knowledge and skill base" [1] while communicating and advocating for the needs of patients and families. The child life professional coordinates information regarding assessments and care plans with other members of the health care team, especially psychosocial team members, through documentation in the medical record as well as participation in clinical rounds and family care conferences.

Child Life in the Pediatric Intensive Care Unit

The Pediatric Intensive Care Unit (PICU) provides care to the most acutely ill pediatric patients. The patients in this setting are admitted for life-altering and life-threatening diagnoses such as a traumatic brain injury, complex genetic disorders, and congenital heart defects. Many of these patients require life-sustaining medical interventions including intubation and sedation rendering them unable to benefit from the usual patient support activities provided by child life on less acute units. However, when patients are awake and alert, Child Life Professionals may provide developmentally appropriate diagnosis education, psychosocial preparation for medical interventions, and therapeutic play opportunities.

When patients are not in a clinical position to participate in these types of direct activities, psychosocial support can continue to be provided to

- parents,
- other adult family member,
- siblings of the patient,
- peers and other members of the community.

When a child or adolescent is admitted to the PICU, families often request guidance and support in sharing medical information and addressing psychosocial issues for siblings, other family members, and friends. Child life professionals offer diagnosis education, psychosocial preparation for bedside visits, bereavement support, and memory-making activities.

Child life professionals are consulted to assess the multisensory environment of a PICU patient room to ensure it provides a family-centered physical setting to promote comfort, familiarity, and encouragement toward wellness. It is known that 5% of PICU patients do not survive their admission [10]. Together with other members of the psychosocial support team including but not limited to chaplaincy and social work, child life specialists play an integral role in guiding families through the process and grief of losing a child.

Child Life in the Adult Intensive Care Unit

In a predictable transition from pediatric to adult health care, child life professionals began developing programs providing services to the children and family members of seriously ill adults. In the 1990s, many child life specialists worked in large, tertiary-level hospitals and although assigned to pediatrics, found themselves responding to requests for assistance from adult care providers. Often these requests were initiated as a result of highly distressed or emotional children visiting a seriously ill adult inpatient. (For suggestions of ways that health care staff can further assist the children of adult patients, see Fig. 14.1) Because staff for adult patients often had no training or resources to assist these children, they reached out to the one professional group available that was specifically trained to deal with such issues. Very little literature was available on this topic, and a child life specialist ([11], rev. 2011) published the first book guiding both parents and professionals in dealing with a parent's illness. A publication by a physician [12] became available next, addressing the needs of children who have a parent with cancer. More recently, a pilot program [13] described child life consultation with staff and families when a parent is seriously ill. In this cohort, 25% of cancer patients had underage children in the home, and between 3.5% and 5% of children under the age of 18 experienced the death of a parent.

One of the most common concerns of adult family members when a parent is seriously ill is how to help the children in the family. Although most research has involved cancer patients, there are data on both the short and long-term negative impact of serious illness among adults on children. Phillips and Prezio [14] and Phillips et al. [15] summarize this literature and describe an intervention program for families facing adult cancer. The program utilized child life specialists and resulted in significant amelioration of children's issues, including improved communication skills, reduced anxiety, increased feelings of security, and improved

When talking to parents or family members about children:

- Determine what children in the life of the patient might be impacted by hospitalization
- Ask open-ended questions about the children; their knowledge, emotional status, etc.
- Find out exactly what concerns the adult has about the children in the family
- Stress the importance of honesty and age-appropriate information to children
- Teach parents signs to watch for that may indicate problematic reactions of children
- Offer visitation and other services as available at your hospital
- Identify resources for children beyond the hospital, and provide written material

When interacting with children directly:

- Use language that is appropriate for the age and developmental level of the child.
- Find out from the child what he/she knows and thinks about the medical situation.
- Talk about emotions and reactions as much as about facts.
- Help the child to talk! Ask him or her about themselves, their friends, school, pets, etc.
- Use play and art to illustrate information or to allow expression of emotion.
- Explain what will be happening in the most immediate time frame, and plan to add additional information as the medical situation evolves and changes.
- Provide opportunities for diversional play and art. Have simple materials like markers and paper, small toys, something for building, something for hugging.
- Assure the child that the parent is being well cared for and you are all doing everything you can to help with recovery. However, be very careful about saying anything that could be construed later by the child as a lie.
- Avoid overwhelming children with too many facts at one time.

Fig. 14.1 Tips for hospital professionals to help children of adult patients

school performance. A pilot program reported by Cross and Bruce [16] describes the outcome of adding child life services to adult intensive care units and reports a high level of both family and staff agreement that child life specialists had a positive impact on parent's and family's ability to cope. Literature on needs and guidelines for child visitation to the adult ICU was summarized in this chapter.

At the present time, there are child life specialists providing interventions to adult patients, their children, and other family members in many hospitals. The services may be provided on a consultation basis, or child life may be an integral component of an adult patient unit with a dedicated child life professional available at all times in that particular service. Child life is most often found in intensive care services, cancer centers, and palliative care and hospice services. The remainder of this chapter will focus on the needs of children of adult patients in the intensive care unit, the role that child life can play in assisting these families, and tools for other care providers to support children in critical care environment.

Before going into specific detail regarding the services provided by child life in the adult intensive care unit, it would be useful to give an overview of the different categories of interventions that are available to patients, families, and the health care team. Obviously, each service category is individualized to the family situation in which it is provided. All considered services are offered in a collaborative manner with the other members of the health care team and are based on the issues and needs that are identified by the family. The following list (Fig. 14.2) provides a summary of general interventions available by child life professionals. To better

- Explanation of the medical situation to children and other family members
- Ongoing support for children and family members during acute hospitalization, with special attention to maintenance of normal routines and activities, such as school, work and family relationships
- Assistance to adult family members in dealing with high stress behaviors and other problematic behaviors in children
- Direct work with children through play, therapeutic art and counseling to manage emotional reactions to the intense medical situation
- Plans and preparation for children/family visitation and support during such visiting episodes. See Appendix B for further information on visitation
- Preparation for status change of patient, such as procedures, change in appearance, change in mental status
- Preparation of children and family members for patient discharge, especially when discharge includes significant change in family function or the patient's role in the family
- Acknowledgement of and assistance in planning family milestone events, such as birthdays and holidays
- Legacy work with patients and other adult caregivers
- Wide range of services and interventions to assist all family members, especially children, with end-of-life situations.
- Consultation regarding child/family oriented physical environment in the ICU, and the impact of sensory experiences on children
- Provision of appropriate resources, both within the hospital and after discharge or death, to continue to assist children and families in coping with the ICU experience

Fig. 14.2 child life interventions and services in an adult intensive care unit

conceptualize these interventions provided by child life specialists in the adult ICU, two examples of patient and family scenarios are introduced below. The remainder of this section will describe in detail interventions relevant to each case.

Patient and Family Scenario 1

Mr. Smith is a 57-year-old male admitted to the neuro intensive care unit with a traumatic brain injury sustained in a motor vehicle crash (MVC). His prognosis at this time is unclear, and he remains intubated and sedated. Prior to this accident, Mr. Smith was an active and healthy husband, father, and grandfather. He has a wife and two sons ages 10 and 12 years old. From a previous marriage, he has a 31-year-old daughter who is mother to his 3-year-old granddaughter. Mr. Smith provides child care to his granddaughter 3 days a week while her mother works. In addition to his immediate family, Mr. Smith is a beloved member of the local little league program and has been a volunteer baseball coach for many years.

Patient and Family Scenario 2

Mrs. Garcia is a 38-year-old female admitted to the medical intensive care unit with complications and severe pain related to advancing metastatic ovarian cancer. She is on heavy pain medications and has limited energy to engage with family or staff. Mrs. Garcia along with her husband and 8-year-old daughter immigrated to the United States less than a year ago. Mr. Garcia presents as a distraught and overwhelmed husband and father trying to balance work, his daughter, and time at the hospital. He has expressed reluctance to share information about his wife's condition with his daughter, although she has been present at the bedside during this and previous hospitalizations. Mr. and Mrs. Garcia speak primarily Spanish, but their daughter speaks both Spanish and English.

Child Life Services to Adult Family Members

When child life provides services in the pediatric arena, the initial contacts are typically with children themselves even when a family member is present. However, when working with the children of adult patients, the first steps in assessment always involve some discussion with an available parent or other adult family member. In Family Scenario 1, the initial assessment would reveal the wide range of children impacted by Mr. Smith's injury and hospitalization.This initial assessment process by child life would focus on the developmental level and current needs and understanding of each child related to the health situation of Mr. Smith. Mrs. Smith would probably be the primary informant regarding the needs of her two sons and could assist with any additional contacts needed in relationship to the other children in Mr. Smith's life, specifically the children he coaches in Little League.

This initial assessment with appropriate adult family members is the cornerstone of the planning for services for both adults and children by child life. Information to children about Mr. Smith's diagnosis and prognosis, plans for the children's visitation, and interventions related to specific emotional, social, and behavioral issues the children may develop would all be dependent on collaboration with adult family members and with the health care team.When a parent is seriously ill or injured, one of a well parent's first concerns is "How do I tell my children about this, and what do I say?" Child life is in a unique role to provide information to adults in order to empower them to appropriately inform their children about a critical medical situation in the family. Rather than asking a parent "How are your children?" which usually elicits a response of "Fine," child life will ask such open-ended questions as "What have you told your children?", "What were their emotional reactions?", and "What specific questions did they have?". It will be very important to know if Mr. Smith's two pre-teen sons tend to be significantly anxious, if they show their emotions openly, if they have a good social support network, if they have had any recent losses or negative medical experiences themselves, and if they are experiencing success or problems in school and other life activities. Only a parent can provide this information, and it will guide the path of future family interventions, to both the adults and the children.

Sometimes, distraught parents and other adult family members need assistance in talking to children about the medical situation. Fear and distress can negatively impact providing an accurate, supportive message to children. These tough conversations can happen at the hospital, via phone or Internet connections, or occasionally in person in the family's home. Child life often functions in the role of support person to assist the parent with the words and questions needed to enhance a child's ability to cope. Mr. Smith's two sons might accompany their mother into the hospital for a meeting with child life, social work, pastoral care, nursing, and/or other medical staff, to receive the details of their father's condition. While it is likely not appropriate for the Little League team to visit the ICU, child life could provide the script needed for coaches or other fathers to explain the situation in a manner that would reduce the children's anxiety. The mother of the 3-year-old granddaughter would need a special plan based on the developmental level of her child, in order to maximize understanding. In all these situations, child life would provide parents and family care givers with written information on helping these children emerge from this experience with trust and safety intact, and with the knowledge and coping skills to face difficult times and proceed through them successfully.

There is probably nothing more distressing to adults than the knowledge that a life-threatening disease in self or spouse is progressing, and that their children may have to grow up without the love, support, and teaching that the parent assumed they would be present to provide. In Family Scenario 2, Mr. Garcia is in an unimaginable state of angst, trying to balance his family responsibilities. Just as in the situation with Mrs. Smith, a thorough assessment of his daughter's knowledge and emotional status will guide the next steps in child life intervention. It may be possible and preferable to include Mrs. Garcia in this assessment if the medical situation allows to get a sense of her wishes related to her daughter. Building a trusting relationship with Mr. Garcia will hopefully reduce the barriers that might interfere with providing the daughter with the support and education she needs.

In situations of advancing disease, it is important for child life to help parents learn how to be both honest and hopeful with children at the same time. Many parents are afraid to allow children to think about a negative outcome or a death when an adult family member is critically ill (see Fig. 14.3). However, the practice of child life, based on both child development theory and empirical data, makes it clear that children proceed through stress, trauma and loss best when prepared for probably outcomes, even sad outcomes. Helping Mr. Garcia to understand that his daughter will cope best and move forward in her life best if he can be honest with her now is foundational to working with this family. Case examples, written material, and evenencouragement from other parents with similar experiences may help Mr. Garcia allow more open communication with his daughter.

Birth - 2 years	Beginning awareness of separation
2 years – 4 years	Beginning cognitive awareness; minimal emotional response, usually imitation of adults
4 years – 6 years	Increasing cognitive understanding; beginning personal emotions, including denial, empathy
6 years – 9 years	Understands fully, and is fascinated; strong emotional reactions, worries and wants to avoid
9 years – 12 years	Acceptance, working on spiritual meanings
12+ years	Personal responses developing; emotions may be open or hidden; may reject family religion

Children's Responses to Death by Developmental Level

Infants/Toddlers

- Cannot "understand" a family crisis cognitively
- Will show distress behaviorally
- Respond to emotional distress in adult care givers
- Distress behaviors often follow changes in routine

School age children

- Performance decline, especially at school
- Compensatory behavior, being "extra" good
- Mood discrepancy, irritability, unpredictable
- Behavior change or problem
- Psychosomatic complaints

Preschoolers

- Withdrawal
- Anxious attachment
- Denial
- Thematic Play
- Fears
- Regression

Adolescents

- Acting out, especially with drugs or alcohol
- Self-criticism and low self-esteem
- Sudden or unusual school problems
- Misdirected anger
- Loss of interest in usual activities

Fig. 14.3 Children's developmental understanding of death by age

Another frequent task of child life in end-of-life situations is to assist either the ill or well parent with plans for legacy activities. Planning connections and messages for children even after a parent has died is painful but important work. Although very emotional, most parents find peace and comfort in preparing some sort of legacy for their children, in the event that they do not survive. These messages can take the form of cards or letters, video and audio recordings, gifts, instruction lists, and more. Mrs. Garcia may be in a position to begin this process and may need a support person by her side as she decides what messages she wants to leave for her daughter.

In summary, child life services to adult family members of an adult ICU patient always begin with a thorough assessment of the children involved. Trusting relationships with the patient, when possible, and with well family members will open the door to interventions with the children. Providing parents and others with the information they need on children's reactions to acute medical situations may empower parents to work with their children themselves, or parents may request that child life assist or take the lead in educating and supporting the children of an adult intensive care unit patient. As the critical care experience unfolds and changes, child life will monitor the family and be available to assist in helping children manage any new issues that may arise. If end-of-life becomes a reality for the family, child life can begin working on issues of grief and loss, can provide useful materials, and can make community referrals for continued support for the children in the family.

Child Life Services to Child Family Members

After a child life specialist has completed an assessment with the adult family members and the choice is made to involve children in further intervention, the specialist would begin the process of coordinating with other members of the medical and psychosocial team. It is important to take into consideration such factors as the patient's current medical status, any planned medical procedures, the atmosphere of the unit, and available space to meet with children. In one university medical setting [16] a child life specialist developed a "Safety Assessment" that included key stakeholders from the ICU as well as the adult family members and children related to the patient. This practice was created to ensure optimal safety and dignity for the patient, child, and unit. If for example, the unit was running a code in the vicinity of the patient at the time of the scheduled visit, the key stakeholders would make plans to postpone the visit to a less stressful time on the unit.

Often the first intervention involves a visit to the hospital by the children. This visit may or may not include seeing the patient. It is vital that a plan is in place for where the initial meeting will occur, who will be present, and what goals the family has for the visit. A specialist would identify a neutral place, preferably outside of the patient's room and away from medical equipment and personnel, and attempt to create a low-stress environment. The specialist may bring developmentally appropriate activities such as art supplies or toys to the room as both a means of cognitive and emotional assessment as well as a visual cue that normalizes the hospital setting. To begin the intervention, the child life specialist would build rapport with the child while simultaneously assessing his or level of comfort, anxiety, and knowledge of the reason for this visit. Often child life specialists will introduce their role as similar to a teacher, but one who teaches children about medical experiences and having a family member in the hospital. "Tell me what you already know about why you are here today," or "tell me what brought your father to the hospital," the specialist might ask. While the specialist likely already has this information from an adult family member, the child's perception of the visit is often different, and it is beneficial to hear the child's point of view. For more information on preparing children for a visit to an ICU, see Fig. 14.4.

From: How to Help Children Through a Parent's Serious Illness Kathleen McCue, MA, LSW, CCLS

General Rule: If the child wants to visit a sick adult, and the hospital staff says it is allowed, it usually can be a positive event for both the child and the adult, with appropriate preparation and support.

Considerations to decide if the visit is appropriate:

- Does the child want to go?
- Does the sick adult want a visit from the child?
- Can the sick adult tolerate a visit medically?
- Will the hospital permit a visit by a minor child?
- Check the hospital rules, then talk to the doctors and nurses about special arrangements

1. **Why should the child visit?**
   - ☐ Opportunity to see that the adult is alive and being cared for
   - ☐ Opportunity to achieve closure
   - ☐ Reduce the fearful magical thinking and misunderstandings a child may have
   - ☐ Reduce post hospitalization anger and regret, especially in situations that are life-threatening
2. **Preparation at home for the visit**
   - ☐ Allows child to have first reactions in a safe place, away from the ICU
   - ☐ Share pictures or drawings, and/or describe in detail what the child will see, smell, feel, hear
   - ☐ Emphasize the emotions the child may experience; anxiety, fear, caution, sadness
   - ☐ Practice the visit: What can the child take for the adult, what can be said, can a hand be held, will the person be able to respond, what exactly will the child do when the actual visit takes place?
   - ☐ Things the child can do at the hospital: tell sick adult about his/her life, school, friends, activities, pets, etc.; give the adult a picture, drawing, poem or something else created by the child; arrange the adult's cards on the wall, table or in a book; bring and distribute cookies or candy to the hospital staff; create a communication book so that visitors can leave messages for the sick adult
3. **The visit itself**
   - ☐ Keep the focus of the visit on the child
   - ☐ Keep the visit short so the child doesn't sit around worrying or imagining
   - ☐ Help facilitate the conversation with open-ended questions to the child, or prompting about the conversation or activities.
   - ☐ If the child is old enough, give him/her some private time with the adult
   - ☐ Help the child say "good-bye," either for this visit, or as a final good-bye.
4. **After the visit**
   - ☐ Review with the child how the visit went. Help the child to feel good about anything he said or did that might have been helpful to the sick adult
   - ☐ Have a picture of the adult looking healthy, to remind the child of the adult he/she will want to hold in mind
   - ☐ Make a plan for any future visits or activities
5. **If the child doesn't want to visit**
   - ☐ Do not force a child to visit an adult in ICU
   - ☐ Help the child to create something that can be sent to the hospital, a letter, poem or picture
   - ☐ Assure the child that the decision not to visit is O.K., no need for guilt

Fig. 14.4 Preparing children for a visit to a seriously ill adult in ICU

Once this in-person assessment has been completed and basic rapport has been established, the child life specialist will proceed with any number of appropriate activities. One such intervention includes medical education through facilitated play. In the case of Mr. Smith, while his sons may have received verbal information from their mother about the life-sustaining equipment being used in his care, the words and descriptions may not make sense without additional visual, verbal, and tactile information. For school-age children, the child life specialist can provide developmentally appropriate education utilizing a medical teaching puppet and real medical supplies (i.e., endotracheal tube, intracranial pressure monitoring supplies, and intravenous catheters and tubing). Photographs of larger equipment such as ventilators, VEEG monitors, and IV pumps can also be used to provide concrete visual information to the child.

During such a session, equipment would be introduced individually and using simple, nonmedical explanations. For example, an ET tube can be described as a "special tube or straw used to give your dad's lungs the air that they need," and the ventilator is a "machine used to make sure he gets the perfect amount of air into his lungs and the perfect amount of air out." Children would be given the option to manipulate the equipment and ask questions at their own level of comfort. This type of activity could be simply educational or used as a psychological preparation for visitation at Mr. Smith's bedside.

In the case of Mrs. Garcia, a direct assessment with the 8-year-old daughter is also important as she has been present at the bedside during this and previous admissions, likely having overheard medical conversations in English between staff but receiving little information from her father on her mother's condition. An important aspect of this intervention will include identifying misconceptions about her mother's condition, current clinical status, and prognosis. These misconceptions should be noted and discussed with Mr. Garcia before corrections or disclosures are made to his daughter. To ensure that communication is clear and culturally sensitive, the use of a medical interpreter in conversations with both Mr. Garcia and his daughter is preferred.

When children are unable to come to the hospital for direct interaction with a child life specialist, technology (i.e., phone, Internet, video conferencing) can be employed to provide similar assessments and interactions. Additionally, medical play supplies and supportive resources can be shared with the family to be used at home. Some child life specialists have the ability in their practice to make home or school visits, as approved by the children's parents, or refer to private practice specialists or community agencies with support services.

Families of ICU patients are often faced with the realization that their loved one will not return home immediately following discharge or may not survive this diagnosis or hospitalization. If Mr. Smith is moved to a rehabilitation facility, a child life specialist can prepare his children and grandchild for physical, cognitive, and functional differences. Furthermore, they can assist with making plans to negotiate the changes to routine at home that will be perpetuated during his continued recovery process. Although Mrs. Garcia's prognosis is unknown, memory-building activities can be initiated during her current hospitalization. Her daughter, with the assistance of a child life specialist, could engage in art activities including hand prints, photography, or journaling projects that create a positive memory in the hospital as well as lasting artifacts in the event of Mrs. Garcia's death. When a parent or grandparent dies during admission to the hospital, a child life specialist can provide opportunities for memory-building activities pre- or post-mortem as a way on processing the event and memorializing the patient.

In an even more innovative approach, one hospital is beginning to use Child Life Professionals to provide nonpharmacological coping support services to adult cardio-thoracic surgery patients in the same manner as those provided to children [17]. An initial review of this program appears to demonstrate that child life is a desirable service from both patient and staff perspectives. More research is needed to assess the generalizability and expansion of such programs.

Conclusion

Although all members of an ICU patient's family are vulnerable to risk from this syndrome, the constellation most likely to be underserved are the children, grandchildren, and other minors that are significant in the patient's life. This particular group not only suffers from the immediate impact of a critical hospitalization of a loved adult but also, due to their susceptible stages of development and dependence, may carry the negative sequelae of these experiences into their later childhood and adulthood. Addressing Family Intensive Care Unit Syndrome is not only about reducing immediate negative emotional responses but also about providing a preventive service to minimize mental health challenges in the future. The professional group most able to reduce the morbidity of Family Intensive Care Unit Syndrome for these children is child life. In order to plan for child life services in an adult intensive care setting, consultation with the Association of Child Life Professionals (www.childlife.org) is the logical place to begin. Not only can child life provide the interventions and services needed by the children and their parents, but child life specialists can also support staff in the often-emotional interactions with children who are coping with the serious illness or injury of an adult patient. With child life on the health care team, children impacted by adult critical illness will not only avoid possible emotional and developmental pathology but can gain psychosocial skills to manage future life crises.

References

1. Child Life Council (2011) Official documents of the child life council. Arlington, VA: Child Life Council. https://www.childlife.org/child-life-profession/mission-values-vision
2. American Academy of Pediatrics. Child life services. Pediatrics. 2014;133(5) Retrieved from http://pediatrics.aappublications.org/content/133/5/e1471.full

3. Wolfer J, Gaynard L, Goldberger J, Laidley LN, Thompson R. An experimental evaluation of a model child life program. Child Health Care. 1988;16(4):244–54.
4. Brewer S, Gleditsch SL, Syblik D, Tiejens ME, Vacik HW. Pediatric anxiety: child life intervention in day surgery. J Pediatric Nurs. 2006;21(1):13–22.
5. Claridge A, Hajec L, Montgomery L, Knapp B. Child and parent psychosocial experiences of hospitalization: an examination of the role of child life specialists. J Child Life Psychosoc Theory Pract. 2020;1(1):3–14. https://doi.org/10.55591/001c.22518.
6. Fein JA, Zempsky WT, Cravero JP. Relief of pain and anxiety in pediatric patients in emergency medical systems. Pediatrics. 2012;130(5):e1391.
7. Gursky B, Kestler LP, Lewis M. Psychosocial intervention on procedure-related distress in children being treated for laceration repair. J Dev Behav Pediatr. 2010;31(3):217–22.
8. Madhok M, Milner D, Teele M, Finkelstein M. Child life services and patient satisfaction in emergency department. Pediatric Emerg Care. 2007;23(10):764.
9. Shea T, Athanasakos E, Cleeve S, Croft N, Gibbs D. Pediatric medical traumatic stress. J Child Life: Psychosoc Theory Pract. 2021;2(1):42–54. https://doi.org/10.55591/001c.22525.
10. Tilford JM, Simpson PM, Green JW, Lensing S, Fiser DH. Volume-outcome relationships in pediatric intensive care units. Pediatrics. 2000;106:289–94.
11. McCue. How to help children through a parent's serious illness. New York: St. Martin's Press; 1994. (rev. 2011)
12. Harpham W. When a parent has cancer: a guide to caring for your children. New York: HarperCollins Publishers; 1997.
13. Sutter C, Reid T. How do we talk to the children? Child life consultation to support the children of seriously ill adult inpatients. J Palliative Med. 2012;15(12):1–7.
14. Phillips F, Prezio EA. Wonders & Worries: evaluation of a child centered psychosocial intervention for families who have a parent/primary caregiver with cancer. Psycho-Oncology. 2016;26:1006. https://doi.org/10.1002/pon.4120.
15. Phillips F, Prezio EA, Panisch LS, Jones BL. Factors affecting outcomes following a psychosocial intervention for children when a parent has cancer. J Child Life Psychosoc Theory Pract. 2021;2(2) https://doi.org/10.55591/001c.28322.
16. Cross J, Bruce J. Child life services in an adult setting: a quality improvement initiative and implementation effort in a university hospital. Child Life Focus. 2015;33(3):13–7.
17. Piazza J, Heering L, Peters SL, White M, Baker M, Baello C, Schwenzer C, Deeb GM. Child life-facilitated coping support with adult patients undergoing cardiac surgery: a pilot program. J Child Life Psychosoc Theory Pract. 2022;3(2) https://doi.org/10.55591/001c.38502.

Chapter 15
Family Engagement in the Neonatal Intensive Care Unit (NICU)

Ashlee J. Vance, Clayton J. Shuman, Ashleigh B. Harlow, and Kathryn Malin

Introduction

Healthcare providers recognize the importance of the family system to patient health and wellbeing, as evidenced by the development and implementation of family-centered care models in healthcare delivery settings. Yet, only in the past few decades has there been an explicit shift within healthcare settings to welcome and include families during hospitalization of their sick child. Family-centered care is a philosophy used across the lifespan, from pediatrics to older adults, and in many healthcare settings (e.g., rehabilitation, family medicine, and palliative care) [1]. The philosophy of family-centered care contends that family members and healthcare providers must create partnerships for addressing the medical and psychosocial health needs of an individual receiving care.

Family-centered care is intended to be an inclusive care philosophy and, as such, it is important to use an inclusive definition of family. Families are complex and diverse, with interconnected members [2, 3]. The definition of "family" adapted from family systems theory is widely accepted by family researchers and clinicians

A. J. Vance (✉)
Henry Ford Health, Detroit, MI, USA
e-mail: avance2@hfhs.org

C. J. Shuman
University of Michigan, Ann Arbor, MI, USA
e-mail: clayshu@med.umich.edu

A. B. Harlow
Duke University, Durham, NC, USA
e-mail: Ashleigh.harlow@duke.edu

K. Malin
Marquette University, Milwaukee, WI, USA
e-mail: kathryn.malin@marquette.edu

© The Author(s), under exclusive license to Springer Nature Switzerland AG 2025

A. J. Vance et al. (eds.), *Families in the Intensive Care Unit*,
https://doi.org/10.1007/978-3-031-83786-9_15

and encourages the view of "family" as being defined "by the patient, or in the case of minors, their surrogates." This may mean that identified family members may not be of blood relation; whomever the patient or surrogate has a significant relationship with is considered a part of their family system.

The purpose of this chapter is to review the history of family-centered care, describe family engagement practices, interventions, and potential benefits on outcomes in the context of the Neonatal Intensive Care Unit (NICU) and summarize implementation strategies to support family engagement. We will also address special considerations and situations that may be unique to the neonatal hospital environment.

Overview of Family Engagement

History of Family-Centered Care

The first hospital for children opened in Paris in 1802 and, for a time, children were cared for by nurses, doctors, and their families. In the pre-World War I era, nursing care considered the emotional and psychological needs of children in tandem with their physical or medical concerns. However, by the 1920s, medical and nursing care had changed from a focus on emotional and psychological needs in a home-like environment to more industrialized hospital environments that were grim and stark for children. Routines in hospital wards were for the benefit of staff and not necessarily the benefit of the children in their care. Parents relinquished the responsibility of their child's care and treatment to the hospital staff, based on the belief that parents posed a risk of infection, even though studies showed that infection rates did not increase if parents remained with their infants [4]. Healthcare during this time attended to the physical and medical needs of children but not their emotional or social needs. In the aftermath of World War II, a perceptible shift in this thinking provided the catalyst for change. The grief and suffering associated with the separation of children from families during war prompted psychologists to study and document the effects of separation and trauma [5].

Elements of the family-centered-care philosophy can be traced back to John Bowlby and James Roberson's theoretical work on parent/child attachment in the 1940s [6, 7]. Their work illuminated the traumatic effects of separating parents and children, which can lead to separation anxiety and subsequent grief and trauma associated with separation. They were among the first advocates of parental presence during a child's hospitalization. At this first attempt to bring children and parents back together in the hospital setting, nursing and medical disciplines were reticent to adopt this care philosophy. A prevailing thought that a "known way" of providing nursing care existed, and clinicians felt this way should be unquestioned and unchallenged [7].

The publication of the landmark Platt Report ushered in a major shift in the social and cultural norms around pediatric hospital care [8]. The Platt report detailed the inhumane treatment of children in hospitals and recommended that children should have unlimited and unrestricted access to their parents while ill [9]. Based on findings in this report, care in both the United States and the United Kingdom began to change; organizations were formed to lobby governments about the level of parental involvement in hospital care. Healthcare consumers became more empowered and informed, and soon parents became the most influential advocates for family participation in the care of hospitalized children. The Association for the Care of Children's Health (ACCH) was formed in 1965 and initially included healthcare professionals only, and excluded parents for fear that "if parents became involved, the health disciplines would lose control"(p. 167) [7]. Not until 1978 were parents invited to join ACCH. With the dissolution of this organization several years later, many of the organization's founders were instrumental in the subsequent creation of the Institute for Patient and Family-Centered Care (IPFCC) in 1992 [4, 10].

The IPFCC established goals for healthcare delivery, and the tenants of family-centered care (FCC) were developed and defined. The core principles of family-centered care (FCC) as outlined by the IPFCC include: (1) dignity and respect, (2) information sharing, (3) participation, and (4) collaboration. The goal of these core principles is to shift healthcare providers' behavior from doing *to* or *for* patients to *working with* patients and their families. The first introduction of FCC into the NICU setting was in 1993 by Helen Harrison, a parent of a NICU survivor and author who advocated for more family-centered healthcare policies: "all of us share the belief that parents should be able to participate more fully in caring for and making decisions for their hospitalized newborns." [11] Since the early 1990s, NICUs have implemented FCC practices, with varied success, to create a more family-centered environment. These include policies or practices such as 24/7 visitation rights for parents and multidisciplinary medical rounds where parents are encouraged to participate.

Since the establishment of the FCC philosophy in 1992 and introduction into clinical settings, there has been much written about how to interpret and operationalize the model into healthcare settings. FCC's operationalization and adoption are complicated by the myriad ways FCC can be interpreted and implemented in different contexts [12]. However, at the core of the FCC philosophy is the belief that patients' family members are more than visitors. Rather, parents and/or caregivers in the pediatric clinical setting are allies in care essential for provision of safe, high-quality care. Those who advocate for more inclusive language assert that families should not be viewed as visitors given their status as *essential* members of the child's care team [13–15]. The use of the word *visitor* or *visitation* implies a sense of 'otherness' and reflects a transient encounter, which is misaligned with the role of a parent/caregiver. Many hospitals continue to use *visit*-related language in their policies; however, there is some momentum towards revising policies that focus more on parent presence and collaboration. For example, using language like family presence or parent presence for policies.

Despite efforts to bring parents and children together in the hospital setting, elements of "gatekeeping" persist within healthcare [16, 17]. Healthcare providers have long utilized their expertise to exert influence over families, both explicitly and implicitly. The resulting imbalance of power is what family-centered care practices aim to diminish. Generally, there is an understanding that FCC is the best mechanism for promoting a hospitalized child's wellbeing, with a corresponding commitment on the part of health professionals to act in the child's best interest [18]. This view does not claim that an individual child's welfare is indistinguishable from that of his or her family.

Some have expressed concern that too much emphasis on families as the "unit of care" [12] may distract from the healthcare goals or needs of the infant or child during hospitalization. For example, consider a child going home with a newly placed tracheostomy tube, requiring two adult caregivers to complete education and training on tracheostomy care and emergency management. One of the child's parents has completed training, but the second caregiver, a grandparent, has been unable to attend training sessions at the hospital due to conflicts with their work schedule. FCC principles would encourage a flexible training schedule to ensure the involvement of the child's family members in their care, rather than relying on home healthcare workers to provide 24/7 tracheostomy care in the absence of a second trained caregiver. Should providers delay a child's discharge home for a secondary caregiver to complete tracheostomy care training, in greater support of a family-centered care model? Or should the focus be on efforts to expedite the child's discharge from the hospital and back into a supportive home environment? This is just one example of how thoughtful inclusion of family in decision-making and provision of care is not always straightforward; thus, tailored, individualized conversations are necessary to meet families where they are at so they can best support the child's treatment and recovery. This may also help to mitigate the disruptive and distressing experience of parenting in the NICU for neonatal patients and families alike.

Care Models Based on FCC Philosophy

To address the difficulty of implementing family-centered care, clinicians and researchers have developed different care models focused on increasing family presence and engagement in care during a child's hospitalization. Unfortunately, given the variation between these models, it has been very difficult to test these interventions and compare outcomes across studies and hospital settings. A Cochrane review of FCC interventions [19] found only one study eligible for inclusion that met criteria as an actual FCC intervention (i.e., care model), highlighting the significant struggle to replicate across settings and understand the effect of FCC practices on infant and family outcomes. Even so, we have identified a few FCC models for reference, which are outlined in Table 15.1.

Table 15.1 NICU care models supporting parenting in the NICU

Care model name	Citation(s)/ location	Target population/ objective	Core elements	Dedicated staff necessary for program adoption
Family nurture intervention (FNI)	Welch [33, 34] *United States*	Preterm infants *To counteract adverse effects of separation of mothers and infants*	• Nurture specialists facilitate mother-infant calming cycle sessions (e.g., emotional connections) • Calming cycle meant to encourage reciprocal physical, sensory, and emotional experiences, that includes scent cloths, calming touch, & holding	Yes, family nurture specialist (e.g., nurse, former NICU parent, social worker)
Family integrated care (FICare)	O'Brien [29, 30] *Canada*	Infants in a neonatal intensive care unit *To include parents as an integral part of the NICU team so that they could provide active care for their infant.*	• Parents learned how to provide all care (except for intravenous fluid & medication administration) for their infants in the NICU • Commit to being presence for >8 h per day and daily educational sessions • Nurses take on the role of educators and coaches for the parents	Yes, resource nurse and/or former NICU parent
Close collaboration	Ahlqvist-Bjorkroth [36] He [36] *Finland*	Infants in a neonatal intensive care unit *To change neonatal care culture, targeting the entire healthcare team, using experiential learning methods including bedside mentoring and reflective discussions*	• Staff desire to increase parent presence and improve skills with parent communication *Core elements* 1. Preterm infant behaviors 2. Acknowledging parents' intuitive capacity for parenting 3. Supporting parents' emotional bond with infant	No, unit-level training for all NICU professionals

(continued)

Table 15.1 (continued)

Care model name	Citation(s)/ location	Target population/ objective	Core elements	Dedicated staff necessary for program adoption
Neonatal parenting unit (NIPU)	Hall [60] *United States*	Infants in a neonatal intensive care unit *To promote interdisciplinary collaboration with caregivers in equal partnership to create a culture where everyone is concerned with the Well-being of each other*	*Potentially better practices* 1. Family-centered developmental care 2. Peer-to-peer family support 3. Mental health professionals 4. Palliative & bereavement care 5. Post-discharge follow-up 6. Staff education & support	Maybe, some better practices call for dedicated staff (e.g., mental health providers, palliative care specialists)
Neonatal integrative developmental care model	Altimier [61] *United States*	Infants in a neonatal intensive care unit *To create a healing environmental centered around the parent/caregiver to optimize synaptic neural connections by promoting neuroprotective interventions*	*7 Core measures* 1. Healing environment 2. Partnering with families 3. Positioning and handling 4. Safeguarding sleep 5. Minimizing stress and pain 6. Protecting skin 7. Optimizing nutrition	No, unit policies should be created to support developmental care practices in the NICU
Newborn individual development care and assessment program (NIDCAP)	Als [62, 63] Wallin [64] *United States*	Preterm infants *To provide adequate stimulation to preterm infants adapted to their degree of neurological maturity* (e.g., *gestational age)*	• Observation & assessment of infant (e.g., reading behavioral cues) • Care plan recommendations • Parents essential for co-regulatory support	Yes, training and certification for nurses, psychologist or other NICU professionals

(continued)

Table 15.1 (continued)

Care model name	Citation(s)/ location	Target population/ objective	Core elements	Dedicated staff necessary for program adoption
Eat, sleep, console	Grisham [65] Young [66] *United States*	Substance-exposed infants *To give the family both place and purpose within the NICU, creating collaborative relationships by using strategies to maximize nonpharmacologic interventions*	• Eat: Infant is given appropriate amounts of food depending on age, chest-feeding encouraged • Sleep: Undisturbed sleep for a minimum of 1 h; holding is encouraged to support sleep • Console: Assess if infant can be consoled within 10 min; encourage second caregiving attempts to console, then assess for pharmacologic intervention	No, structure of care fits within nursing care and supportive family presence. No dedicated staff necessary

Supporting Engagement in the NICU

Broadly speaking, parent involvement is conceptualized as a one-way process where healthcare providers inform parents and caregivers of the child's status and needs and may invite them to participate in care. Involvement is more likely to include delegation of basic tasks with no transfer of knowledge required, and these tasks do not extend to more complex activities like decision-making. Similarly, parent participation implies a transfer of knowledge between the nurse and parent. This requires a willingness of providers, such as nurses, to relinquish some control and form a working relationship with parents. Parent collaboration implies joint parent-provider involvement in intellectual activities and is based on cooperative endeavors between patient and nurse. Like parent participation, the goal of collaboration is to improve the working relationship between parents and providers, although parent participation is considered a more comprehensive definition. Lastly, parent participation is not about competence, rather whether there is a willingness from parents to engage in activities and or if the nurse is willing to teach and engage families in care. For additional reading and information regarding similarities and differences among these concepts, please refer to these concept analyses [20–23].

In contrast to parental involvement, parental participation, and collaboration, which describe actions parents take or relationships among parents and healthcare providers, parental engagement reflects a parent's internal state. This internal state represents a parents' readiness to concern themselves with their child's health,

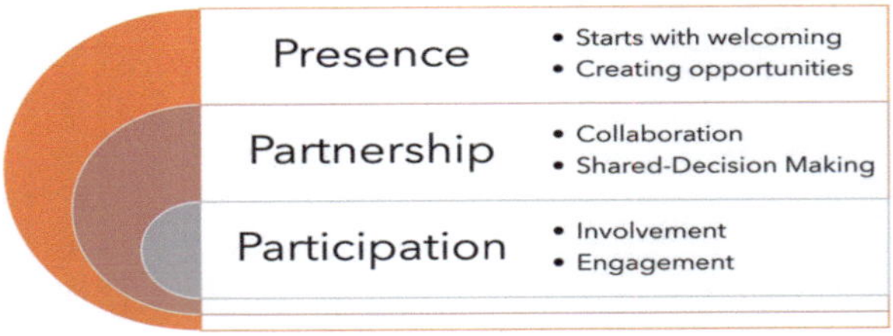

Fig. 15.1 Terms related to engagement in the NICU

healthcare, and health outcomes [24]. Though engagement may be operationalized via certain behaviors or actions exhibited by parents such as speaking during bedside rounds or learning how to safely hold their baby while intubated, some components of engagement are not readily observable. This is a major consideration for healthcare providers, who may not have tools to assess engagement that is not readily observed. Regardless of what term is used (i.e., engagement, involvement, participation, collaboration) (see Fig. 15.1), presence from caregivers is necessary first and foremost; presence can be encouraged, welcomed, and supported by NICU professionals. We advocate that parent presence benefits and creates positive outcomes for families, infants, and staff alike.

Uniquely, effective parent engagement only exists in the context of trusting relationships and must be a priority of healthcare providers. As such, it is the responsibility of those who work in the hospital (i.e., clinical and support staff) to welcome and normalize the experience of hospitalization for the families with whom we interact. Especially in the NICU, staff have a direct effect on whether care or interactions are family-centered by supporting and encouraging (or through indirect omission) parent engagement in their infant's care. In the unique context of the NICU, staff are uniquely positioned to help guide parents in their transition to parenthood and help them build confidence in their parental role at such an early stage of parenting. Provision of family-centered care affords an opportunity for parents to develop trusting partnerships with NICU staff to support them in their parental role development and to offer education and guidance in navigating the foreign world of parenting in the NICU, thus enabling parents the ability to fully engage in their child's care.

Clinicians should strive to provide the key elements needed for parental engagement, first and foremost, through effective and respectful communication. Communication should include information and education related to the infant's care and treatment during hospitalization but should also extend to include anticipatory guidance about their care needs after discharge. Parent engagement exists in the space of trusting relationships and respectful partnerships. It is in this sense that we are *fighting together* for the common goal of this infant's wellbeing. The opportunity exists for clinicians to recognize that, while they bring technical skill and medical knowledge, parents can teach them an immense amount about their family, themselves, and their child.

In sum, the essential components of family engagement in the NICU include the following:

1. Closeness and interaction with infant.
2. Good communication with the healthcare team.
3. Information and education related to care needs during and after hospitalization.
4. Individualized emotional support.

When the culture of the NICU holds family-centered care and parent engagement as core values, then the care delivery will reflect these essential components.

Infant and Parent Outcomes Secondary to Family Engagement

The evidence is clear that the presence of caregivers and family benefits patient safety, experiences, and outcomes. NICU staff consistently identify family-centered care as necessary [25] and despite challenges, nurses describe satisfaction in providing family support and the ability to participate in, and witness as, infants and families develop [26]. While some may believe the myth that interacting with parents or caregivers, or providing family-centered care is too time consuming, the majority of neonatal and pediatric clinicians recognize the importance of the investment in the family and more opportunities for engagement ease the transition to parenthood and can shorten hospitalizations [27, 28]. Interventions with the purpose of improving family engagement, such as the Family Integrated Care program (FICare) [29–32] and the Family Nurture Intervention (FNI) [33] are associated with improved infant weight gain [30], increased exclusive breastfeeding at time of discharge [30], increased brain activity at term [34] and improved infant motor development at 18 months corrected age [31]. Other programs such as Close Collaboration [35, 36] focus on systematic changes and enhancements to the unit culture through staff education and empowerment that lead to improved outcomes for parents and infants.

Of all the possible interventions, one of the central elements of family-centered care in the NICU is the provision of developmentally supportive care. Figure 15.2 illustrates an organizational approach to understanding how developmental care practices may influence infant outcomes [37]. When an infant is admitted to the NICU they are at greater risk for poor neurobehavioral outcomes, especially if those experiences do not support the infant's developing neurological system [38]. Developmental care practices that support development such as family engagement and presence have the potential to improve outcomes. These practices may be considered neuroprotective, especially if they take advantage of a preterm infant's neuroplasticity [39]. Yet, neuroprotection is not only for preterm infants, rather for all

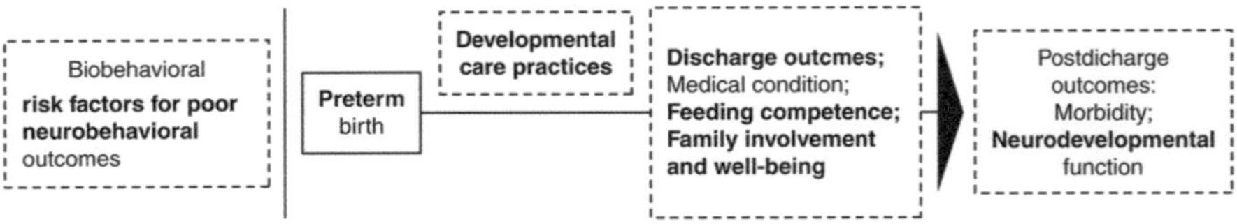

Fig. 15.2 Organizational model to understand outcomes

infants in the NICU. The improvements resulting from these practices often are seen at discharge, particularly improvements in medical condition, feeding competence, and parenting behaviors and confidence. Improved long-term outcomes of developmental care practices are more difficult to demonstrate; however, some evidence supports the effects of developmental care interventions and programs on long-term morbidity, neurodevelopmental function, and family well-being [40].

Parents of infants requiring NICU hospitalization benefit from targeted family engagement strategies. When parents are provided family-centered care during their infant's hospitalization, they are more likely to report higher satisfaction [41], decreased mean stress scores, and lower mean anxiety scores [30]. Interventions supporting parent engagement can be divided into three levels: (1) interventions to support parents, (2) parent-delivered interventions, and (3) interventions integrating parents as full partners in the NICU [42]. Interventions to support parents include activities such as psychoeducation, journaling, and peer support. These activities are associated with improved parental knowledge and confidence and with decreased psychological distress. Parental-delivered interventions, such as skin-to-skin contact, chest-milk feedings, infant massage, and parent-led infant assessments, are associated with decreased parent-reported stress, worry, and depression [43, 44]. Finally, interventions that facilitate family engagement through creation of full partnerships between parents and NICU staff are also associated with improved parental outcomes [42]. The environment and policies of the NICU can either facilitate or diminish parental engagement. Single-family NICU rooms [45], dedicated in-hospital parent space [46], family rounding [47], and unrestricted access to the NICU [13] provide structural assurances aimed at promoting family engagement.

The benefits achieved from family engagement in the NICU are dependent on the quality of the engagement practices and their successful implementation. It is imperative that support for family engagement practices come from all levels of the healthcare systems. Healthcare providers report challenges in staffing and unpredictable workloads as barriers providing family-centered care [48]. Special attention to individualized support of parents, inclusion of all family members, and integration of support programs into both internal and external health systems are needed to help assure quality parental engagement and improved long-term outcomes [49]. Infants requiring NICU care consistently demonstrate improved neurodevelopmental and physiologic outcomes when family engagement is prioritized, thus, the significance of parent and family presence cannot be overstated.

Implementing FCC Models or Practices in the NICU to Increase Family Engagement

Implementing FCC in the NICU is critically important to ensure that patients, families, clinicians, and organizations achieve the benefits of FCC practices. Although implementation can be challenging and difficult to achieve, efforts to implement can be supported by evidence and recommendations discovered and tested through implementation science [50]. Implementation science is the study of methods and strategies that contribute to the use of evidence-based practices (EBPs) in clinical settings [51], such as FCC models and interventions. Implementation scientists have investigated and described unique combinations of barriers and facilitators (at various levels both internal and external to an organization) that contribute to the relative success or difficulty in implementing and sustaining the use of EBPs. Barriers are defined as factors that may make it more difficult to implement EBPs and facilitators are defined as factors that may make it easier to implement EBPs [52, 53]. Levels of implementation refer to the various agents/actors of implementation [51]. For example, barriers and facilitators to implementation likely occur at the innovation level (e.g., ease of use, fit with workflow); individual level (e.g., clinician knowledge, clinician self-efficacy), and organizational level (e.g., policies within the NICU).

Since clinical settings and patient populations are diverse and vary from one setting to the next, there are nearly an unlimited number of possible combinations of barriers and facilitators that may impact successful implementation. As such, numerous theories, frameworks, and models were developed and tested to guide scientists and practitioners in identifying barriers and facilitators related to implementation. These implementation models aim to bridge the gap between research and clinical uptake by supporting individuals in selecting appropriate implementation strategies to address barriers (and/or bolster facilitators) for their unique context [54–56].

For the purposes of this chapter, the RE-AIM framework, a common framework used to implement EBP in healthcare settings, is used to discuss implementation of new FCC practices in the NICU setting. RE-AIM consists of five main domains, (1) Reach, (2) Effectiveness, (3) Adopters, (4) Implementation, and (5) Maintenance, which are considered critical to successful implementation and sustainability of EBPs [57–59].

Reach

In RE-AIM, *reach* refers to the individuals and populations receiving the EBP. For FCC, this is specific to the patients and families who receive care in the NICU. When planning to implement FCC practices or other family engagement interventions in the NICU, it is important to identify and describe the patient and family populations benefiting from these practices. Consider characteristics and demographics of the general family population served by the NICU while paying particular attention to potentially harder-to-reach populations, such as those with limited ability to be present with their infants and those representing diverse family structures. Considering subgroups or hard-to-reach populations can contribute to improving health equity. Additionally, evaluate and describe demographic differences between the original family populations included in previous research and the intended population and setting for your implementation. This is important because the families and populations included in previous clinical trials or quality improvement projects may be different from the families and populations in the NICU where FCC is intended to be implemented.

Effectiveness

In RE-AIM, *effectiveness* refers to evaluating specific and measurable individual outcomes related to the use of the intervention—both related to individual outcomes as well as broader outcomes (e.g., quality of life, economic outcomes). FCC primary RE-AIM outcomes might focus on comparing patient outcomes to national standards or pre-implementation metrics. Secondary outcomes might focus on robustness of effects or attrition across subgroups. In terms of monitoring and evaluating, it will be important to define your outcomes to be observable and measurable (e.g., minutes of parents reading to infants in the NICU). FCC practices have previously demonstrated efficacy and effectiveness and if implemented successfully and delivered as intended, a NICU can expect to achieve these intended benefits. If these benefits are not realized, the problem may not be related to the FCC practices but may be due to implementation issues such as limited uptake by clinicians, reduced or failed delivery of FCC practices at the bedside, or other context or population-specific characteristics.

Adoption

Adoption refers to the individuals and groups who are intended to deliver the EBPs. FCC models and practices must be adopted and delivered by members of the NICU healthcare team. Implementation of a unit-specific care model requires involvement from all disciplines (i.e., medicine, nursing, pharmacy, respiratory therapy, social work, etc.) in the NICU setting, although each discipline may have varying responsibilities in delivering FCC. During the *adoption* phase, the healthcare workers involved in FCC delivery must be identified, characterized, and their roles specified. For example, by identifying educational and training needs, evaluating attitudes (positive or negative) about FCC, and examining the social context (e.g., roles and relationships) for facilitators and barriers to implementation.

Implementation

Implementation is a coordinated and planned effort to integrate the delivery of EBPs, like FCC practices, with fidelity, by using a combination of strategies informed by the EBP and the barriers and facilitators specific to the setting. It is recommended that those facilitating implementation select a model or framework to guide their efforts and evaluation. The RE-AIM model is one option, but many other models and frameworks are available. After selecting a framework to guide implementation, consider any adaptations to the original FCC model or practice that must be made to better fit the specific context and audience where implementation occurs. A challenge to implementing FCC is that the original contexts in which effectiveness was demonstrated may differ from the intended implementation context. For example, the original study may have tested FCC in a 75-bed Level IV NICU in an academic medical center, but the context for implementation is a 15-bed Level II NICU in a rural hospital. These settings differ in unit size, acuity level, geographic region, and hospital type and staffing model. Therefore, implementation facilitators must evaluate the intervention's fit considering these differences, and adaptations may be needed. It is important to carefully consider adaptations and ensure that key, core components of the intervention are not changed to preserve the effectiveness of the intervention and achieve its intended benefits.

Identifying barriers and facilitators to implementation is often the key to successful uptake of EPBs, such as FCC. Barriers to implementing FCC may include clinician "gatekeeping" attitudes, visitor restriction policies, or low levels of family presence due to transportation issues or other barriers. Facilitators may include leadership support, active and engaged parent-peer support groups, and positive interdisciplinary team dynamics. Upon identifying barriers and facilitators, implementation strategies should be selected to address such barriers and bolster identified facilitators. For example, a nurse identifies a family who is experiencing transportation challenges and collaborates with a unit-based social worker who can provide bus or taxi vouchers to eligible families. Additionally, parents may be bolstered by support from peer coaches who can engage them early in the implementation process and seek their feedback regularly. These peer support groups may encourage parent visitation and engagement in infant care.

Maintenance

Maintenance, often referred to as sustainability, is what is needed to keep the innovation or intervention in use beyond the initial implementation period. Implementation champions are encouraged to describe what aspects of FCC they would like to sustain. Similar to approaches that guide planning for implementation, consider potential barriers and facilitators to sustainability, and identify strategies to support ongoing delivery of FCC practices. Implementation of FCC in NICU settings can be challenging but is critical to improve patient and organizational outcomes. There are numerous implementation resources available to help plan for and guide implementation of FCC. Utilizing available resources while engaging a diverse team of collaborators will contribute to successful implementation of FCC in the NICU.

Future Directions and Conclusion

In conclusion, we have reviewed the history of family-centered care, discussed the essential components of FCC care models and practices, outcomes of family engagement, and detailed the ways implementation science can help achieve greater effectiveness and sustainability of FCC models and practices into NICU settings. Family-centered care facilitates family engagement by acknowledging the importance of their presence and involvement during a child's hospitalization. When FCC is implemented and supported, the model and practices help providers provide optimal care, with the goal of achieving better outcomes for infants and families.

We acknowledge there may be many institutional or interpersonal barriers for improving family-centered care practices that require additional investment in human and capital resources (Frank 2021); thus, buy-in from leadership and administration is vital. We recommend that NICU clinicians and staff conduct assessments of FCC values and practices in their own unit, by identifying strengths, weaknesses, resources, and gaps so that solutions can be developed in partnership with parent advisors. Using implementation science and quality improvement science in the RE-AIM framework to guide these first steps, provides support and direction to successfully implement, improve, and/or sustain FCC models and practices (e.g., resources, team dynamics, culture, and attitudes). FCC is more than a conglomeration of single practices or strategies used by individual healthcare providers; but a shared vision or collective value system where the NICU team works together to support the care and treatment needs of infants in their care, while supporting their caregivers. The principles and practices of family-centered care can be implemented in many different configurations to enable and enhance parental engagement and achieve FCC's core goals: partnership between parents and healthcare providers, shared decision-making, and caregiving competence and confidence so that infants receive safe and high-quality care while in the NICU, and that families have a foundation in which to grow and thrive after discharge.

References

1. Kokorelias KM, Gignac MAM, Naglie G, Cameron JI. Towards a universal model of family centered care: a scoping review. BMC Health Serv Res. 2019;19(1):564.
2. Rothbaum F, Rosen K, Ujiie T, Uchida N. Family systems theory, attachment theory, and culture. Fam Process. 2002;41(3):328–50.

3. Coontz S. Historical perspectives on family studies. J Marriage Fam. 2000;62(2):283–97.
4. Gooding JS, Cooper LG, Blaine AI, Franck LS, Howse JL, Berns SD. Family support and family-centered Care in the Neonatal Intensive Care Unit: origins, advances. Impact Semin Perinatol. 2011;35(1):20–8.
5. Zahra T. The lost children: reconstructing Europe's families after world war II. Cambridge, MA: Harvard University Press; 2011.
6. Bowlby J. Grief and mourning in infancy and early childhood. Psychoanal Study Child. 1960;15(1):9–52.
7. Jolley J, Shields L. The evolution of family-centered care. J Pediatr Nurs. 2009;24(2):164–70.
8. Platt H. The welfare of children in hospital, vol. 273. London; 1959. p. 475.
9. Shields L, Nixon J. "I want my mummy". Changes in the care of children in hospital. Collegian. 1998;5(2):16–23.
10. Malusky SK. A concept analysis of family-centered care in the NICU. Neonatal Netw. 2005;24(6):25–32.
11. Harrison H. The principles for family-centered neonatal care. Pediatrics. 1993;92(5):643–50.
12. Uniacke S, Browne TK, Shields L. How should we understand family-centred care? J Child Health Care. 2018;22(3):460–9.
13. Vance AJ, Malin KJ, Benjamin A, Shuman CJ, Moore TA, Costa DK. Pandemic visitor policies: parent reactions and policy implications. Acta Paediatr. 2022;111(3):604–6.
14. Association of Women's Health Obstetric and Neonatal Nurses, National Association of Neonatal Nurses, National Perinatal Association. Essential Care in the NICU during the COVID-19 Pandemic. https://nann.org/position-statements/. Published 2021. Accessed March 15, 2021.
15. Griffin T. Family-centered care in the NICU. J Perinat Neonatal Nurs. 2006;20(1):98–102.
16. Lupton D, Fenwick J. "They've forgotten that I'm the mum" constructing and practicing motherhood in special care nurseries. Soc Sci Med. 2001;53(8):1011–21.
17. Roden J. The involvement of parents and nurses in the care of acutely-ill children in a non-specialist paediatric setting. J Child Health Care. 2005;9(3):222–40.
18. Coyne I. Families and health-care professionals' perspectives and expectations of family-centred care: hidden expectations and unclear roles. Health Expect. 2015;18(5):796–808.
19. Shields L, Zhou H, Pratt J, Taylor M, Hunter J, Pascoe E. Family-centred care for hospitalised children aged 0–12 years. Cochrane Database Syst Rev. 2012;10:Cd004811.
20. Cahill J. Patient participation: a concept analysis. J Adv Nurs. 1996;24(3):561–71.
21. Coyne I. Parent particpiation: a concept analysis. J Adv Nurs. 1996;23:733–40.
22. Harlow AB, Ledbetter L, Brandon DH. Parental presence, participation, and engagement in paediatric hospital care: a conceptual delineation. J Adv Nurs. 2023;80:2758.
23. Vance AJ, Brandon DH. Delineating among parenting confidence, parenting self-efficacy, and competence. ANS Adv Nurs Sci. 2017;40(4):E18–37.
24. Vittner D, Butler S, Smith K, et al. Parent engagement correlates with parent and preterm infant oxytocin release during skin-to-skin contact. Adv Neonatal Care. 2019;19(1):73–9.
25. Franck LS, Cormier DM, Hutchison J, et al. A multisite survey of NICU healthcare Professionals' perceptions about family-centered care. Adv Neonatal Care. 2021;21(3):205–13.
26. Turner M, Chur-Hansen A, Winefield H. The neonatal nurses' view of their role in emotional support of parents and its complexities. J Clin Nurs. 2014;23(21–22):3156–65.
27. North K, Whelan R, Folger LV, et al. Family involvement in the routine care of hospitalized preterm or low birth weight infants: a systematic review and meta-analysis. Pediatrics. 2022;150(Suppl. 1)
28. Powers SA, Taylor K, Tumin D, Kohler JA Sr. Measuring parental presence in the neonatal intensive care unit. Am J Perinatol. 2020;39:134.
29. O'Brien K, Bracht M, Macdonell K, et al. A pilot cohort analytic study of family integrated care in a Canadian neonatal intensive care unit. BMC Pregnancy Childbirth. 2013;13(Suppl. 1):S12.
30. O'Brien K, Robson K, Bracht M, et al. Effectiveness of family integrated care in neonatal intensive care units on infant and parent outcomes: a multicentre, multinational, cluster-randomised controlled trial. Lancet Child Adolesc Health. 2018;2(4):245–54.

31. Synnes AR, Petrie J, Grunau RE, et al. Family integrated care: very preterm neurodevelopmental outcomes at 18 months. Arch Dis Child Fetal Neonatal Ed. 2022;107(1):76–81.
32. Franck LS, Gay CL, Hoffmann TJ, et al. Neonatal outcomes from a quasi-experimental clinical trial of family integrated care versus family-centered care for preterm infants in U.S. NICUs. BMC Pediatr. 2022;22(1):674.
33. Welch CD, Check J, O'Shea TM. Improving care collaboration for NICU patients to decrease length of stay and readmission rate. BMJ Open Qual. 2017;6(2):e000130.
34. Welch MG, Grieve PG, Stark RI, et al. Family nurture intervention increases term age forebrain EEG activity: a multicenter replication trial. Clin Neurophysiol. 2022;138:52–60.
35. Ahlqvist-Bjorkroth S, Boukydis Z, Axelin AM, Lehtonen L. Close collaboration with parents intervention to improve parents' psychological well-being and child development: description of the intervention and study protocol. Behav Brain Res. 2017;325(Pt B):303–10.
36. He F, Axelin A, Ahlqvist-Björkroth S, Raiskila S, Löyttyniemi E, Lehtonen L. Effectiveness of the close collaboration with parents intervention on parent-infant closeness in hospital. 2020.
37. Kenner C, McGrath JM, editors. Developmental care of newborns & infants: a guide for health professionals. 3rd ed. St. Louis, MO: Wolters Kluwer Health, Inc; 2022.
38. Soleimani F, Azari N, Ghiasvand H, Shahrokhi A, Rahmani N, Fatollahierad S. Do NICU developmental care improve cognitive and motor outcomes for preterm infants? A systematic review and meta-analysis. BMC Pediatr. 2020;20(1):67.
39. Pickler RH, McGrath JM, Reyna BA, et al. A model of neurodevelopmental risk and protection for preterm infants. J Perinat Neonatal Nurs. 2010;24(4):356–65.
40. Griffiths N, Spence K, Loughran-Fowlds A, Westrup B. Individualised developmental care for babies and parents in the NICU: evidence-based best practice guideline recommendations. Early Hum Dev. 2019;139:104840.
41. Davidson JE, Aslakson RA, Long AC, et al. Guidelines for family-centered care in the neonatal, pediatric, and adult ICU. Crit Care Med. 2017;45(1):103–28.
42. Franck LS, O'Brien K. The evolution of family-centered care: from supporting parent-delivered interventions to a model of family integrated care. Birth Defects Res. 2019;111(15):1044–59.
43. Holditch-Davis D, White-Traut RC, Levy JA, O'Shea TM, Geraldo V, David RJ. Maternally administered interventions for preterm infants in the NICU: effects on maternal psychological distress and mother-infant relationship. Infant Behav Dev. 2014;37(4):695–710.
44. Sweeney S, Rothstein R, Visintainer P, Rothstein R, Singh R. Impact of kangaroo care on parental anxiety level and parenting skills for preterm infants in the neonatal intensive care unit. J Neonatal Nurs. 2017;23(3):151–8.
45. Vohr B, McGowan E, Keszler L, et al. Impact of a transition home program on Rehospitalization rates of preterm infants. J Pediatr. 2017;181:86–92.
46. White RD, Smith JA, Shepley MM. Committee to establish recommended standards for newborn ID. Recommended standards for newborn ICU design, eighth edition. J Perinatol. 2013;33(Suppl. 1):S2–16.
47. Harris GM. Family-centered rounds in the neonatal intensive care unit. Nurs Womens Health. 2014;18(1):18–27.
48. Benzies KM, Shah V, Aziz K, Lodha A, Misfeldt R. The health care system is making 'too much noise' to provide family-centred care in neonatal intensive care units: perspectives of health care providers and hospital administrators. Intensive Crit Care Nurs. 2018;50:44.
49. Treyvaud K, Spittle A, Anderson PJ, O'Brien K. A multilayered approach is needed in the NICU to support parents after the preterm birth of their infant. Early Hum Dev. 2019;139:104838.
50. Zullig LL, Deschodt M, De Geest S. Embracing implementation science: a paradigm shift for nursing research. J Nurs Scholarsh. 2020;52(1):3–5.
51. Bauer MS, Damschroder L, Hagedorn H, Smith J, Kilbourne AM. An introduction to implementation science for the non-specialist. BMC Psychol. 2015;3(1):32.
52. Mirlashari J, Brown H, Fomani FK, de Salaberry J, Zadeh TK, Khoshkhou F. The challenges of implementing family-centered care in NICU from the perspectives of physicians and nurses. J Pediatr Nurs. 2020;50:e91–8.

53. Toivonen M, Lehtonen L, Ahlqvist-Björkroth S, Axelin A. Key factors supporting implementation of a training program for neonatal family-centered care—a qualitative study. BMC Health Serv Res. 2019;19(1):394.
54. Moullin JC, Dickson KS, Stadnick NA, et al. Ten recommendations for using implementation frameworks in research and practice. Implement Sci Commun. 2020;1(1):42.
55. Moullin JC, Sabater-Hernández D, Fernandez-Llimos F, Benrimoj SI. A systematic review of implementation frameworks of innovations in healthcare and resulting generic implementation framework. Health Res Policy Syst. 2015;13:16.
56. Albers B, Mildon R, Lyon AR, Shlonsky A. Implementation frameworks in child, youth and family services—results from a scoping review. Child Youth Serv Rev. 2017;81:101–16.
57. Pineda R, Roussin J, Kwon J, Heiny E, Colditz G, Smith J. Applying the RE-AIM framework to evaluate the implementation of the supporting and enhancing NICU sensory experiences (SENSE) program. BMC Pediatr. 2021;21(1):137.
58. Glasgow RE, Harden SM, Gaglio B, et al. RE-AIM planning and evaluation framework: adapting to new science and practice with a 20-year review. Front Public Health. 2019;7:64.
59. Kwan BM, McGinnes HL, Ory MG, Estabrooks PA, Waxmonsky JA, Glasgow RE. RE-AIM in the real world: use of the RE-AIM framework for program planning and evaluation in clinical and community settings. Front Public Health. 2019;7:345.
60. Hall SL, Hynan MT, Phillips R, et al. The neonatal intensive parenting unit: an introduction. J Perinatol. 2017;37(12):1259–64.
61. Altimier L, Phillips R. The neonatal integrative developmental care model: advanced clinical applications of the seven core measures for neuroprotective family-centered developmental care. Newborn Infant Nurs Rev. 2016;16(4):230–44.
62. Als H, Lawhon G, Duffy FH, McAnulty GB, Gibes-Grossman R, Blickman JG. Individualized developmental care for the very low-birth-weight preterm infant. Medical and neurofunctional effects. JAMA Pediatr. 1994;272(11):853–8.
63. Als H, McAnulty GB. The newborn individualized developmental care and assessment program (NIDCAP) with kangaroo mother care (KMC): comprehensive care for preterm infants. Curr Womens Health Rev. 2011;7(3):288–301.
64. Wallin L, Eriksson M. Newborn individual development care and assessment program (NIDCAP): a systematic review of the literature. Worldviews Evid-Based Nurs. 2009;6(2):54–69.
65. Grisham LM, Stephen MM, Coykendall MR, Kane MF, Maurer JA, Bader MY. Eat, sleep, console approach: a family-centered model for the treatment of neonatal abstinence syndrome. Adv Neonatal Care. 2019;19(2):138–44.
66. Young LW, Ounpraseuth ST, Merhar SL, et al. Eat, sleep, console approach or usual care for neonatal opioid withdrawal. N Engl J Med. 2023;388(25):2326–37.

Chapter 16
Family-Centered Care in the Cardiac Intensive Care Unit

Jonathan Ludmir

Introduction

Cardiovascular critical care delivery involves multiple clinical stakeholders, use of mechanical circulatory support devices, and patients who often require prolonged lengths of stay. Effectively supporting family members in a cardiac intensive care unit (CICU) and other ICUs with critically ill cardiac patients is challenging, and evidence-based approaches to family-centered care are lacking. The 2022 American Heart Association (AHA) Statement ("Engaging Families in Adult Cardiovascular Care") highlights suggestions for supporting families in acute cardiac care settings in order to "decrease the residual trauma that can be associated with these hospitalizations" [1]. Similar to the Society of Critical Care Medicine guidelines [2], the AHA statement stresses the importance of providing open visitation, being present during procedures and resuscitation, participating in family-centered rounds, and having families contribute to direct care [1].

Overview

CICU patients experience an array of clinical, physical, and emotional challenges throughout admission. Modern-day CICUs support a variety of cardiovascular patients; some units exclusively have nonsurgical cardiovascular patients, some have cardiothoracic and/or vascular surgery patients, some have mechanical circulatory support (MCS) patients, and others contain a combination of surgical,

---

J. Ludmir (✉)
Corrigan Minehan Heart Center, Cardiology Division, Massachusetts General Hospital, Harvard Medical School, Cambridge, MA, USA
e-mail: JLUDMIR@mgh.harvard.edu

© The Author(s), under exclusive license to Springer Nature Switzerland AG 2025

A. J. Vance et al. (eds.), *Families in the Intensive Care Unit*,
https://doi.org/10.1007/978-3-031-83786-9_16

nonsurgical, and MCS patients. Postoperative cardiac surgery patients may develop significant complications—some of whom require temporary support devices and a prolonged ICU course with respiratory, renal, and cardiovascular support. Patients with underlying depressed left ventricular ejection fraction, kidney injury, and those with a nonelective surgical status have the highest risk of prolonged ICU lengths of stay [3, 4]. Furthermore, quaternary academic medical centers assume care of higher risk patients, and thus likely have a higher rate of postoperative morbidity and longer ICU lengths of stay. CICU teams should therefore be prepared and equipped to effectively support family members. Moreover, anticipatory guidance as part of the informed consent process should highlight all potential complications and prepare not only the patients but also their families for a potential long and complex postoperative journey [5].

Some CICU patients may require mechanical circulatory support devices as a bridge to myocardial recovery or more definitive durable therapy such as an left ventricular assist device (LVAD) or transplant [6]. Temporary support devices may assist the left ventricle, right ventricle, both ventricles, and/or the lungs. Examples of these devices include: the intra-aortic balloon pump, Impella (left sided and right sided), Protek Duo (right-sided support device), and extracorporeal membrane oxygenation (VA-ECMO or VV-ECMO). Patients on mechanical circulatory support typically have longer lengths of stay, require highly specialized multidisciplinary care, and are prone to significant complications—such as extensive bleeding and/or thromboses [7]. Consequently, families may develop anxiety, PTSD, and depressive symptoms while their loved ones are on MCS [8]. What's more is the potential for a prolonged MCS course (weeks or months), which can lead to further anxiety, depression, and avoidance behaviors [9]. Thus, it becomes critical to provide daily family-centered care through open communication, inclusive rounds, and frequent family meetings [10].

Temporary Mechanical Circulatory Support Devices

The Impella is one of the most commonly used temporary support devices, often remaining in place for days, weeks, or even months. The Impella (left-sided device) may be used electively in high-risk percutaneous coronary interventions, acute cardiogenic shock (most commonly in the setting of myocardial infarction), as an left ventricular vent strategy with concomitant VA-ECMO, or in the setting of decompensated heart failure as a bridge to decision, durable LVAD, or transplant [11, 12]. The American Heart Association recommends early involvement of palliative care specialists when considering escalating to a temporary support device, such as the Impella, as well as when deescalating [7]. In the absence of emergent procedures, placement and removal of temporary devices require careful and thoughtful communication with the patient and family highlighting all of the potential outcomes, in particular, the multitude of possible complications and the risk of not being able to wean the device [13, 14]. The International Society for Heart and Lung

Transplantation (ISHLT) as well as the Heart Failure Society of America (HFSA) recommends setting expectations with families and using the N-U-R-S-E mnemonic for communicating (Naming, Understanding, Respecting, Supporting, Exploring) to help frame discussions surrounding support devices [14]. Establishing early goals of care with the patient and family is key as is the involvement of palliative care. Unfortunately, few temporary support device patients receive palliative care consultations. One 2018 National Inpatient Sample study of 10,930 patients with support devices revealed that only 20% received palliative care services [15]. While the downstream effect of palliative care in temporary MCS patients has not been extensively studied, a randomized control trial of advanced heart failure patients demonstrated that palliative care involvement led to an improvement in patient quality of life, anxiety, depression, and spiritual well-being [16]. Similarly, we can extrapolate the finding to patients and families with temporary support devices by offering early palliative care consultations, which is in line with AHA, ISHLT, and HFSA recommendations. We can also learn from Indiana University which successfully implemented a multidisciplinary protocol for early palliative care involvement in all patients being considered for MCS implantation. The protocol involved effective communication between the cardiology team and palliative care team as well as palliative care participation in weekly cardiovascular meetings. The implementation resulted in an increase in palliative care consults for MCS patients from 17.2% to 96.6% [17].

Venoarterial ECMO is another form of temporary support device used for left-sided, right-side, or biventricular failure. Additionally, VA-ECMO is unique as it is the only device used in the setting of cardiac arrest through extracorporeal cardiopulmonary resuscitation (E-CPR) [18]. Hence, it is often implemented in emergent situations using implied consent, sometimes without knowledge of family members. And, thus it becomes even more important to not only focus on optimal ECMO management but also "preventing and relieving suffering and providing emotional support to the patients and their families" [19]. Similar to other temporary support device patients, ECMO patients also benefit from early palliative care involvement. One recent ECMO registry review revealed that only 44.9% of patients received palliative care consultation with higher proportion of consults occurring when the ICU attending physician was from a medical specialty (versus surgical specialty) [20]. Similar to other temporary support device patients, VA-ECMO patients typically have a shorter run time as decisions need to be made regarding potential decannulation, transitioning to other devices, or terminal decannulation [7]. Withdrawal of ECMO support is indicated with catastrophic events (such as a massive intracranial bleed resulting in brain death) or if the patient has no exit strategy [21, 22]. In a single center study of 460 VA-ECMO patients, early palliative care consultation resulted in a significantly shorter duration of VA-ECMO use, reflecting the effective goals of care conversations with families [22]. As noted above, a standardized approach to early palliative care involvement for all temporary device patients, but in particular, VA-ECMO patients, is crucial.

Durable LVAD Support

CICU patients, in particular those with durable LVADs, require significant family support post-discharge. Family involvement in care tasks and partnership with the medical team has demonstrated positive overall benefits for caregivers [23]. One ICU study found that more than 80% of family members preferred being involved with daily grooming, communication, and education [24]. Family members may experience emotional distress, a heavy feeling of responsibilities, and often lack coping strategies with their love ones post-LVAD or transplant [25]. In one study of 50 caregivers of patients receiving LVAD therapy, a high level of strain existed within the first month which gradually improved by 6 months [26]. Yet, in another study of 41 caregivers of LVAD patients, depression and anxiety symptoms showed no improvement in the first 3 months postimplantation [27]. However, with appropriate support and eventual understanding and acceptance of the caregiver's new role, adjustment and emotional improvement is feasible [28–30]. Family support and discussion regarding expectations throughout the ICU stay perhaps can help mitigate some of the psychological symptoms. At many institutions, both the nurses and LVAD specialists spend ample time teaching family members about daily VAD care. Furthermore, one study of a nationally distributed training course designed to teach LVAD clinicians on how best to support caregivers showed promising results. The 10 LVAD clinicians who completed the training and used the program to support caregivers were deemed "caregiver coaches," and were successfully able to assist family members in LVAD care [31]. At MGH, the LVAD coordinators and cardiac nurses educate family members on LVAD care and ensure that the caregivers are comfortable with all aspects of LVAD care such as driveline changes prior to discharge.

Institutional Experience

At the Massachusetts General Hospital, a 999-bed urban quaternary care academic medical center with two CICUs totaling 34 beds, certain key family-centered care principles have been implemented. This includes at least weekly multidisciplinary family meetings, daily updates (either during family-centered rounds or at other parts of the day), nursing-led family instruction and environmental orientation, family recuperation space, and open visitation for the most critically ill. Additionally, all patients on VA-ECMO automatically receive an ethics consultation [32]. Beginning in 2013, the MGH ethics team has been consulting on all patients cannulated for VA-ECMO to provide overall support for family and staff by focusing on two main issues: patient goals of care and to assist with decision regarding duration/goal of ECMO [32]. Furthermore, all patients considered for transplantation are evaluated by palliative care, social work, and psychiatry. Palliative care specialists can effectively support patients and their families, assist with decision-making, and aid with end-of life care when needed [10, 33, 34]. During the tumultuous time that a patient is on MCS, extra family support is necessary to mitigate psychological symptoms. Benefits of these support systems have yet to be carefully explored in the CICU, yet the positive benefits can be deduced from general adult and pediatric ICU data [2].

CICU Clinical Stakeholders

Another unique feature of the CICU is the multidisciplinary clinical team approach (Fig. 16.1). Many patients in the ICU are managed or co-managed by an ICU team, heart failure/transplant team, and a cardiac surgery team [35, 36]. In some institutions, all stakeholders round together to ensure all teams come up with a unified plan. For example, at our institution, the ICU team rounds together with the heart failure/transplant cardiology team on all patients in the peri-transplant period as well as most patients with temporary support devices. The cardiac surgery team is also involved daily in the overall care plan through frequent communication. Given the multiple stakeholders, it is critical to deliver consistent and united messages to the family to minimize confusion and cause further stress. Thus, we have implemented weekly multidisciplinary meetings (which must include at least the ICU team and the cardiac surgeons) for patients on VA-ECMO and any patient remaining in the ICU > 7 days. Furthermore, ensuring the stakeholders are skilled in serious illness conversations as well as using preset evidence-based protocols, such as Dr. Curtis' VALUE (validate, acknowledge, listen, understand, elicit) algorithm can be useful [36, 37]. In a randomized, multicenter study using the mnemonic VALUE to guide family conversations decreased anxiety, depression, and PTSD symptoms among caregivers at 90 days post-intervention [38]. Our institution is in the process of studying a standardized family meeting approach in our CICUs and exploring caregiver perceptions.

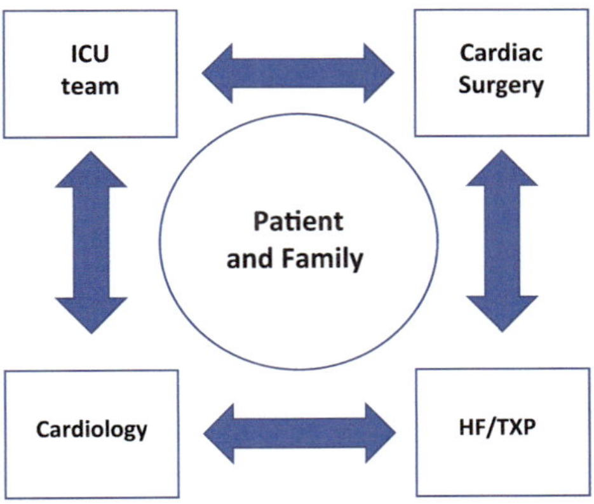

Fig. 16.1 Key stakeholders in the cardiac ICU

Family-Centered Rounds

Few data exist surrounding the role of family-centered rounds (FCR) in the CICU. One national survey found that a majority of cardiologists believed that FCR in the CICU benefits families and improves overall communication, but also may reduce workflow efficiency and result in longer duration of rounds [39]. A recent 2023 survey study from the Critical Care Cardiology Trials Network of 39 North American CICUs found that only 25% of sites fully adopted family-centered rounds [40]. Additionally, the survey noted significant variability in CICU attending interest in family-centered care practices, including FCR, making it challenging to standardize family support practices [40]. Multiple non-CICU-based studies have solidified the benefits of family-centered rounds—through reduction of family member stress and anxiety, improving family-clinician communication, and augmenting overall satisfaction [2, 41]. Furthermore, some studies also suggest that rounds do not increase in duration and by including families less time may actually be needed during the day for updates [41, 42]. While family-centered rounds in the CICU may be more challenging given the multiple stakeholders and unique patient population, data are lacking to prove its efficacy. Given the paucity of data, our institution recently analyzed the role of virtual family-centered rounds over the course of one year. During the course of the one year of study, 82 family members participated in FCR, and 75% of post-discharge survey respondents perceived the highest level of trust, communication, and compassion with the medical team [43]. Despite the high level of family satisfaction and improvement in communication, standardizing FCR in our institution, like in others, remains challenging. Significant variations in family involvement in rounds exist amongst the team, prompting the need for further optimal implementation strategies.

Novel Approaches—Child Life

Given the paucity of family support intervention studies in the adult CICU, we can learn from our pediatric colleagues [44]. The importance of acknowledging and addressing children's emotional needs has been recognized for a century and was formalized into the field of Child Life [41]. Child Life specialists provide support through providing play experiences, presenting developmentally appropriate medical information, and establishing therapeutic relationships with the child and family [45]. Child Life has been demonstrated to improve the experience for pediatric patients and their respective families and should be considered for adult patients [46]. A pilot study at Michigan Medicine incorporated Child Life in the overall care of cardiac surgery patients. In this study, 11 cardiac surgery patients were randomized to either receive routine care or a total of five sessions with a Child Life specialist throughout the cardiac surgery journey (preop, ICU, and on the stepdown). Child life involvement was well received by patients and their families and resulted in a

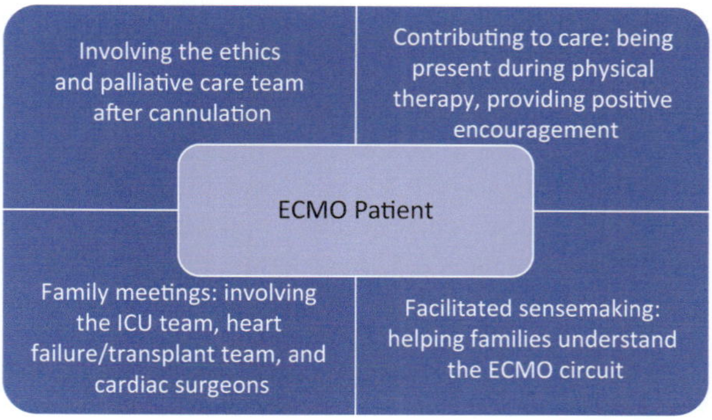

Fig. 16.2 Family support strategies for ECMO patients

positive experience [47]. Participants completed a qualitative follow-up phone survey after discharge. One patient reported the following: "I benefited greatly from talking with the comfort coach. From simple distraction, things like a glitter wand to guided imagery" [47]. While Child Life support is standard in pediatrics, it remains novel in adult medicine and certainly merits further investigation as a patient and family-centered support tool. Moreover, as many cardiac ICU patients, in particular those with temporary support devices, have long lengths of stay, effective patient/family support strategies are necessary to mitigate downstream psychological symptoms (Fig. 16.2).

Teaching Families

Throughout an ICU admission, family members are exposed to learning more about their loved one's disease process and recovery. This process may spark conversations about preventative measures in hopes of avoiding further illness both for the patient and caregiver. The 2022 AHA family support statement also highlights how families are often willing to be referred for cardiovascular screening [1]. In one study of acute coronary syndrome patients admitted to a CICU, patients were given a letter for family members to obtain cardiovascular screening. A total of 51 patients referred 101 family members for screening, demonstrating the success of a patient-led referral strategy [48]. While the exact timing and logistics of when to approach patients with screening letters is unclear, perhaps it makes sense prior to transferring out of the ICU. One suggested approach is for a medical team member (nurse or physician) to discuss family cardiovascular screening during a family update or meeting, and to provide a letter toward the end of the ICU stay and also after hospital discharge. Often, family cardiovascular screening is discussed throughout the ICU stay, in particular, when patients suffer from early onset myocardial infarction, acute aortic dissection, or familial cardiomyopathy (among other conditions).

Conclusions

The cardiovascular ICU poses unique communication and family support challenges. Utilizing the SCCM guidelines and guidance from the recent AHA family support statement—CICUs can learn to optimize the delivery of family-centered care. Further research is needed to understand the efficacy of family-centered care interventions in the CICU in order to create standardized supportive approaches.

References

1. Goldfarb MJ, Bechtel C, Capers Q, et al. Engaging families in adult cardiovascular care: a scientific statement from the American Heart Association. J Am Heart Assoc. 2022;11(10):e025859. https://doi.org/10.1161/JAHA.122.025859.
2. Davidson JE, Aslakson RA, Long AC, et al. Guidelines for family-centered care in the neonatal, pediatric, and adult ICU. Crit Care Med. 2017;45(1):103–28. https://doi.org/10.1097/CCM.0000000000002169.
3. Barili F, Barzaghi N, Cheema FH, et al. An original model to predict intensive care unit length-of stay after cardiac surgery in a competing risk framework. Int J Cardiol. 2013;168(1):219–25. https://doi.org/10.1016/j.ijcard.2012.09.091.
4. Almashrafi A, Elmontsri M, Aylin P. Systematic review of factors influencing length of stay in ICU after adult cardiac surgery. BMC Health Serv Res. 2016;16:318. https://doi.org/10.1186/s12913-016-1591-3.
5. Isenberg SR, Aslakson RA, Dionne-Odom JN, et al. Family companions' involvement during pre-surgical consent visits for major cancer surgery and its relationship to visit communication and satisfaction. Patient Educ Couns. 2018;101(6):1066–74. https://doi.org/10.1016/j.pec.2018.01.011.
6. Shreenivas SS, Rame JE, Jessup M. Mechanical circulatory support as a bridge to transplant or for destination therapy. Curr Heart Fail Rep. 2010;7(4):159–66. https://doi.org/10.1007/s11897-010-0026-4.
7. Geller BJ, Sinha SS, Kapur NK, et al. Escalating and de-escalating temporary mechanical circulatory support in cardiogenic shock: a scientific statement from the American Heart Association. Circulation. 2022;146(6):e50–68. https://doi.org/10.1161/CIR.0000000000001076.
8. Onrust M, Lansink-Hartgring AO, van der Meulen I, Luttik ML, de Jong J, Dieperink W. Coping strategies, anxiety and depressive symptoms in family members of patients treated with extracorporeal membrane oxygenation: a prospective cohort study. Heart Lung. 2022;52:146–51. https://doi.org/10.1016/j.hrtlng.2022.01.002.
9. Goetzinger AM, Blumenthal JA, O'Hayer CV, et al. Stress and coping in caregivers of patients awaiting solid organ transplantation. Clin Transpl. 2012;26(1):97–104. https://doi.org/10.1111/j.1399-0012.2011.01431.x.
10. Grouls A, Dobbie K, Neuendorf K, et al. Top 10 tips palliative care clinicians should know about working with adults receiving extracorporeal membrane oxygenation. J Palliat Med. 2023;26:1270. https://doi.org/10.1089/jpm.2023.0017.
11. Zein R, Patel C, Mercado-Alamo A, Schreiber T, Kaki A. A review of the impella devices. Interv Cardiol. 2022;17:e05. https://doi.org/10.15420/icr.2021.11.
12. Amin AP, Spertus JA, Curtis JP, et al. The evolving landscape of impella use in the United States among patients undergoing percutaneous coronary intervention with mechanical circulatory support. Circulation. 2020;141(4):273–84. https://doi.org/10.1161/CIRCULATIONAHA.119.044007.

13. Oren D, Zilinyi R, Lotan D, Uriel M, Uriel N, Sayer G. The role of temporary mechanical circulatory support as a bridge to advanced heart failure therapies or recovery. Curr Opin Cardiol. 2022;37(5):394–402. https://doi.org/10.1097/HCO.0000000000000976.
14. Bernhardt AM, Copeland H, Deswal A, et al. The international society for heart and lung transplantation/heart failure society of America guideline on acute mechanical circulatory support. J Heart Lung Transplant. 2023;42(4):e1–e64. https://doi.org/10.1016/j.healun.2022.10.028.
15. Khdeir O, Atluri R, Krishan S, Yalamanchili S. Utilization of palliative care services inhospitalizations with cardiogenic shock on temporary mechanical circulatory support. J Soc Cardiovasc Angiogr Intervent. 2022;1:5.
16. Rogers JG, Patel CB, Mentz RJ, et al. Palliative care in heart failure: the PAL-HF randomized, controlled clinical trial. J Am Coll Cardiol. 2017;70(3):331–41. https://doi.org/10.1016/j.jacc.2017.05.030.
17. Sinha S, Belcher C, Torke A, et al. Development of a protocol for successful palliative care consultation in population of patients receiving mechanical circulatory support. J Pain Symptom Manag. 2017;54(4):583–8. https://doi.org/10.1016/j.jpainsymman.2017.07.021.
18. Kruit N, Burrell A, Tian D, et al. Expert consensus on training and accreditation for extracorporeal cardiopulmonary resuscitation an international, multidisciplinary modified Delphi study. Resuscitation. 2023;192:109989. https://doi.org/10.1016/j.resuscitation.2023.109989.
19. Padilla M. The sooner the better: initiating palliative care in extracorporeal membrane oxygenation. Am J Crit Care. 2023;32(3):175. https://doi.org/10.4037/ajcc2023919.
20. Peeler A, Davidson PM, Gleason KT, et al. Palliative care utilization in patients requiring extracorporeal membrane oxygenation: an observational study. ASAIO J. 2023;69(11):1009–15. https://doi.org/10.1097/MAT.0000000000002021.
21. Godfrey S, Sahoo A, Sanchez J, et al. The role of palliative care in withdrawal of venoarterial extracorporeal membrane oxygenation for cardiogenic shock. J Pain Symptom Manag. 2021;61(6):1139–46. https://doi.org/10.1016/j.jpainsymman.2020.10.027.
22. Carey MR, Tong W, Godfrey S, Takeda K, Nakagawa S. Withdrawal of temporary mechanical circulatory support in patients with capacity. J Pain Symptom Manag. 2022;63(3):387–94. https://doi.org/10.1016/j.jpainsymman.2021.10.007.
23. Liput SA, Kane-Gill SL, Seybert AL, Smithburger PL. A review of the perceptions of healthcare providers and family members toward family involvement in active adult patient care in the ICU. Crit Care Med. 2016;44(6):1191–7. https://doi.org/10.1097/CCM.0000000000001641.
24. Hetland BD, McAndrew NS, Kupzyk KA, et al. Family caregiver preferences and contributions related to patient care in the ICU. West J Nurs Res. 2022;44(3):214–26. https://doi.org/10.1177/01939459211062954.
25. Cicolini G, Cerratti F, Della Pelle C, Simonetti V. The experience of family caregivers of patients with a left ventricular assist device: an integrative review. Prog Transplant. 2016;26(2):135–48. https://doi.org/10.1177/1526924816640648.
26. Bidwell JT, Lyons KS, Mudd JO, et al. Patient and caregiver determinants of patient quality of life and caregiver strain in left ventricular assist device therapy. J Am Heart Assoc. 2018;7(6):e008080. https://doi.org/10.1161/JAHA.117.008080.
27. Bidwell JT, Lyons KS, Mudd JO, et al. Quality of life, depression, and anxiety in ventricular assist device therapy: longitudinal outcomes for patients and family caregivers. J Cardiovasc Nurs. 2017;32(5):455–63. https://doi.org/10.1097/JCN.0000000000000378.
28. Marcuccilli L, Casida JJ, Bakas T, Pagani FD. Family caregivers' inside perspectives: caring for an adult with a left ventricular assist device as a destination therapy. Prog Transplant. 2014;24(4):332–40. https://doi.org/10.7182/pit2014684.
29. Akbarin M, Aarts C. Being a close relative of a patient with a left ventricular assist device. Eur J Cardiovasc Nurs. 2013;12(1):64–8. https://doi.org/10.1177/1474515111432996.
30. Marcuccilli L, Casida JM. From insiders' perspectives: adjusting to caregiving for patients with left ventricular assist devices. Prog Transplant. 2011;21(2):137–43. https://doi.org/10.1177/152692481102100209.

31. Pfahl J, Thompson JS, Matlock DD, et al. ENABLE-LVAD: development and implementation of a novel training program for clinicians supporting family caregivers of patients with a left ventricular assist device. J Cardiovasc Nurs. 2023;39:E136. https://doi.org/10.1097/JCN.0000000000001065.
32. Courtwright AM, Robinson EM, Feins K, et al. Ethics committee consultation and extracorporeal membrane oxygenation. Ann Am Thorac Soc. 2016;13(9):1553–8. https://doi.org/10.1513/AnnalsATS.201511-757OC.
33. Wordingham SE, McIlvennan CK. Palliative care for patients on mechanical circulatory support. AMA J Ethics. 2019;21(5):E435–42. https://doi.org/10.1001/amajethics.2019.435.
34. van Diepen S, Katz JN, Albert NM, et al. Contemporary management of cardiogenic shock: a scientific statement from the American Heart Association. Circulation. 2017;136(16):e232–68. https://doi.org/10.1161/CIR.0000000000000525.
35. Quien M, Thomas A, Ludmir J, Miller PE. Staffing models in the cardiac intensive care unit. Curr Opin Crit Care. 2022;28(4):453–9. https://doi.org/10.1097/MCC.0000000000000958.
36. Metkus TS, Lindsley J, Fair L, et al. Quality of heart failure care in the intensive care unit. J Cardiac Fail. 2021;27(10):1111–25. https://doi.org/10.1016/j.cardfail.2021.08.001.
37. Curtis JR, White DB. Practical guidance for evidence-based ICU family conferences. Chest. 2008;134(4):835–43. https://doi.org/10.1378/chest.08-0235.
38. Lautrette A, Darmon M, Megarbane B, et al. A communication strategy and brochure for relatives of patients dying in the ICU. N Engl J Med. 2007;356(5):469–78. https://doi.org/10.1056/NEJMoa063446.
39. Ludmir J, Liu X, Gupta A, et al. Cardiologist perceptions of family-centred rounds in cardiovascular clinical care. Open Heart. 2018;5(2):e000834. https://doi.org/10.1136/openhrt-2018-000834.
40. Goldfarb M, Alviar C, Berg D, et al. Family engagement in the adult cardiac intensive care unit: a survey of family engagement practices in the cardiac critical care trials network. Circ Cardiovasc Qual Outcomes. 2023;16(9):e010084. https://doi.org/10.1161/CIRCOUTCOMES.123.010084.
41. Ludmir J, Netzer G. Family-centered care in the intensive care unit-what does best practice tell us? Semin Respir Crit Care Med. 2019;40(5):648–54. https://doi.org/10.1055/s-0039-1697957.
42. Rappaport DI, Ketterer TA, Nilforoshan V, Sharif I. Family-centered rounds: views of families, nurses, trainees, and attending physicians. Clin Pediatr. 2012;51(3):260–6. https://doi.org/10.1177/0009922811421002.
43. Ramirez P, Mueller A, Shelton K, et al. Family perceptions of virtual family-centered rounds in a quaternary cardiac intensive care unit. J Intensive Care Med. 2024;39:8850666241233495. https://doi.org/10.1177/08850666241233495.
44. Ludmir J, Small AJ. The challenge of identifying and addressing psychological comorbidities. J Am Coll Cardiol. 2018;71(14):1590–3. https://doi.org/10.1016/j.jacc.2018.02.042.
45. American Academy of Pediatrics. Committee on hospital care. Child Life Serv Pediatr. 2000;106(5):1156–9.
46. Bruce Je MK. Child life in the adult ICU: including the youngest members of the family. In: Families in the intensive care unit: a guide to understanding, engaging, and supporting at the bedside. Springer; 2018.
47. Piazza J, Heering L, Peters SL, et al. Child life-facilitated coping support with adult patients undergoing cardiac surgery: a pilot program. J Child Life Psychosoc Theory Pract. 2022;3(2) https://doi.org/10.55591/001c.38502.
48. Castiel J, Chen-Tournoux A, Thanassoulis G, Goldfarb M. A patient-led referral strategy for cardiovascular screening of family and household members at the time of cardiac intensive care unit admission. CJC Open. 2020;2(6):506–13. https://doi.org/10.1016/j.cjco.2020.06.014.

Chapter 17
Supporting Families of Patients in Neuroscience Intensive Care Units

Andrew P. Huang and David Y. Hwang

Introduction

In the clinic for survivors of severe, acute brain injury, the patient sat down slowly with his walker, 3 months after suffering anoxic brain injury from sudden cardiac arrest. In the neuroscience intensive care unit (NICU), he had been in a coma, and his note had read: poor neurologic prognosis. “I never thought we could get to this,” his wife said. “He is getting stronger and stronger every day, but he is different.”

In addition to anoxic brain injury in the vignette above, common examples of severe, acute brain injury include ischemic stroke, intracerebral hemorrhage, traumatic brain injury, and subarachnoid hemorrhage. The experience of families for severe, acute brain injury patients—many admitted to dedicated NICUs—can differ from those for patients with non-neurologic diseases with regard to prognostic uncertainty, threat to a patient’s personal identity, and varying opinions regarding patient quality of life with cognitive and functional impairment.

Patients with acute brain injury experience a sudden and severe deterioration that prompts NICU admission. They lose neurologic function rapidly, contrasting other illness trajectories (Fig. 17.1a, b) [1, 2]. *Hyperacutely* over the first couple of days or so in the NICU, many families experience shock while patients are evaluated for emergent interventions (e.g., thrombolysis, thrombectomy, craniotomy or

A. P. Huang
Division of Neuropalliative Care, Department of Neurology, University of Rochester Medical Center, Rochester, NY, USA
e-mail: Andrew_Huang@urmc.rochester.edu

D. Y. Hwang (✉)
Division of Neurocritical Care, Department of Neurology, University of North Carolina School of Medicine, Chapel Hill, NC, USA
e-mail: David_hwang@med.unc.edu

© The Author(s), under exclusive license to Springer Nature Switzerland AG 2025

A. J. Vance et al. (eds.), *Families in the Intensive Care Unit*,
https://doi.org/10.1007/978-3-031-83786-9_17

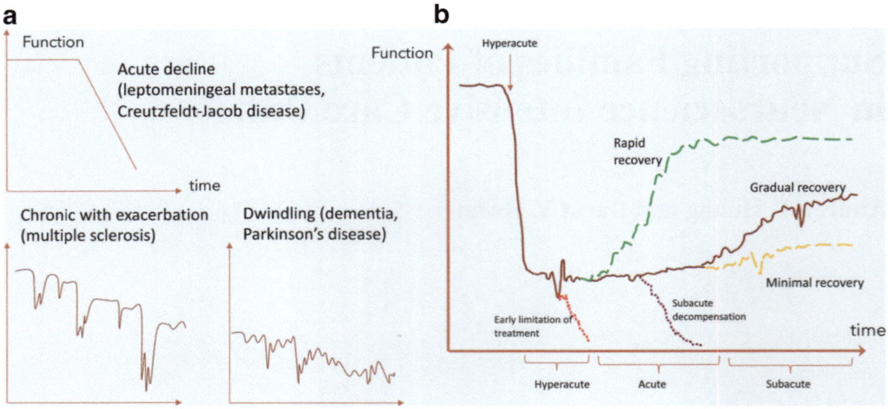

Fig. 17.1 Illness trajectories of severe, acute brain injury. (**a**) Other illness trajectories. (**b**) Severe, acute brain injury

craniectomy, anticoagulation reversal, intraventricular drain placement), if the initial goal is determined to be patient survival. *Acutely* over their first days to a week or so, many brain injury patients are stabilized from secondary and subsequent brain injuries (e.g., seizures, intracranial hemorrhage, elevated intracranial pressure, herniation, delayed cerebral ischemia). For some patients, *subacutely* over days to weeks, families and clinical teams assess long-term quality-of-life outcomes and arrive at decisions regarding life-sustaining therapies like tracheostomy or gastrostomy and optimal rehabilitation settings. Depending on goals-of-care discussions, patients may transition out of the NICU to an uncertain future or a natural death.

In this chapter, we discuss topics related to supporting NICU families using these archetypal phases of a typical admission, recognizing that many patients facing brain injury may shift between phases. Within each phase, we emphasize the NICU clinician's approach to family communication as an organized procedure during discussions of specific considerations; such as early limitation of life-sustaining therapies, brain death discussions, and decision-making regarding tracheostomy and gastrostomy [3, 4].

General Approaches to NICU Communication

Communication skill in the NICU can be learned like procedural skills [5, 6]. Just as clinicians can learn procedures through step-by-step processes, they can also learn communication with families in NICUs through practice [7]. Typical steps of a family meeting include a pre-brief (meeting before the meeting to discuss goals of the meeting), orienting the meeting (introducing participants, setting an agenda), sharing information, making a plan, and a debrief afterward. These steps allow clinicians to evaluate patient and family values and allow families to understand medical circumstances from clinical teams [8]. They can give clinicians the opportunity to respond to strong emotions that may arise in meeting participants [7] and help tackle challenging decisions such as whether a patient should undergo tracheostomy and gastrostomy.

Hyperacute Period

The Family Experience

Hyperacutely over the first few days (Fig. 17.1b), family members of brain injury survivors can experience terrible situations of shock and urgent decisions. They can feel overwhelmed with emotional, cognitive, social, and spiritual distress [9] that can cause prolonged grief and post-traumatic stress later [10, 11]. Families must serve as proxies in high-stakes decision-making [12] because brain injury survivors frequently lack decisional capacity. They must forecast what their loved one would want, which may be unknown. As a result, families (and clinicians) can fall prey to a host of cognitive biases when making rapid and early decisions based on forecasts of prognosis; e.g., biases of confirmation (favoring information confirming previous belief), anchoring (favoring initial conclusions drawn from initial data), and framing (favoring information given in either a positive or negative context) [13].

Meeting Family Needs

Decision-making support. Healthcare staff can support families with decision-making by using established communication strategies. For example, the skill of "being explicit" [8] ("your loved one is experiencing a large stroke") can help clinicians shorten verbose explanations ("the CT angiogram we just obtained showed a tandem, proximal occlusion of the middle cerebral artery"). Being explicit can reduce the effort required by families in shock to understand the situation and allow more time deciding how to move forward. Clinical teams need to identify the patient's named proxy or legal surrogate. While clinicians assess how proxies approach decisions—i.e., to what degree a proxy wants to be the decision-maker or defer to the clinical team—proxies need to understand the medical circumstances.

Sometimes, strong emotions and cognitive biases can impede communication and deliberation. Strong emotions in families can arise from hearing serious news. Clinicians can help families with strong emotions by communication skills such as empathy ("I can only imagine what it is like to hear this") and empowerment ("It is incredible how hard you are working to honor your loved one's wishes"). Cognitive biases can be ameliorated by pre-brief time-outs, which are a mindful practice and akin to intentional pauses prior to procedures [14]. Such pauses can draw attention to missed facts, unvoiced moral distress, and cognitive pitfalls [15].

Early Limitations of Life-Sustaining Therapy

Limiting life-sustaining therapy in the first days after admission can create ethical concerns for brain injury patients. Outcomes after severe brain injury range widely from neurologically devastated to full recovery, and our ability to predict outcome is limited. When patients die from limiting life support in the first days after admission, one concern is that such deaths may be a result of overly nihilistic perceptions of a patient's prognosis and quality of life by family or clinical teams [16, 17], when the patient could have possibly had acceptable recovery. Outcome studies of brain injury have become biased to some degree by including patient deaths from limiting life support [18], potentially coloring the information clinicians use to advise patients and families who face brain injury. This fear—described as a 'self-fulfilling prophecy' [19]—has led guidelines for several types of brain injuries to recommend generally avoiding early limitation of life-sustaining therapy in the first 48–72 h [17, 20, 21].

On the other hand, prolonging life-sustaining therapy in certain situations may disrespect a patient's interests and values. Early limitation of life-sustaining therapy is appropriate when advance care directives or conversations with proxies paint a clear and convincing preference to limit prolonging life in the setting of clear poor prognosis or long uncertain recovery.

Acute Period

The Family Experience

In the acute period (Fig. 17.1b), families of the typical acute brain injury patient witness the aftermath of neurologic injury. Clinical teams stabilize the patient from complications (e.g., seizures, secondary ischemia or hemorrhage, increased intracranial pressure, paroxysmal autonomic storming, hemodynamic compromise, delirium). Families can experience moral distress wondering about the future and whether their loved one will remain severely disabled [22]. Surrogate perceptions of patient values are often incomplete or indeterminate [23]. They may wonder "who am I" to decide on goals-of-care and feel reluctant to "let" their loved one pass away. They may struggle to achieve family consensus or predict how the potential cost of long-term care might impact family members' own lives. [24] In surveys of hypothetical circumstances of having a loved one face brain injury [25], top concerns include family agreement, prognostic accuracy, religion, and cost of care.

Meeting Family Needs

Build the clinical relationship. Families in the NICU need assistance in the clinical relationship to make healthcare decisions for their loved one. Clinical relationships require trust and effective communication between parties. Unlike the hyperacute period, the acute period allows clinical teams to build the clinical relationship with the patient and family.

Evaluating the psychosocial determinants of the survivor and family is essential in decision-making. While some family members may be overwhelmed by shock, others may desire information. While many families are highly involved in decisions, others may be more deferential to the clinical team [25]. Premature closure of investigating surrogates' decision-making concerns is similar to premature closure in diagnosis. Assessments in the prior hyperacute period may have missed religious beliefs against limiting life support or regret from previous healthcare decisions of family members.

Anchor prognosis with clinical humility. Clinical humility, which is a psychological care attitude embracing uncertainty [26, 27], is important toward the current science of prognostication in brain injury. In one study on patients with moderate to severe traumatic brain injury, 82% of patients who initially were comatose later regained consciousness in the short term. In total, 40% of patients comatose during post-acute care rehabilitation regained *functional independence* by the end of rehabilitation [28]. Studies of cardiac arrest survivorship show disparities in outcome and frequency of limiting life support based on location between specialized "hub" cardiac arrest centers [29, 30] and "spoke" centers. Prognostic scales in stroke may be biased by early limitation of life-sustaining therapy, with outcome studies showing significant variability due to delivery settings [15, 31]. While families need clinical humility in their clinicians regarding discussions of prognosis, they also need a ballpark of potential outcomes to anchor forecasts of the future.

Death by Neurologic Criteria

Patients with the most severe of brain injuries may progress to brain death or death by neurologic criteria, despite best efforts of the NICU team. In the United States, brain death is defined as the permanent and irreversible cessation of all functions of the entire brain, including the brain stem [32]. An individual no longer has the legal rights of the living once fulfilling death by neurologic criteria. The clinical determination of brain death involves lack of arousal/awareness, absent brainstem reflexes (nonreactive pupils, lack of corneal, oculocephalic, oculovestibular, cough, gag reflex, no brain mediated motor response in the face or limbs to noxious stimuli), and no spontaneous respiration, as well as formal testing for apnea. Ancillary testing, such as a nuclear medicine cerebral perfusion study, may supplement clinical determination in circumstances of uncertainty or clinical limitation (e.g., if apnea testing is not possible).

Communicating with families about brain death is challenging due to its emotionally charged nature, organ donation, and how life-sustaining therapy will be addressed. The clinical determination and laws regarding brain death can come into conflict with the diversity of cultural and societal perceptions around death. Families find the BD/DNC diagnosis counter-intuitive because their loved one's body is warm with a beating heart. The risk of family distrust is high [33], especially given the parallel process of organ donation.

Family meetings to communicate with families about BD/DNC should include a pre-brief for the clinical team (and organ procurement organization, if involved) to plan what content will be discussed. Communication programs have been specifically developed to practice communicating about brain death in a simulated, low-stakes environment [34]. Important topics to discuss include acknowledgment of brain death as a legal construct; broad acceptance of the clinical examination; and ventilator withdrawal with respect to time needed for family closure.

Subacute to Chronic Period

The Family Experience

In the weeks and months after brain injury, family can experience fatigue regarding the patient's debilitated state, cautious hope from slow recovery, or new shock from clinical decompensation. Families can experience moral distress wondering about the patient's future, their assumptions about the patient's wishes, and the impact of prolonged rehabilitation or skilled nursing facility admission [22, 25]. Surrogates can have trouble separating what they want for the patient and what the patient would want for themselves. Conflicts can develop within family, within healthcare teams, or between healthcare team and family. Healthcare staff can feel distressed as well when the care plan goes against their values [35].

Meeting Family Needs

Cultivate the clinical relationship. To tackle challenging decisions about life-sustaining therapy in the subacute and chronic period, families need guidance through the clinical relationship. One important topic is communicating explicitly about conflicting goals. While most families hope for approaches that will simultaneously pursue neurorecovery and minimize suffering, individuals vary on how much one is willing to allow a patient to through for the prospect of uncertain recovery. As time increases after the initial brain injury, families and clinical teams can feel stuck between these goals, as more data clarify a patient's trajectory.

One useful concept to foster the clinical relationship is using a time-limited trial, which is an agreement between the clinical team and family to use time without decision to collect more information before re-engaging deliberation about the issue at hand [36]. Time-limited trials are correlated with improved quality of family meetings and reduced intensity and duration of ICU treatments [37]. The agreement includes a statement of the purpose of the trial (e.g., to see if a patient has more neurologic recovery over a month), a plan for subsequent meetings and decision timeline, as well as the risks of not making a decision. These time trials can help surrogates feel that their loved one was given the chance to recover and that the surrogates themselves were given an opportunity to perceive clinical trajectory.

Discuss prognosis and clinical trajectory. NICU clinicians may unconsciously be biased toward more negative outcomes compared to rehabilitation clinicians, who may experience a range of positive patient outcomes in their day-to-day work [38, 39]. On the other hand, in one cohort study of family care goals for brain injury patients, many participants set patients' minimally acceptable cognitive recovery at "able to think and communicate" (82%) or physical independence (66%) or better, while most patients survived below that level (64% and 80%, respectively) at 6 months. After discussing prognosis in the acute period with initial ranges and guard rails, additional time and data can help refine [40] prognostic estimate ranges. Prognosis should be expressed with "best, worst, and most likely case"' scenarios, depicting a range of outcomes, which complement the range of timelines of recovery (Fig. 1).

Tracheostomy and Gastrostomy

NICU patients in the subacute/chronic period frequently face the need for permanent tracheostomy and or gastrostomy (trach/PEG). Impaired mental status from brain injury commonly precludes safe swallowing or ventilation beyond the safe duration of temporary feeding or endotracheal tube (skin and airway mucosal breakdown). Many individuals have strong preferences about being on permanent life-sustaining therapy. Many patients and families need multiple conversations, trust, and exploration of preferences to decide about tracheostomy and gastrostomy. Families should know that it is ethically permissible to stop either form of life-sustaining treatment in the future, though it can be challenging logistically for nursing facilities and morally for families.

In one study of time-limited trials about life-sustaining therapy in the NICU [22], families incorporated patients' pre-stroke health and stated views of treatment preferences into their decisions following such trials. If a patient had already discussed hypothetical life-threatening illness and had deteriorating health, time-limited trials reinforced the plan to limit care. If a patient was moderately independent before injury, families tended to give their loved one more time, limiting care only later if poor prognosis was confirmed. If treatment preferences were unknown and the patient was independent, families tended to continue treatments without limits.

NICU decision-making regarding trach/PEG and life-sustaining treatment in general is centered upon the idea of goal concordance. Such concordance often assumes fidelity of personal identity amongst an incapacitated patient's decision-makers. However, for NICU patients, personal identity may be forevermore altered. When assessing and respecting goal concordance, a patient's surrogate and/or family may need to factor in their own perceptions of long-term ability to care for patients once a trach/PEG has been performed, whether plans for a longer time-limited trial have been established or not. In studies, limiting life-sustaining therapy occurred less in patients with high religiosity, certain racial backgrounds, or who underwent surgery, and more in settings of delirium [18, 41–44].

Future Areas of Importance

Families of NICU patients with brain injury face a roller coaster of experiences. Hyperacutely, families need support to make urgent, life-death care decisions, especially toward limiting life support. Acutely, families and clinical teams may need space and time via which they can exchange information about clinical courses, potential complications, and patients as persons before illness. Subacutely, families may need help in navigating possible fluctuating goals of care, such as to rehabilitate and preserve life or to move away from life-sustaining therapy.

Future directions to support NICU families include strengthening care transitions between intensive care, hospital floor, and discharge, evidenced by the rise of post-ICU clinics [45, 46]. The post-NICU clinic population needs additional clinical research to determine optimal care structures, especially patients with persistent disorders of consciousness who can undergo months or years of admission [23, 47, 48].

References

1. Creutzfeldt CJ, Longstreth WT, Holloway RG. Predicting decline and survival in severe acute brain injury: the fourth trajectory. Br Med J. 2015;351:h3904. https://doi.org/10.1136/bmj.h3904.
2. Goostrey K, Muehlschlegel S. Prognostication and shared decision making in neurocritical care. Br Med J. 2022;377:e060154. https://doi.org/10.1136/bmj-2021-060154.
3. Frontera JA, Curtis JR, Nelson JE, et al. Integrating palliative care into the care of neurocritically ill patients: a report from the improving palliative care in the ICU project advisory board and the center to advance palliative care. Crit Care Med. 2015;43(9):1964–77. https://doi.org/10.1097/ccm.0000000000001131.
4. Holloway RG, Arnold RM, Creutzfeldt CJ, et al. Palliative and end-of-life care in stroke. A statement for healthcare professionals from the America Heart Association/American Stroke Association. Stroke. 2014;45:1887–916.

5. Zulman DM, Haverfield MC, Shaw JG, et al. Practices to Foster physician presence and connection with patients in the clinical encounter. JAMA. 2020;323(1):70–81. https://doi.org/10.1001/jama.2019.19003.
6. Lakin JR, Tulsky JA, Bernacki RE. Time out before talking: communication as a medical procedure. Ann Intern Med. 2021;174(1):96–7. https://doi.org/10.7326/m20-4223.
7. Back AL, Arnold RM, Baile WF, et al. Efficacy of communication skills training for giving bad news and discussing transitions to palliative care. Arch Intern Med. 2007;167(5):453–60. https://doi.org/10.1001/archinte.167.5.453.
8. Horowitz RK, Hogan LA, Carroll T. MVP-medical situation, values, and plan: a memorable and useful model for all serious illness conversations. J Pain Symptom Manag. 2020;60(5):1059–65. https://doi.org/10.1016/j.jpainsymman.2020.07.022.
9. Creutzfeldt CJ, Engelberg RA, Healey L, et al. Palliative care needs in the neuro-ICU. Crit Care Med. 2015;43(8):1677–84. https://doi.org/10.1097/ccm.0000000000001018.
10. Anderson WG, Arnold RM, Angus DC, Bryce CL. Posttraumatic stress and complicated grief in family members of patients in the intensive care unit. J Gen Intern Med. 2008;23(11):1871–6. https://doi.org/10.1007/s11606-008-0770-2.
11. Wendlandt B, Olm-Shipman C, Ceppe A, et al. Surrogates of patients with severe acute brain injury experience persistent anxiety and depression over the 6 months after ICU admission. J Pain Symptom Manag. 2022;63(6):e633–9. https://doi.org/10.1016/j.jpainsymman.2022.02.336.
12. Wendler D, Rid A. Systematic review: the effect on surrogates of making treatment decisions for others. Ann Intern Med. 2011;154(5):336–46. https://doi.org/10.7326/0003-4819-154-5-201103010-00008.
13. Hammond MEH, Stehlik J, Drakos SG, Kfoury AG. Bias in medicine: lessons learned and mitigation strategies. JACC Basic Transl Sci. 2021;6(1):78–85. https://doi.org/10.1016/j.jacbts.2020.07.012.
14. Lee JY, Szulewski A, Young JQ, Donkers J, Jarodzka H, van Merriënboer JJG. The medical pause: importance, processes and training. Med Educ. 2021;55(10):1152–60. https://doi.org/10.1111/medu.14529.
15. Gao L, Zhao CW, Hwang DY. End-of-life care decision-making in stroke. Front Neurol. 2021;12:702833. https://doi.org/10.3389/fneur.2021.702833.
16. Becker KJ, Baxter AB, Cohen WA, et al. Withdrawal of support in intracerebral hemorrhage may lead to self-fulfilling prophecies. Neurology. 2001;56(6):766–72. https://doi.org/10.1212/wnl.56.6.766.
17. Souter MJ, Blissitt PA, Blosser S, et al. Recommendations for the critical care management of devastating brain injury: prognostication, psychosocial, and ethical management: a position statement for healthcare professionals from the neurocritical care society. Neurocrit Care. 2015;23(1):4–13. https://doi.org/10.1007/s12028-015-0137-6.
18. Mark NM, Rayner SG, Lee NJ, Curtis JR. Global variability in withholding and withdrawal of life-sustaining treatment in the intensive care unit: a systematic review. Intensive Care Med. 2015;41(9):1572–85. https://doi.org/10.1007/s00134-015-3810-5.
19. Hwang DY. Patients' families, physicians, and nurses: trying to see eye-to-eye regarding prognosis in neurocritical care. Neurocrit Care. 2022;37(1):10–1. https://doi.org/10.1007/s12028-022-01503-5.
20. Turgeon AF, Dorrance K, Archambault P, et al. Factors influencing decisions by critical care physicians to withdraw life-sustaining treatments in critically ill adult patients with severe traumatic brain injury. CMAJ. 2019;191(24):E652–e663. https://doi.org/10.1503/cmaj.190154.
21. Steinberg A, Abella BS, Gilmore EJ, et al. Frequency of withdrawal of life-sustaining therapy for perceived poor neurologic prognosis. Crit Care Explor. 2021;3(7):e0487. https://doi.org/10.1097/cce.0000000000000487.
22. Visvanathan A, Mead GE, Dennis M, Whiteley WN, Doubal FN, Lawton J. The considerations, experiences and support needs of family members making treatment decisions for patients admitted with major stroke: a qualitative study. BMC Med Inform Decis Mak. 2020;20(1):98. https://doi.org/10.1186/s12911-020-01137-7.

23. Fins JJ, Bernat JL. Ethical, palliative, and policy considerations in disorders of consciousness. Neurology. 2018;91(10):471–5. https://doi.org/10.1212/wnl.0000000000005927.
24. de Boer ME, Depla M, Wojtkowiak J, et al. Life-and-death decision-making in the acute phase after a severe stroke: interviews with relatives. Palliat Med. 2015;29(5):451–7. https://doi.org/10.1177/0269216314563427.
25. Hwang DY, Knies AK, Mampre D, et al. Concerns of surrogate decision makers for patients with acute brain injury: a US population survey. Neurology. 2020;94(19):e2054–68. https://doi.org/10.1212/wnl.0000000000009406.
26. Ruberton PM, Huynh HP, Miller TA, Kruse E, Chancellor J, Lyubomirsky S. The relationship between physician humility, physician–patient communication, and patient health. Patient Educ Counsel. 2016;99(7):1138–45. https://doi.org/10.1016/j.pec.2016.01.012.
27. Huynh HP, Dicke-Bohmann A. Humble doctors, healthy patients? Exploring the relationships between clinician humility and patient satisfaction, trust, and health status. Patient Educ Counsel. 2020;103(1):173–9. https://doi.org/10.1016/j.pec.2019.07.022.
28. Kowalski RG, Hammond FM, Weintraub AH, et al. Recovery of consciousness and functional outcome in moderate and severe traumatic brain injury. JAMA Neurol. 2021;78(5):548–57. https://doi.org/10.1001/jamaneurol.2021.0084.
29. Elmer J, Rittenberger JC, Coppler PJ, Guyette FX, Doshi AA, Callaway CW. Long-term survival benefit from treatment at a specialty center after cardiac arrest. Resuscitation. 2016;108:48–53. https://doi.org/10.1016/j.resuscitation.2016.09.008.
30. Sunde K, Pytte M, Jacobsen D, et al. Implementation of a standardised treatment protocol for post resuscitation care after out-of-hospital cardiac arrest. Resuscitation. 2007;73(1):29–39. https://doi.org/10.1016/j.resuscitation.2006.08.016.
31. Maas MB, Francis BA, Sangha RS, Lizza BD, Liotta EM, Naidech AM. Refining prognosis for intracerebral hemorrhage by early reassessment. Cerebrovasc Dis. 2017;43(3–4):110–6. https://doi.org/10.1159/000452679.
32. Greer DM, Shemie SD, Lewis A, et al. Determination of brain death/death by neurologic criteria: the world brain death project. JAMA. 2020;324(11):1078–97. https://doi.org/10.1001/jama.2020.11586.
33. Stahl D, Tomlinson T. Death by neurological criteria: caring for families amid tragedy. Linacre Q. 2019;86(4):394–403. https://doi.org/10.1177/0024363919874957.
34. Kramer NM, O'Mahony S, Deamant C. Brain death determination and communication: an innovative approach using simulation and standardized patients. J Pain Symptom Manag. 2022;63(6):e765–72. https://doi.org/10.1016/j.jpainsymman.2022.01.020.
35. Atashzadeh-Shoorideh F, Tayyar-Iravanlou F, Chashmi ZA, Abdi F, Cisic RS. Factors affecting moral distress in nurses working in intensive care units: a systematic review. Clin Ethics. 2021;16(1):25–36. https://doi.org/10.1177/1477750920927174.
36. Quill TE, Holloway R. Time-limited trials near the end of life. JAMA. 2011;306(13):1483–4. https://doi.org/10.1001/jama.2011.1413.
37. Chang DW, Neville TH, Parrish J, et al. Evaluation of time-limited trials among critically ill patients with advanced medical illnesses and reduction of nonbeneficial ICU treatments. JAMA Intern Med. 2021;181(6):786–94. https://doi.org/10.1001/jamainternmed.2021.1000.
38. Turner-Stokes LSN, Silber E, Khatri A, Sutton L, Young E. From diagnosis to death: exploring the interface between neurology, rehabilitation and palliative care in managing people with long-term neurological conditions. Clin Med. 2007;7:129–36.
39. Rogge A, Witt VD, Valdueza JM, Borzikowsky C, Buyx A. Experience in rehabilitation medicine affects prognosis and end-of-life decision-making of neurologists: a case-based survey. Neurocrit Care. 2019;31(1):125–34. https://doi.org/10.1007/s12028-018-0661-2.
40. Tetlock PE, Gardner D. Superforecasting: the art and science of prediction. Superforecasting: the art and science of prediction. Crown Publishers/Random House; 2015. p. 340.
41. Diringer MN, Edwards DF, Aiyagari V, Hollingsworth H. Factors associated with withdrawal of mechanical ventilation in a neurology/neurosurgery intensive care unit. Crit Care Med. 2001;29(9):1792–7. https://doi.org/10.1097/00003246-200109000-00023.

42. Kelly AG, Hoskins KD, Holloway RG. Early stroke mortality, patient preferences, and the withdrawal of care bias. Neurology. 2012;79(9):941–4. https://doi.org/10.1212/WNL.0b013e318266fc40.
43. Reznik ME, Moody S, Murray K, et al. The impact of delirium on withdrawal of life-sustaining treatment after intracerebral hemorrhage. Neurology. 2020;95(20):e2727–35. https://doi.org/10.1212/wnl.0000000000010738.
44. Gambhir S, Grigorian A, Ramakrishnan D, et al. Risk factors for withdrawal of life-sustaining treatment in severe traumatic brain injury. Am Surg. 2020;86(1):8–14.
45. Santhosh L. Beyond "In the Red": building the business case for a post-COVID-19 clinic. Ann Am Thorac Soc. 2022;19(8):1257–9. https://doi.org/10.1513/AnnalsATS.202111-1270PS.
46. Karlic KJ, Valley TS, Cagino LM, et al. Identification of patient safety threats in a post-intensive care clinic. Am J Med Qual. 2023;38(3):117–21. https://doi.org/10.1097/jmq.0000000000000118.
47. Fins JJ. Rights come to mind: brain injury, ethics, and the struggle for consciousness. Cambridge University Press; 2015.
48. Giacino JT, Katz DI, Schiff ND, et al. Practice guideline update recommendations summary: disorders of consciousness: report of the guideline development, dissemination, and implementation Subcommittee of the American Academy of neurology; the American congress of rehabilitation medicine; and the National Institute on Disability, Independent Living, and Rehabilitation Research. Neurology. 2018;91(10):450–60. https://doi.org/10.1212/wnl.0000000000005926.

Chapter 18
The Integrative Approach to Supporting Families in the ICU

Delia Chiaramonte

Integrative Medicine Defined

Integrative medicine emphasizes the care of the whole person and uses multiple therapeutic approaches to support optimal health and wellbeing. It incorporates conventional medical treatments, complementary therapies, and all aspects of lifestyle management. Defining principles of integrative medicine include [1]:

- Patient and practitioner are partners in the healing process.
- Integrates conventional and complementary methods for treatment and prevention.
- Engages mind, body, spirit, and community to facilitate healing.
- Supports the body's innate healing response.
- Less invasive interventions should be used when safe and appropriate.
- Maintains that healing is always possible even when curing is not.
- It neither rejects conventional medical approaches nor unquestioningly accepts complementary approaches.
- Practitioners of integrative medicine should actively practice self-development and self-care.

The label "alternative medicine" is generally avoided as it suggests using complementary modalities, such as acupuncture or massage, in lieu of conventional approaches rather than alongside them. Integrative medicine is used to facilitate both physical [2] and psychological [3] health.

D. Chiaramonte (✉)
Integrative Palliative Institute, Baltimore, MD, USA

University of Maryland, Baltimore, MD, USA
e-mail: dchiaramonte@integrativepalliative.com; dchiaramonte@umaryland.edu

© The Author(s), under exclusive license to Springer Nature Switzerland AG 2025

A. J. Vance et al. (eds.), *Families in the Intensive Care Unit*,
https://doi.org/10.1007/978-3-031-83786-9_18

The Healing Encounter

Creating an optimal healing encounter, for patients and families, requires more than the accurate implementation of pharmaceuticals or procedures. It includes a focus on collaborative and relationship-centered care, attention to the treatment environment, a healing intention, and clinicians who attend to their own wellbeing [4]. Establishing a therapeutic relationship with the patient and family is crucial. Psychiatrists with strong patient relationships using placebo medication for depression have better outcomes than psychiatrists rated lower on relationship skills administering active drugs [5]. Thus, the clinician him or herself contributes directly to the healing encounter.

The Need for Physician as Mentor for Health

Practitioner self-care is a tenet of the integrative approach to the care of patients and families. Yet the culture of medical and nursing training may encourage physicians and nurses to ignore their hunger, fatigue, elimination needs, and psychological stress. Thus, ironically, healthcare providers who are tasked with shepherding people to health often fail to attend to their own health and wellbeing.

Prolonged psychological stress can lead to burnout, which is significantly more common in physicians than in the general population [6]. Intensive care unit clinicians are at particularly high risk of burnout, particularly since the COVID-19 pandemic [7]. Burnout syndrome results from chronic stressors, often work-related, and it can result in emotional exhaustion, feelings of cynicism, and a reduced sense of personal accomplishment [8]. Medical students experiencing burnout may use alcohol and other drugs to facilitate coping [9]. Burned-out physicians may have less satisfied patients [10] and provide lower quality care [11]. ICU clinicians who practice wellness behaviors, such as exercise, mindfulness, self-reflection, and group support, may decrease their risk of burnout [12, 13].

Integrative Medicine in the Intensive Care Unit

The integrative approach prioritizes wellness of the mind, body, and spirit and is appropriate for patients, families, and clinicians. A patient might use acupuncture to address neuropathic pain, a family member might be taught diaphragmatic breathing to help initiate sleep, and an ICU clinician might use yoga as part of a burnout prevention plan. Adding integrative medicine services into intensive care units can benefit patients, families, clinicians, and ICU staff. Family caregivers of seriously ill patients experience significant stress [14] and are likely to benefit from stress reduction techniques.

Integrative Approaches to Enhance Family Wellbeing in the ICU

Mind-Body Medicine

The stress experienced by family members of patients in the ICU results in negative physical and emotional outcomes [15]. Mind-body techniques have been shown to decrease perceived stress and improve symptoms of anxiety, depression [16], and PTSD [17]. They are easy to learn, generally considered safe [18], accessible, and often without cost. Even telephone-based [19] and online mind-body skill programs have shown benefits in improving psychological distress, decreasing perceived stress, and increasing mindfulness, empathy, and resilience [20].

Breathing for Relaxation

Breathing can be used therapeutically to decrease the stress response and elicit the relaxation response. Therapeutic breathing may involve altering the speed of breathing or the muscles associated with breathing, and it may be linked with relaxing imagery. The relaxation response is essentially the opposite of the fight-flight-freeze stress response, and it is characterized by decreased blood pressure, respiratory rate, heart rate, and metabolic rate [21]. It has been described as a "hypometabolic state of parasympathetic activation" [22]. Breathing that focuses the inhalation into the lower abdomen, commonly called diaphragmatic breathing, can stimulate the relaxation response as evidenced by decreased anxiety, heart rate, and respiratory rate [23]. In addition, diaphragmatic breathing has been shown to decrease negative effects and levels of cortisol [24]. Shallow breathing into the chest may be associated with feelings of anxiety [25]. Family members can be instructed to use breath to stimulate the relaxation response. Instruction usually includes direction to "breathe deeply into the belly" and to slow down the rate of breathing, while slightly prolonging the exhalation. One simple breathing exercise that can easily be taught to family members is called "counting breaths" (Table 18.1).

Meditation/Mindfulness

Meditation is the intentional and nonjudgmental focus of attention on something in the present moment. It does not require belief in any religious or spiritual system. The attentional focus can be almost anything, including a sound, a word or phrase, a picture, a behavior (such as breathing or walking), a candle flame, or simply the experience of being in the present moment. When the mind wanders, the meditator simply brings attention, without judgment, back to the meditative focus. This refocusing of attention will likely occur repeatedly, which is to be expected. Some people believe that they "can't meditate" because their attention frequently wanders.

Table 18.1 Counting breaths

Count steps	When to count breaths
As you breathe in, think to yourself "one"	First thing in the morning
As you breathe out, think to yourself "calm"	Before a meal
As you breathe in, think to yourself "two"	When you're feeling agitated or frustrated
As you breathe out, think to yourself "calm"	Every hour on the hour while you're in the hospital room
As you breathe in, think to yourself "three"	After anyone enters/leaves the hospital room
As you breathe out, think to yourself "calm"	As you lie in bed at night
Continue this pattern until you reach "ten"	

This is a misconception as it is the repeated refocusing of attention that trains the mind in a way that may explain some of the benefits of meditation. Just as repeatedly lifting weights creates stronger muscles, repeatedly noticing one's thoughts and choosing not to get carried away by them trains mindfulness, which results in multiple health improvements including decreased anxiety and depression [26]. Mindfulness-Based Stress Reduction (MBSR) was shown to be as effective in the treatment of anxiety as Escitalopram, a selective serotonin reuptake inhibitor [27].

"Mindfulness" is the ability to retain one's focus on the present moment without judgment. It involves intentional awareness of one's moment-by-moment thoughts, feelings, environment, and bodily sensations. Mindfulness can be achieved through a formal meditation practice and/or via an informal cognitive practice of refocusing attention to the present moment when attention wanders either to the past or the future. Anxious thinking requires that attention be focused in the future—imagining the many terrible things that might happen. Depressive thinking tends to be focused in the past, ruminating on negative experiences or slights. Thus, intentionally focusing on the present moment can counteract a tendency toward anxious or depressive thinking. The greater one's ability to remain focused on the present moment, the higher one's mindfulness. There are validated metrics to assess level of mindfulness, such as the Five Facet Mindfulness Questionnaire (FFMQ) [28]. The practice of meditation, with its repeated focus on attending to something in the present moment, trains the skill of mindfulness. However, it is not necessary to practice meditation in order to achieve a mindful perspective. Cognitive skills can be implemented to identify when attention has wandered to the future or the past and intentionally bring the focus back to the present moment. It can be helpful to use an anchor such as taking a deep breath, rubbing the hands together, or pressing the thumb and forefinger firmly together. Mindfulness interventions have been shown to improve data-driven information processing [29], which could be helpful for family members facing difficult medical decisions. These interventions are acceptable to multiple populations including African American women with PTSD [30].

The Western, secular practice of mindfulness was introduced and championed by Jon Kabat-Zinn at the University of Massachusetts Medical School in 1979. He created MBSR, a well-researched mindfulness and meditation training program that is widely available in the USA [31]. MBSR is a standardized 8-week mind-body training program that includes 8 2.5-h classes, a full-day retreat, and at least 45 min per day of home meditation practice. It is offered in many communities and can be recommended to family members who are interested in intensive mind-body training. In addition to effectively treating anxiety [27], practicing MBSR has been shown to improve sleep [32], reduce biomarkers of stress [33], and improve pain [34].

Guided Imagery

Guided imagery is the intentional use of imagination to facilitate positive health and wellness outcomes. The term is used to describe a variety of techniques that support physical and psychological relaxation, including visualization and imagery-based suggestion. It has been shown to reduce preoperative anxiety and postoperative pain [35]. In family-centered ICU care, guided imagery can be used for patients and family members simultaneously. Guided imagery can be delivered live or from a recording, and once a particular script is listened to repeatedly, patients or family members can replicate the images in their mind without outside assistance. Potential images are unlimited and may include progressive relaxation of the muscles, being in a relaxing location, wrapping painful body parts in bubble wrap or white light or stimulating an activated immune system to attack cancer cells. Patients with pain may benefit from an imagery involving an "inner sanctuary," while families facing difficult medical decisions might be offered an imagery of a wise "inner advisor."

Creative Arts

Creative arts such as therapeutic music, visual arts, and writing for wellness can be used in the ICU setting to help support family members who are struggling with anxiety, anticipatory grief, and difficulty coping with a seriously ill loved one. These techniques can facilitate mindfulness, stimulate the relaxation response, enhance self-awareness, and help the family member to find meaning in a difficult experience.

Therapeutic Music

Therapeutic music and music therapy are distinct interventions. Music therapy is a professional, research-based healthcare field that applies science to the use of music for health [36].

The approach to therapeutic music may be considered in three categories:

1. Music therapy certification requires a 4-year college degree and over 1000 h of clinical training. It is generally impractical as a family intervention in the ICU setting.
2. Therapeutic music is offered by Certified Music Practitioners (CMPs), or similarly trained musicians, and focuses on meeting patient and family immediate need for relaxation, support, or a healing environment. Live therapeutic music is performed by musicians who have special training in providing care to patients with serious illness and their families. CMPs are trained to choose the music played based on the current needs of the patient or family member and to modify the music as needed. Training programs include the Music for Healing and Transition Program [37] and the International Harp Therapy Program [38]. Patients in the intensive care unit who received live therapeutic music had reductions in respiratory rate, heart rate, pain and anxiety [39].
3. Recorded music has also been used in ICU settings. Structured music listening time has been shown to decrease cortisol in ICU patients [40] as well as blood pressure and pulse during weaning from mechanical ventilation [41]; family members could be expected to benefit as well if the music is played aloud in the hospital room. The vibrational quality of live music coupled with the healing presence of the therapeutic musician may offer some advantage over recorded music.

Therapeutic sound is another low-cost option that can be provided to both patients and family members in the ICU setting. Playing live Tibetan singing bowls resulted in decreased tension, anger, fatigue, and depressed mood and enhanced feelings of spiritual well-being [42].

Visual Arts

Formal art therapy is not practical for family members in the ICU setting, but therapeutic art can be used to enhance coping skills and facilitate coping. Art-based activities have been shown to decrease anxiety in parents of hospitalized infants [43] and help hospitalized children improve communication with healthcare providers and develop more effective coping skills [44]. Mindfulness-based art therapy decreased anxiety and depression in breast cancer patients [45]. Simple techniques such as coloring and mandalas are inexpensive, portable, and easy to provide to family members. Mandalas, geometric drawings that may be seen to represent universal concepts, can be used to focus attention and to facilitate relaxation and meditation. Therapeutic visual art interventions can also be used to identify coping strategies and personal strengths. One exercise involves having the participant draw a "hole" that represents a difficulty with which they are coping and then asking them to draw how they would traverse this hole. The therapeutic artist reviews the drawing with the participant, using the discussion to identify the strategies chosen to overcome the difficulty. Examples might include recruiting the help of others, using animals for support, using personal creative skills to build a bridge, etc. Thus, the art exercise can be used to facilitate a discussion about personal strengths and resources.

Writing for Wellness

Journaling may reduce anxiety, depression, and suffering in patients with serious illness [46], help manage negative thoughts, and assist with problem-solving. Journaling techniques are varied and can be targeted to the wishes of the family member and the situation. Examples of patient journaling techniques include:

Dumping Journal

In this form of journaling, the writer's goal is simply to release thoughts and concerns about which they are ruminating. The technique involves writing quickly, without stopping or censoring and without attention to punctuation or spelling. It may be particularly helpful for family members with sleep dysfunction caused by rumination about stressful events. The journal may be kept at the side of the bed and used as a repository for thoughts that are contributing to insomnia.

Writing to a Symptom

In this form of journaling, family members choose a symptom that is bothering them such as headache, sleeplessness, back pain, or anxiety. The writer writes first as themselves and then as their symptom, continuing this written dialogue back and forth for approximately 10 min. They then review what they have written looking for insights that have emerged. For example, in response to the question "anxiety, why won't you leave me alone?" the response might be "I'm just trying to keep you safe."

Responding to Prompts

Family members may be offered writing prompts to facilitate self-discovery and identification of personal resources. Examples of writing prompts include:

- Words I like to live by are….
- Things I can do to be kind to myself include….
- Things that inspire me and give me hope include….
- Ways that I cope effectively with difficult things are….
- Supportive people in my life include….
- My personal strengths include….
- I don't like ______, but at least _______.
- Things that give my life meaning are….

Gratitude Journaling

Developing a regular gratitude practice has been shown to increase positive affect, happiness and life satisfaction, and reduce negative affect and depression symptoms [47]. Gratitude journaling can be both a daily practice and an intervention to facilitate coping with a difficult experience. For daily gratitude journaling, the participant writes 3–5 things every day for which they are grateful in a dedicated gratitude journal. The most important instruction is that each day the list must be different from what was written the day before. This trains the cognitive skill of identifying things for which one is grateful even on difficult days. It is important to emphasize that listing things for which the family member is grateful does not in any way minimize the sadness, worry, or grief that they feel for their loved one in the ICU. Another method of gratitude journaling involves listing, in one sitting, a full page of things for which a person is grateful. The list should include large things ("my family"), small things ("a seat heater in my car"), conveniences ("air conditioning"), and personal traits ("my sense of humor").

Intensive care diaries, in which healthcare staff (and sometimes family members) document daily notes and pictures in a document presented to the patient after discharge, have been shown to reduce incidence of post-traumatic stress disorder [48].

Biofield Therapy

Biofield therapy, sometimes referred to as energy medicine, has been defined as "noninvasive, practitioner-mediated therapies that explicitly work with the biofield of both the practitioner and client to stimulate a healing response in the client" [49]. These therapies are controversial, with many passionate advocates and equally passionate critics. Many cultures use the concept of "energy" in discussions of health and wellness, using terms such as life energy, chi, prana, and others. There are varied approaches to energy medicine, including healing touch, Reiki, zero balancing, and many others. The evidence base for biofield therapies is small but growing. A review of studies published between 2008 and 2013 concluded that biofield therapies may be effective in improving quality of life, pain, well-being, and stress in palliative care patients [50], although not all reviews have found benefit [51].

Seated Massage and Touch Therapy

Seated massage therapy has shown benefits in family caregivers, including relaxation, comfort, distraction, relief from anxiety, and an increase in well-being [52]. Full body massage is not practical for family members in the ICU, but seated massage or structured touch techniques, such as M technique, may be both beneficial and feasible. Seated massage requires a massage chair, as well as the services of a licensed massage therapist; thus, there may be barriers to implementation. In contrast, the M technique can be offered to family members in the patient's room. M technique is a method of structured light touch, provided in a set pattern, sometimes just to the hands and feet. It can be easily learned by licensed healthcare providers and even family caregivers. Family members can offer the M technique to each other and to the patient. M technique is often used in hospital and hospice settings, although it cannot be provided on abraded skin or open wounds. A study of hand and foot massage provided to family caregivers showed positive outcomes, including feeling "cared for" and experiencing "body vitality" and "peace of mind." Participants were able to temporarily put aside their worries and experience simply "being" [53].

Emotional Freedom Technique (EFT)

Emotional freedom technique, also called "tapping," can be thought of as a combination of acupressure, exposure therapy, and cognitive therapy. It involves the participant tapping on predetermined acupressure points while verbally acknowledging negative emotions. Proponents believe that this allows for acceptance and resolution of these negative emotions. Evidence supports the benefit of EFT in PTSD [54], anxiety [55], fatigue [56], physiologic markers of stress [57], and reducing depressive symptoms [58]. One study of cancer patients and caregivers showed that EFT led to improved marital functioning and improved patients' experience of caregiver empathic care.[59]

The process involves identifying a specific issue to work on, for example, a disagreement the previous week with a sister over treatment decisions for their mother. Then, while tapping the lateral edge of one hand, the participant speaks a "set up statement" out loud. For example, "even though my sister and I don't agree on what to do with mom…I am open to us finding a resolution." The participant then taps approximately 5–7 times on a series of eight predetermined acupressure points:

- Top of the head.
- Medial eyebrow.
- Side of the eye.
- Under the eye.
- Under the nose.
- Chin crease.
- Under the clavicle.
- Under the axilla.

While tapping the participant restates and expands upon the problem: "my sister and I don't agree," "I hate that we're fighting," "she's so unreasonable," "I just want to do the right thing," and "I just want to help mom." After going through two cycles of tapping, the participant takes a deep breath and assesses if their level of distress has decreased. If not, they repeat the cycle.

EFT is easy to learn, requires no equipment, and can be done anywhere. It can either be guided by a therapist or it can be used as a self-care tool by patients and family members without the assistance of a practitioner. Licensed healthcare providers can easily learn EFT and teach it to patients, or they can refer patients to online education resources.

Summary

Complementary and integrative approaches can effectively help family members of ICU patients manage their stress and distress. A sample stress reduction plan is presented in Table 18.2. Teaching mindfulness, providing stress management skills,

Table 18.2 A sample stress reduction plan

Step	Activities
Elicit the relaxation response	Meditation, guided imagery, diaphragmatic breathing
Choose a movement plan	Walking, yoga, tai chi, aerobics, dancing
Sleep plan	Try to get 7–8 h of sleep most nights
Start a gratitude practice	At the end of the day, call to mind 3–5 things that you are grateful for from the day Make them different each day
Spend time doing things that enrich you	Nature, animals, friends, family, learning, music, reading, volunteering, etc.
Become an observer of your thoughts	*"That was an anxious thought"* *"That was a negative thought"*
Ask positive questions	"What will help me find strength?" "What can I learn from this experience?" "How can I use this experience to help someone else?"

and offering techniques to support self-reflection can facilitate coping and resilience. ICUs may choose to hire dedicated practitioners to provide modalities such as massage and Reiki if funding is available. If funding is not available, nurses, physicians, nurse practitioners, physician assistants, social workers, and chaplains can pursue training in complementary modalities and provide these services as part of their standard interactions with family members. Facilities that offer integrative medicine patient consultation in the ICU can include care of the family members as part of the consultation.

References

1. https://awcim.arizona.edu/about/definition.html. Accessed January 14, 2023.
2. Hillinger MG, Wolever RQ, McKernan LC, Elam R. Integrative medicine for the treatment of persistent pain. Prim Care. 2017;44(2):247–64. https://doi.org/10.1016/j.pop.2017.02.008.
3. Shah AK, Becicka R, Talen MR, Edberg D, Namboodiri S. Integrative medicine and mood, emotions and mental health. Prim Care. 2017;44(2):281–304. https://doi.org/10.1016/j.pop.2017.02.003.
4. Rakel D. Integrative medicine. 3rd ed. Elsevier; 2012. p. 15.
5. McKay KM, Imel ZE, Wampold BE. Psychiatrist effects in the psychopharmacological treatment of depression. J Affect Disord. 2006;92(2–3):287–90.
6. Ibar C, Fortuna F, Gonzalez D, Jamardo J, Jacobsen D, Pugliese L, Giraudo L, Ceres V, Mendoza C, Repetto EM, Reboredo G, Iglesias S, Azzara S, Berg G, Zopatti D, Fabre B. Evaluation of stress, burnout and hair cortisol levels in health workers at a university hospital during COVID-19 pandemic. Psychoneuroendocrinology. 2021;128:105213. https://doi.org/10.1016/j.psyneuen.2021.105213.
7. Fumis RRL, Costa ELV, Dal'Col SVC, Azevedo LCP, Pastore Junior L. Burnout syndrome in intensive care physicians in time of the COVID-19: a cross-sectional study. BMJ Open. 2022;12(4):e057272. https://doi.org/10.1136/bmjopen-2021-057272.
8. Maslach C, Leiter MP. Understanding the burnout experience: recent research and its implications for psychiatry. World Psychiatry. 2016;15(2):103–11. https://doi.org/10.1002/wps.20311.
9. Erschens R, Loda T, Herrmann-Werner A, Keifenheim KE, Stuber F, Nikendei C, Zipfel S, Junne F. Behaviour-based functional and dysfunctional strategies of medical students to cope with burnout. Med Educ Online. 2018;23(1):1535738. https://doi.org/10.1080/10872981.2018.1535738.
10. Anagnostopoulos F, Liolios E, Persefonis G, Slater J, Kafetsios K, Niakas D. Physician burnout and patient satisfaction with consultation in primary health care settings: evidence of relationships from a one-with-many design. J Clin Psychol Med Settings. 2012;19(4):401–10. https://doi.org/10.1007/s10880-011-9278-8.
11. Hodkinson A, Zhou A, Johnson J, Geraghty K, Riley R, Zhou A, Panagopoulou E, Chew-Graham CA, Peters D, Esmail A, Panagioti M. Associations of physician burnout with career engagement and quality of patient care: systematic review and meta-analysis. Br Med J. 2022;378:e070442. https://doi.org/10.1136/bmj-2022-070442.
12. Dyrbye LN, Satele D, Shanafelt TD. Healthy exercise habits are associated with lower risk of burnout and higher quality of life among U.S. medical students. Acad Med. 2017;92(7):1006–11. https://doi.org/10.1097/ACM.0000000000001540.
13. Horn DJ, Johnston CB. Burnout and self care for palliative care practitioners. Med Clin North Am. 2020;104(3):561–72. https://doi.org/10.1016/j.mcna.2019.12.007.
14. Schandl A, Ringborg C, Mälberg K, Johar A, Lagergren P. Caregiver burden and health-related quality of life among family caregivers of oesophageal cancer patients: a prospective

nationwide cohort study. Acta Oncol. 2022;61(10):1186–91. https://doi.org/10.1080/0284186X.2022.2119098.
15. Netzer G, Sullivan DR. Recognizing, naming, and measuring a family intensive care unit syndrome. Ann Am Thorac Soc. 2014;11(3):435–41. https://doi.org/10.1513/AnnalsATS.201309-308OT.
16. Gotink RA, Chu P, Busschbach JJ, Benson H, Fricchione GL, Hunink MG. Standardised mindfulness-based interventions in healthcare: an overview of systematic reviews and meta-analyses of RCTs. PLoS One. 2015;10(4):e0124344. https://doi.org/10.1371/journal.pone.0124344.eCollection2015.
17. Polusny MA, Erbes CR, Thuras P, Moran A, Lamberty GJ, Collins RC, et al. Mindfulness-based stress reduction for posttraumatic stress disorder among veterans: a randomized clinical trial. JAMA. 2015;314(5):456–65. https://doi.org/10.1001/jama.2015.8361.
18. https://www.nccih.nih.gov/health/meditation-and-mindfulness-what-you-need-to-know. Accessed January 14, 2023.
19. Cox CE, Porter LS, Buck PJ, Hoffa M, Jones D, Walton B, et al. Development and preliminary evaluation of a telephone-based mindfulness training intervention for survivors of critical illness. Ann Am Thorac Soc. 2014;11(2):173–81. https://doi.org/10.1513/AnnalsATS.201308-283OC.
20. Kemper KJ, Khirallah M. Acute effects of online mind-body skills training on resilience, mindfulness, and empathy. J Evid Based Complementary Altern Med. 2015;20(4):247–53. https://doi.org/10.1177/2156587215575816.
21. Benson H. The relaxation response. New York: Morrow; 1975.
22. Benson JBK, Crassweller KD. The relaxation response: a bridge between psychiatry and medicine. Med Clin North Am. 1977;61:929–38.
23. Chen YF, Huang XY, Chien CH, Cheng JF. The effectiveness of diaphragmatic breathing relaxation training for reducing anxiety. Perspect Psychiatr Care. 2017;53(4):329–36. https://doi.org/10.1111/ppc.12184.
24. Ma X, Yue ZQ, Gong ZQ, Zhang H, Duan NY, Shi YT, et al. The effect of diaphragmatic breathing on attention, negative affect and stress in healthy adults. Front Psychol. 2017;8:874. https://doi.org/10.3389/fpsyg.2017.00874.eCollection2017.
25. Conrad A, Müller A, Doberenz S, Kim S, Meuret AE, Wollburg E, et al. Psychophysiological effects of breathing instructions for stress management. Appl Psychophysiol Biofeedback. 2007;32(2):89–98.
26. Goyal M, Singh S, Sibinga EM, Gould NF, Rowland-Seymour A, Sharma R, et al. Meditation programs for psychological stress and Well-being: a systematic review and meta-analysis. JAMA Intern Med. 2014;174(3):357–68. https://doi.org/10.1001/jamainternmed.2013.13018.
27. Hoge EA, Bui E, Mete M, Dutton MA, Baker AW, Simon NM. Mindfulness-based stress reduction vs escitalopram for the treatment of adults with anxiety disorders: a randomized clinical trial. JAMA Psychiatry. 2023;80(1):13–21. https://doi.org/10.1001/jamapsychiatry.2022.3679.
28. Baer RA, Smith GT, Hopkins J, et al. Using self-report assessment methods to explore facets of mindfulness. Assessment. 2006;13(1):27–45.
29. Wimmer L, Bellingrath S, von Stockhausen L. Cognitive effects of mindfulness training: results of a pilot study based on a theory driven approach. Front Psychol. 2016;7:1037. https://doi.org/10.3389/fpsyg.2016.01037.eCollection2016.
30. Dutton MA, Bermudez D, Matas A, Majid H, Myers NL. Mindfulness-based stress reduction for low-income, predominantly African American women with PTSD and a history of intimate partner violence. Cogn Behav Pract. 2013;20(1):23–32.
31. Kabat-Zinn J. Full catastrophe living: using the wisdom of your body and mind to face stress, pain and illness, vol. 1990. New York: Bantam Books; 2013.
32. Rusch HL, Rosario M, Levison LM, Olivera A, Livingston WS, Wu T, Gill JM. The effect of mindfulness meditation on sleep quality: a systematic review and meta-analysis of randomized controlled trials. Ann N Y Acad Sci. 2019;1445(1):5–16. https://doi.org/10.1111/nyas.13996.

33. Hoge EA, Bui E, Palitz SA, Schwarz NR, Owens ME, Johnston JM, Pollack MH, Simon NM. The effect of mindfulness meditation training on biological acute stress responses in generalized anxiety disorder. Psychiatry Res. 2018;262:328–32. https://doi.org/10.1016/j.psychres.2017.01.006.
34. Petrucci G, Papalia GF, Russo F, Vadalà G, Piredda M, De Marinis MG, Papalia R, Denaro V. Psychological approaches for the integrative care of chronic low back pain: a systematic review and metanalysis. Int J Environ Res Public Health. 2021;19(1):60. https://doi.org/10.3390/ijerph19010060.
35. Giacobbi PR Jr, Stabler ME, Stewart J, Jaeschke AM, Siebert JL, Kelley GA, Guided imagery Álvarez-García C, Yaban ZŞ. The effects of preoperative guided imagery interventions on preoperative anxiety and postoperative pain: a meta-analysis. Complement Ther Clin Pract. 2020;38:101077. https://doi.org/10.1016/j.ctcp.2019.101077.
36. https://www.musictherapy.org/about/quotes/. Accessed January 14, 2023.
37. https://www.mhtp.org. Accessed January 14, 2023.
38. https://www.playharp.com/international-harp-therapy-program/. Accessed January 14, 2023.
39. Golino AJ, Leone R, Gollenberg A, Christopher C, Stanger D, Davis TM, Meadows A, Zhang Z, Friesen MA. Impact of an active music therapy intervention on intensive care patients. Am J Crit Care. 2019;28(1):48–55. https://doi.org/10.4037/ajcc2019792.
40. Beaulieu-Boire G, Bourque S, Chagnon F, Chouinard L, Gallo-Payet N, Lesur O. Music and biological stress dampening in mechanically-ventilated patients at the intensive care unit ward-a prospective interventional randomized crossover trial. J Crit Care. 2013;28(4):442–50. https://doi.org/10.1016/j.jcrc.2013.01.007.
41. Jaber S, Bahloul H, Guétin S, Chanques G, Sebbane M, Eledjam JJ. Effects of music therapy in intensive care unit without sedation in weaning patients versus non-ventilated patients [article in French]. Ann Fr Anesth Reanim. 2007;26(1):30–8.
42. Goldsby TL, Goldsby ME, McWalters M, Mills PJ. Effects of singing bowl sound meditation on mood, tension, and Well-being: an observational study. J Evid Based Complementary Altern Med. 2016;22:pii: 2156587216668109. [Epub ahead of print].
43. Mouradian LE, DeGrace BW, Thompson DM. Art-based occupation group reduces parent anxiety in the neonatal intensive care unit: a mixed-methods study. Am J Occup Ther. 2013;67(6):692–700. https://doi.org/10.5014/ajot.2013.007682.
44. Aguilar BA. The efficacy of art therapy in pediatric oncology patients: an integrative literature review. J Pediatr Nurs. 2017;36:173–8. https://doi.org/10.1016/j.pedn.2017.06.015.
45. Jang SH, Kang SY, Lee HJ, Lee SY. Beneficial effect of mindfulness-based art therapy in patients with breast cancer—a randomized controlled trial. Explore (NY). 2016;12(5):333–40. https://doi.org/10.1016/j.explore.2016.06.003.
46. Tan TT, Tan MP, Lam CL, Loh EC, Capelle DP, Zainuddin SI, Ang BT, Lim MA, Lai NZ, Tung YZ, Yee HA, Ng CG, Ho GF, See MH, Teh MS, Lai LL, Pritam Singh RK, Chai CS, Ng DLC, Tan SB. Mindful gratitude journaling: psychological distress, quality of life and suffering in advanced cancer: a randomised controlled trial. BMJ Support Palliat Care. 2021.:bmjspcare-2021-003068;13:e389. https://doi.org/10.1136/bmjspcare-2021-003068.
47. Cunha LF, Pellanda LC, Reppold CT. Positive psychology and gratitude interventions: a randomized clinical trial. Front Psychol. 2019;10:584. https://doi.org/10.3389/fpsyg.2019.00584.
48. Jones C, Bäckman C, Capuzzo M, Egerod I, Flaatten H, Granja C, RACHEL Group, et al. Intensive care diaries reduce new onset post traumatic stress disorder following critical illness: a randomised, controlled trial. Crit Care. 2010;14(5):R168. https://doi.org/10.1186/cc9260.
49. Jain R, Hammerschlag PM, et al. Clinical studies of biofield therapies: summary, methodological challenges, and recommendations. Global Adv Health Med. 2015;4:58–66.
50. Hennaghan AM, Schnyer RN. Biofield therapies for symptomatic management in palliative care and end-of-life. Am J of Hosp Palliat Med. 2015;32(1):90–100.
51. Gonella SG, Garrina L, Dimonte V. Biofield therapies and cancer related symptoms: a review. Clin J Oncol Nurs. 2014;18(5):568–76.

52. Mackereth P, Campbell G, Maycock P, Hennings J, Breckons M. Chair massage for patients and carers: a pilot service in an outpatient setting of a cancer care hospital. Complement Ther Clin Pract. 2008;14(2):136–42. https://doi.org/10.1016/j.ctcp.2007.11.003.
53. Cronfalk BS, Strang P, Ternestedt BM. Inner power, physical strength and existential well-being in daily life: relatives' experiences of receiving soft tissue massage in palliative home care. J Clin Nurs. 2009;18(15):2225–33. https://doi.org/10.1111/j.1365-2702.2008.02517.x.
54. Church D, Stapleton P, Mollon P, Feinstein D, Boath E, Mackay D, Sims R. Guidelines for the treatment of PTSD using clinical EFT (emotional freedom techniques). Healthcare (Basel). 2018;6(4):146. https://doi.org/10.3390/healthcare6040146.
55. König N, Steber S, Seebacher J, von Prittwitz Q, Bliem HR, Rossi S. How therapeutic tapping can alter neural correlates of emotional prosody processing in anxiety. Brain Sci. 2019;9(8):206. https://doi.org/10.3390/brainsci9080206.
56. Ghaderi Z, Nazari F, Shaygannejad V. The effect of emotional freedom technique on fatigue among women with multiple sclerosis: a randomized controlled trial. Iran J Nurs Midwifery Res. 2021;26(6):531–6. https://doi.org/10.4103/ijnmr.IJNMR_188_19.
57. Bach D, Groesbeck G, Stapleton P, Sims R, Blickheuser K, Church D. Clinical EFT (emotional freedom techniques) improves multiple physiological markers of health. J Evid Based Integr Med. 2019;24:2515690X18823691. https://doi.org/10.1177/2515690X18823691.
58. Nelms JA, Castel L. A systematic review and meta-analysis of randomized and nonrandomized trials of clinical emotional freedom techniques (EFT) for the treatment of depression. Explore (NY). 2016;12(6):416–26. https://doi.org/10.1016/j.explore.2016.08.001.

Chapter 19
The Role of Ethics Consultation in Enhancing Family-Centered Care

Henry J. Silverman

The Role and Contribution of Ethics Consultation to Family-Centered Care

Clinical ethics consultation represents a service provided by an individual consultant, team, or committee to address ethical issues that involve patients and various aspects of their medical care. The central purpose of ethics consults is to enhance the process and outcomes of patient care by identifying and analyzing ethical issues.

Several reasons explain how families of patients assume an important role in these dilemmas. For example, patient autonomy represents a guiding ethical principle that characterizes patients as being highly individualistic and independent agents who make rational decisions. However, individuals fundamentally exist in a social web of relationships that help form their identity. This relational account of autonomy imparts a significant role for discussions with others, in general, and with family members, in particular [1].

Another role for families involves them acting as surrogate decision-makers for patients who lack the capacity to make decisions for themselves and for neonates and adolescents. Such treatment decisions are often necessary when patients are critically ill or in end-of-life and beginning-of-life situations. Being involved in such complex decision-making may result in tremendous emotional burdens for families. Undoubtedly, families report desiring a greater role in decision-making to share their unique family values and preferences with healthcare professionals [2–4]. This concept of shared decision-making between patients, families, and healthcare professionals represents a significant aspect of family-centered care [5]. As a result, family-clinician communication becomes a central component of medical decision-making, especially in the adult and pediatric intensive care units (ICUs).

H. J. Silverman (✉)
Department of Medicine, University of Maryland School of Medicine, Baltimore, MD, USA
e-mail: hsilverm@som.umaryland.edu

© The Author(s), under exclusive license to Springer Nature Switzerland AG 2025

A. J. Vance et al. (eds.), *Families in the Intensive Care Unit*,
https://doi.org/10.1007/978-3-031-83786-9_19

However, the evidence is mixed regarding the effect of communication interventions on patient- and family-centered outcomes that include "satisfaction" and decreased "emotional distress" [6, 7]. Furthermore, despite interventions that strive to enhance communications, decision-making, especially at the end-of-life, frequently depends on moral, religious, and cultural viewpoints that may differ broadly in our pluralistic society, and hence, may differ between the perspectives of families and healthcare providers. Accordingly, potentially disparate moral perspectives between families and healthcare providers can result in intractable **conflicts**, which can have profound adverse effects on families and on clinicians. Consequences for families include depression, complicated grief, anxiety, and posttraumatic stress disorder [8–10]. For healthcare providers, conflicts can cause moral distress, disengagement, cynicism, and burnout [11].

Several studies have shown a high prevalence of clinician-surrogate conflicts, ranging between 22% and 48% [12–14]. A recent study demonstrated that either physicians or surrogates reported conflict in 63% of the cases and that physicians reported conflict less frequently than family members (27.8% vs. 42.3%, respectively); concordance between physicians and family reports of conflicts was extremely poor [15]. Clinicians and surrogates agreed to the existence of a conflict in only approximately 26% of the cases.

Conflicts regarding end-of-life decisions may also occur between members of the healthcare team caring for the patient as well as within the family unit itself, which can lead to ethical **uncertainty** regarding the "correct" decision to make. Due to the presence of moral, religious, and culturally disparate factors that influence decision-making at the end of life and the uncertain nature of proactive communication strategies in preventing conflict, the use of "experts" to help resolve conflicts, specifically an ethics or a palliative care consult, can be recommended. One study showed that the presence of conflicts triggered ethics consultation requests more commonly than other ethical concerns [16]. Cho and colleagues performed a qualitative study to explore the range of situations and perceptions of ethical concerns of families when patients are hospitalized [17]. The range included end-of-life care, decision-making capacity, healthcare costs, patient's refusal of treatment or engaged in self-harming behavior (e.g., substance abuse), family disagreements about patients' medical care, perceived suboptimal care/discrimination, and poor communication with healthcare providers [17].

This chapter reviews the role of ethics consultants in addressing moral uncertainty and the presence of conflicts between families and clinicians; the evidence demonstrating the effectiveness of ethics consults in patient medical care, how best to incorporate ethics expertise in decision making, and suggests areas that warrant further investigation to optimize the outcomes of ethics consultation.

Role of Ethics Consults

Ethics consultation represent a set of services provided by an individual ethics consultant, a team, or a committee) in response to questions from patients, families, surrogates, and healthcare professionals who seek to resolve moral **uncertainty** or **conflict** regarding value-laden concerns that emerge in healthcare, especially at the end of life and beginning of life [18, 19]. Although all healthcare professionals engage in ethical decision-making as part of their everyday practice, ethics consultants respond to specific ethical concerns and questions that arise in healthcare. For example, advances in medical science and innovations in healthcare have expanded the scope of medical options across the lifespan. While many options might be appropriate for any given situation, the role of the ethicist is to help facilitate which option might be most appropriate based on the value systems of the involved stakeholders and which options are inappropriate to consider. As such, ethics consultants require a distinctive set of competencies to perform their role effectively. Such competencies fall into the following domains: (1) knowledge of common bioethical issues and concepts; (2) moral reasoning skills; (3) process skills that enable one to communicate and collaborate with different individuals; (4) interpersonal skills; (5) facilitation of meetings; and (6) ethical assessment and analytic skills [20].

Such competencies enable ethics consultants to identify, analyze, and resolve ethical questions or concerns. Also, consultants' knowledge of ethical arguments may help them clarify unrecognized implications of the parties' view, allowing the primary decision-makers to come to more firmly grounded conclusions. Additionally, ethics consultants help promote practices consistent with ethical norms and standards, inform policy development to ensure the institutionalization of such practices, and assist individuals to address future ethical problems by providing education in healthcare ethics.

Ethics issues in healthcare that typically involve families arise in one or more of several broad domains:

- End-of-life care and beginning-of-life situations.
- Determining patient's capacity to make decisions.
- Selection of the appropriate surrogate.
- Tensions and disagreements between family members regarding decisions for patients.
- Balancing family's values and hopes that ground requests for continued treatment vs. professional integrity.
- Determining when treatment might be futile or ethically inappropriate.
- Determination of what constitutes a "safe" discharge for patients.
- The involvement of families when patients refuse recommended treatments.

Examples of specific ethical questions include the following:

- At what point would it be ethically appropriate not to insert a feeding tube in a patient with dementia who keeps pulling out the tube and has a poor prognosis?

- When can a patient with an aspiration syndrome still be fed orally at the patient's or families' request?
- How does one resolve disputes between family members regarding end-of-life or beginning-of-life situations?
- When is it ethically justified to withhold blood products in an unconscious patient with end-stage liver disease?
- How to resolve situations when the healthcare team believes an intervention is required (e.g., leg amputation in a patient with gangrene or ventilator treatment in a patient with respiratory failure), but the patient/surrogate refuses?
- When is a family's request for a tracheostomy inappropriate in a patient with advanced lung cancer and respiratory failure?
- When is continued treatment with ECMO indefensible in a patient who lacks a destination therapy (e.g., lung or heart transplant)?
- When is it inappropriate to allow surrogates to withhold or withdraw life-prolonging treatments in a patient with a spinal cord injury?
- How long is it reasonable to maintain interventions that preserve cardiopulmonary function in a patient who has been declared brain dead?
- How to manage situations when families desire to take mentally incapable patients home when the discharge is considered "unsafe"?

Common examples that highlight cultural and religious perspectives regarding routine intensive care that might lead to conflict families and healthcare professionals include:

- Families of the Jehovah Witness faith refuse blood transfusions for a patient who is not a practicing Jehovah Witness.
- Families who request that their father not be told that he has a terminal condition, as it is not in their culture to tell the elders of their cancer diagnosis.
- Families of the Orthodox Jewish faith refuse to have the ventilator withdrawn in their mother who has been declared brain dead.
- Families who refuse to forgo life-sustaining treatments as their faith believes that only God can decide when a patient will die.

Requests that do not involve ethical concerns should be referred to other departments (e.g., chaplain's department, risk management, patient advocate, or office of general council (e.g., allegations of misconduct or unprofessionalism should be referred to department heads).

What Do the Data Show Regarding the Value of Ethics Consultations?

Studies are limited regarding the value and outcomes of ethics consultation. Such studies have assessed the effects of ethics consults on quality of care, process factors, and clinical factors using surveys, qualitative interviews or focus groups, mixed methods, and medical record reviews [19]. Quality of care domains include length of stay (LOS), perceived usefulness, satisfaction, relief of moral distress, timeliness, and accessibility. Process factors include identification of previously unknown issues, assist in transitioning discharge of patients, impact on patient care, and support interpersonal reflection and collaboration. Clinical factors include achievement of consensus, improvement of quality of patient care, limitation in the degree of minimally beneficial treatment, and minimize suffering [19].

Four studies of diverse methodological quality performed in different populations assessed the effects of ethics consults on LOS [21–24]. In a study involving 99 patients, Dowdy showed that proactive ethics consultation for critically and terminally ill patients who were receiving mechanical ventilation for >96 h had more frequent decisions to forgo life-sustaining treatments and reduced ICU LOS [21]. Schneiderman and colleagues performed a randomized trial involving 74 patients and evaluated routine ethics consultation for patients "in whom value related treatment conflicts arose" [22]. By focusing on improving communications and addressing ethical dilemmas, these investigators showed that ethics consultations reduced the number of days patients spent in the ICU before death and led to reductions in life-sustaining treatments. These investigators conducted a follow-up study involving several centers that randomized 551 patients; ethics consultations were associated with reductions in hospital and ICU days and life-sustaining treatments [23]. Andereck and colleagues performed a single-center randomized-control study that measured the effects of using an ethics consultative model preventively (i.e., before an ethics issue or conflict arose) and showed no effect on LOS between the two study groups [24].

Two of the previous trials examined the effects of ethics consultation on family satisfaction in a controlled intervention study. Results in both studies showed that family satisfaction was greater with ethics consultation. Specifically, in Schneiderman and colleagues' single-center study involving 74 patients that studied the effect of ethics consultation in response to disputes that arose between family members and the healthcare team or within the healthcare team, of the eight families they interviewed, six of eight agreed that the consult helped resolve differences and 7/8 agreed that it was responsive to their personal values.

In their follow-up, multicenter randomized study involving more than 540 patients randomized to an intervention (ethics consultation offered) or to usual care in response to conflicts either within the healthcare team, within the family, or between families and the healthcare team, Schneiderman and colleagues showed in follow-up interviews that 87% of both the nurses and physicians and the patients/surrogates agreed or strongly agreed that ethics consultation were helpful.

In the study performed by Andereck and colleagues that involved a randomized control study examining a preventative ethics intervention for patients in an ICU prior to any recognized ethical conflict, patients', and providers' perceptions of quality of care were not different between the two groups [24].

Based on these studies, a recent guideline concluded that the overall quality of evidence for ethics consultation is low and recommended that ethics consultation should be provided to decrease ICU and hospital LOS among critically ill patients for whom there is a value-related conflict between clinicians and family. Due to the limited data regarding family satisfaction shown in the above-mentioned studies, the guideline did not recommend using ethics consultation with the goal of increasing family satisfaction [25]. A recent systemic review and meta-analysis examined changes in processes and outcomes because of clinical ethics consultation in the ICU. Categories of outcomes included user perception, clinical decision, or conflict resolution and resource utilization. This study showed that clinical ethics consultation decreased ICU length of stay and increased family and healthcare provider satisfaction.

Several studies investigated the effects of a "consultative" model in which specialists (e.g., palliative care and ethics consultants) work with the usual ICU personnel to implement communication interventions, and other studies examined effects of an "integrative model" in which palliative care and ethics principles are embedded into the daily practice of the usual care team. In a paper that performed a systemic review of communication quality improvement interventions, a higher percentage of studies that were consultative in nature as opposed to those that were integrative led to significant improvement in outcomes regarding healthcare utilization [7]. The authors of this study hypothesized that the benefit associated with a consultative model could be due to multiple potential reasons, e.g., consultative teams may focus specifically on communication-related issues as opposed to balancing them with other clinical responsibilities, as must occur with integrative interventions. Additionally, optimization of healthcare utilization represents a culture change in the workplace in which consults who represent "outside agents of such change" might be able to effect change more reliably and/or rapidly effective [7].

Considerations for Implementing the Ethics Consult Team in Clinical Decision-Making

Several aspects of ethics consults should be considered when used to manage end-of-life decisions. One involves the timing of an ethics consult. Since most disagreements in ICUs arise not from conflicts in values, but from breakdowns in communication, it is reasonable to resolve such disagreements through routine communication interventions, e.g., family conferences. However, for disputes that are based on value conflicts, once they become intractable, resolution strategies are likely to be protracted and burdensome. Hence, while commentators recommend the use of ethics consultants when there are value-conflicts causing disputes, the question is when should ethics consultants become involved? On the one hand, there is a concern that such consults are employed in a reactive fashion, whereby ethics consults are requested only after an ethics issue has already caused doubts, confusion, and mistrust. On the other hand, one study showed that when used preventively, i.e., when an ethics concern does not yet exist, there was no difference in quality of care or family satisfaction. Such a "broad application" may be too early, as implied in Andereck's study [24], but waiting for a problem to develop could lead to intractable conflicts. A more helpful process would involve the identification of a specific set of early triggers that foreshadow a value-laden conflict in its early stages.

An issue regarding requests for ethics consultation involves accessibility to ethics services; including who can request an ethics consult; is physician permission required for such requests; are patients and families aware of the process of requesting an ethics consult and how can they be empowered to make such requests within the strict hierarchy of the medical institution? Related to the issue of access is whether requests for ethics consults are associated with racial, ethnic, and gender characteristics of patients. One retrospective study showed that consultation requests for females were initiated earlier in their hospital stays (6.57 days) compared with that for males (16.07 days). For African American patients, the differences in admission-to-request intervals for female patients (5.93 days) and male patients (18.64 days) were greater than for Caucasian male and female patients [26]. Future investigations are warranted to determine whether there are racial and gender disparities in the extent of requests as well as the timing of ethics consultations.

Another aspect of ethics consultations regard the approach taken by ethics consultants. One commentator opined that "on balance, ethics consults may be an inappropriate mechanism to resolve conflict" [27]. The concern is that the extent to which ethics consultants engage the patient or family when addressing concerns is unclear and that "decisions by the ethics service may be rendered in a hierarchical manner with a vote either 'for' or 'against' one of the disputants", voting for the withholding of dialysis or cardiopulmonary resuscitation), resulting in a "win–lose" scenario [19]. Rather than the authoritative or the consensus approach, the ASBH recommends a facilitated approach to ethics consultation [20]. With this approach, the ethics consultant engages all stakeholders respectfully and simultaneously to create a "win–win" solution. The goal is for all stakeholders to leave a meeting feeling their concerns have been recognized and equally considered leading to an actionable resolution. However, not all ethics consultants are trained in principles of negotiation.

A related issue involves whether ethics consultations should be performed by a single-trained ethicist, a small consultative team, or by all the members of the ethics committee. No one model fits all types of cases and an ethics consult service should try to match a particular model to the contextual features of each case; balancing responsiveness and representativeness of the committee [28]. Additionally, when considering the type of ethics consult model to use in any one case, one should consider the potential adverse psychological effects on a family that occurs from an inquiry into patients' preferences and values, which has been recently shown [29]. For example, a team or committee approach might be threatening to a family as opposed to a single ethicist, especially if families believe that their "ethics" are being questioned by the involvement of an ethics consult. That said, it might not be possible to have families explore the preferences and values of their family member who is critically ill and also reduce the emotional burden that occurs with such conversations [30]. However, trade-offs may need to be made between effectiveness of ethics consults and the emotional burden that occurs for families with such consults.

For example, in the two studies that explored the "effects" of ethics consults, both showed that while many surrogates found the ethics process to be "stressful," a greater number of surrogates agreed that the ethics process was more "helpful" and would "seek" it again and "recommend" it to others [22, 23]. Similarly, a recent study compared family meetings led by palliative care specialists and provision of an informational brochure (intervention) compared with provision of an informational brochure and routine family meetings conducted by ICU teams (control) [29]. The results showed no significant difference in anxiety and depression symptoms between surrogate decision-makers in the intervention group and the control group and showed that posttraumatic stress disorder symptoms were higher in the intervention group at 3 months. Hence, somewhat counterintuitive, in attempts to help families/surrogates understand their values and those of the patients when making end-of-life decisions, such communications might enhance unwanted emotional and psychological reactions. However, the palliative care study did not represent of a full palliative care consult, and hence, intensive and broad support is necessary to improve surrogates' psychological outcomes and decision making for patients with chronic critical illnesses [31]. Accordingly, when either ethics or palliative care consultants help families face difficult end-of-life decisions, there should be active management of patients/families' emotional and psychological symptoms is needed, with enlisting the help of social workers and chaplains.

Specific Ethical Issue: Medical Futility

Ethics consultants frequently play a role in "futility disputes" between families and healthcare providers. Such disputes can often be intractable. Surrogates opposed to the withdrawal of life support often appeal to the ethical principle of autonomy or embrace the concept of miracles. Healthcare providers express concern with potential harms that can occur to patients from resuscitative attempts as well as the moral distress that healthcare providers experience with providing CPR that is deemed to be futile [32].

Attempts at reaching consensus on a definition of medical futility have failed, as it became obvious that the concept of futility is very value-laden [33]. As such, commentators have recommended a procedural approach to address futility disputes, rather than giving all decision-making authority to either surrogates or individual clinicians [34]. Although it is generally accepted that surrogates should be allowed to request available treatment options, giving sole authority to surrogates is problematic, as there is no positive right to interventions that are outside the boundaries of accepted practice and surrogates sometimes experience strong emotional and psychological reactions that interfere with accepting decisions to forego life support, even when those decisions are clearly consistent with the patient's values and preferences [34]. Giving sole authority to clinicians is problematic because there is well-documented undue variability between clinicians in their judgments about when it is appropriate to write DNR orders for patients. Additionally, giving all authority to clinicians may also create a disincentive for them to "fully engage in the time-consuming, challenging conversations often required to support surrogates and achieve mutually agreeable decisions" [34].

Instead, a procedural approach will incorporate multiple perspectives to minimize the risk that the values of any one individual or party dominate the discussion and are better with fulfilling transparency, legitimacy, accountability, and opportunity for appeal. Finally, a procedural approach allows mutually agreeable solutions to emerge as the conflict-resolution process occurs over time. Ethics consultants can play an important role as facilitators with such a process-oriented approach. Recently, the American Thoracic Society proposed a seven-step process for addressing requests for inappropriate treatment that remain intractable [34]. Also, the Massachusetts General Hospital developed a "Do No Harm" policy that involved the intervention of the ethics committee in their procedural approach [35]. Reviewing their data collected during the past few years showed that about a third of the surrogates reversed their initial request for CPR and consented to a DNR order (45/134) after a procedural approach. For the remaining surrogates, the ethics committee determined that a CPR order should persist but recommended a DNR order in the remaining 67 cases. The healthcare providers subsequently entered a DNR order in 61 of these patients and most surrogates of these patients agreed, but 19 persisted to request CPR, but were denied by the healthcare team. Although not assessed, it would not be difficult to assume that the surrogates of these patients suffered a range of negative emotions, which begs the question as to how to manage trade-offs between giving priority to surrogates' preferences for CPR versus writing DNR orders to support professional integrity and lessen health caregivers' moral distress albeit with potential greater anxiety, depression, and post-traumatic distress syndrome for surrogates?

Future Themes to Explore Regarding Ethics Consultation at the End-of-Life

Further research is warranted to better understand the ethical concerns of families when a member of their family is hospitalized. Other areas to explore include elucidating the outcomes of ethics consultations, which consultative model is successful in terms of achieving consensus, while reducing or limiting the emotional burden surrogates experience with a process of inquiry, and identification of the patients for whom ethics consultation is most beneficial.

Furthermore, the timing of an ethics consults might prove to be important, as its use after conflicts have become intractable might thwart its effectiveness. As such, determining what early triggers for ethics consults would be useful to prevent intractable disputes without decreasing the cost-effectiveness of such consults. In conclusion, ethics consultations are used as an intervention to address conflicts in shared decision-making and to enhance discussions between providers, patients, and families. Such consults play an important role in clarifying values and obligations, defusing tensions, and refocusing attention on appropriate goals.

References

1. Walter JK, Ross LF. Relational autonomy: moving beyond the limits of isolated individualism. Pediatrics. 2014;133(Suppl. 1):S16–23. https://doi.org/10.1542/peds.2013-3608D.
2. Johnson SK, Bautista CA, Hong SY, Weissfeld L, White DB. An empirical study of surrogates' preferred level of control over value-laden life support decisions in intensive care units. Am J Respir Crit Care Med. 2011;183(7):915–21. https://doi.org/10.1164/rccm.201008-1214OC.
3. Anderson WG, Arnold RM, Angus DC, Bryce CL. Passive decision-making preference is associated with anxiety and depression in relatives of patients in the intensive care unit. J Crit Care. 2009;24(2):249–54. https://doi.org/10.1016/j.jcrc.2007.12.010.
4. Moore B, McDougall R. Exploring the ethics of the parental role in parent-clinician conflict. Hast Cent Rep. 2022;52(6):33–43. https://doi.org/10.1002/hast.1445.
5. Pellikka HK, Axelin A, Sankilampi U, Kangasniemi M. Shared responsibility for decision-making in NICU: a scoping review. Nurs Ethics. 2023;30:462. https://doi.org/10.1177/09697330221134948.
6. Scheunemann LP, McDevitt M, Carson SS, Hanson LC. Randomized, controlled trials of interventions to improve communication in intensive care: a systematic review. Chest. 2011;139(3):543–54. https://doi.org/10.1378/chest.10-0595.
7. Fawole OA, Dy SM, Wilson RF, Lau BD, Martinez KA, Apostol CC, et al. A systematic review of communication quality improvement interventions for patients with advanced and serious illness. J Gen Intern Med. 2013;28(4):570–7. https://doi.org/10.1007/s11606-012-2204-4.
8. Wright AA, Zhang B, Ray A, Mack JW, Trice E, Balboni T, et al. Associations between end-of-life discussions, patient mental health, medical care near death, and caregiver bereavement adjustment. JAMA. 2008;300(14):1665–73. https://doi.org/10.1001/jama.300.14.1665.
9. Gries CJ, Engelberg RA, Kross EK, Zatzick D, Nielsen EL, Downey L, et al. Predictors of symptoms of posttraumatic stress and depression in family members after patient death in the ICU. Chest. 2010;137(2):280–7. https://doi.org/10.1378/chest.09-1291.
10. Pochard F, Azoulay E, Chevret S, Lemaire F, Hubert P, Canoui P, et al. Symptoms of anxiety and depression in family members of intensive care unit patients: ethical hypothesis regarding decision-making capacity. Crit Care Med. 2001;29(10):1893–7.
11. Azoulay E, Timsit JF, Sprung CL, Soares M, Rusinova K, Lafabrie A, et al. Prevalence and factors of intensive care unit conflicts: the conflicus study. Am J Respir Crit Care Med. 2009;180(9):853–60. https://doi.org/10.1164/rccm.200810-1614OC.
12. Abbott KH, Sago JG, Breen CM, Abernethy AP, Tulsky JA. Families looking back: one year after discussion of withdrawal or withholding of life-sustaining support. Crit Care Med. 2001;29(1):197–201.
13. Breen CM, Abernethy AP, Abbott KH, Tulsky JA. Conflict associated with decisions to limit life-sustaining treatment in intensive care units. J Gen Intern Med. 2001;16(5):283–9.
14. Studdert DM, Mello MM, Burns JP, Puopolo AL, Galper BZ, Truog RD, et al. Conflict in the care of patients with prolonged stay in the ICU: types, sources, and predictors. Intensive Care Med. 2003;29(9):1489–97. https://doi.org/10.1007/s00134-003-1853-5.
15. Schuster RA, Hong SY, Arnold RM, White DB. Investigating conflict in ICUs-is the clinicians' perspective enough? Crit Care Med. 2014;42(2):328–35. https://doi.org/10.1097/CCM.0b013e3182a27598.
16. DuVal G, Sartorius L, Clarridge B, Gensler G, Danis M. What triggers requests for ethics consultations? J Med Ethics. 2001;27(Suppl. 1):i24–9.
17. Cho HL, Grady C, Tarzian A, Povar G, Mangal J, Danis M. Patient and family descriptions of ethical concerns. Am J Bioeth. 2020;20(6):52–64. https://doi.org/10.1080/15265161.2020.1754500.
18. Buchanan CA, Bester JC, Bruno B, Delany C, Kennedy KO, Koogler T, et al. Pediatric ethics consultation: practical considerations for the clinical ethics consultant. J Clin Ethics. 2019;30(3):270–83.

19. Bell JAH, Salis M, Tong E, Nekolaichuk E, Barned C, Bianchi A, et al. Clinical ethics consultations: a scoping review of reported outcomes. BMC Med Ethics. 2022;23(1):99. https://doi.org/10.1186/s12910-022-00832-6.
20. American Society for Bioethics and Humanities. Core Competencie for healthcare ethics consultation. 2nd ed. Glenview, IL: ASBH; 2011.
21. Dowdy MD, Robertson C, Bander JA. A study of proactive ethics consultation for critically and terminally ill patients with extended lengths of stay. Crit Care Med. 1998;26(2):252–9.
22. Schneiderman LJ, Gilmer T, Teetzel HD. Impact of ethics consultations in the intensive care setting: a randomized, controlled trial. Crit Care Med. 2000;28(12):3920–4.
23. Schneiderman LJ, Gilmer T, Teetzel HD, Dugan DO, Blustein J, Cranford R, et al. Effect of ethics consultations on nonbeneficial life-sustaining treatments in the intensive care setting: a randomized controlled trial. JAMA. 2003;290(9):1166–72. https://doi.org/10.1001/jama.290.9.1166.
24. Andereck JW, Kipp AM, Ondiek M, Vermund SH. Helminth prevalence among adults in rural Kenya: a stool survey for soil-transmitted helminths and schistosomiasis in Nyanza province. Trans R Soc Trop Med Hyg. 2014;108(12):804–9. https://doi.org/10.1093/trstmh/tru164.
25. Davidson JE, Aslakson RA, Long AC, Puntillo KA, Kross EK, Hart J, et al. Guidelines for family-centered care in the neonatal, pediatric, and adult ICU. Crit Care Med. 2017;45(1):103–28. https://doi.org/10.1097/CCM.0000000000002169.
26. Spielman B, Gorka C, Miller K, Pointer CA, Hinze B. Gender and race in the timing of requests for ethics consultations: a single-center study. J Clin Ethics. 2016;27(2):154–62.
27. Kayser JB, Kaplan LJ. Conflict Management in the ICU. Crit Care Med. 2020;48(9):1349–57. https://doi.org/10.1097/CCM.0000000000004440.
28. Cohen CB. Avoiding "Cloudcuckooland" in ethics committee case review: matching models to issues and concerns. Law Med Health Care. 1992;20(4):294–9.
29. Carson SS, Cox CE, Wallenstein S, Hanson LC, Danis M, Tulsky JA, et al. Effect of palliative care-led meetings for families of patients with chronic critical illness: a randomized clinical trial. JAMA. 2016;316(1):51–62. https://doi.org/10.1001/jama.2016.8474.
30. Wendler D. The theory and practice of surrogate decision-making. Hast Cent Rep. 2017;47(1):29–31. https://doi.org/10.1002/hast.671.
31. White DB. Strategies to support surrogate decision makers of patients with chronic critical illness: the search continues. JAMA. 2016;316(1):35–7. https://doi.org/10.1001/jama.2016.8691.
32. Dodek PM, Jameson K, Chevalier JM. New approach to assessing and addressing moral distress in intensive care unit personnel: a case study. Can J Anaesth. 2022;69(10):1240–47. https://doi.org/10.1007/s12630-022-02307-z.
33. Olmstead JA, Dahnke MD. The need for an effective process to resolve conflicts over medical futility: a case study and analysis. Crit Care Nurse. 2016;36(6):13–23. https://doi.org/10.4037/ccn2016472.
34. Bosslet GT, Pope TM, Rubenfeld GD, Lo B, Truog RD, Rushton CH, et al. An official ATS/AACN/ACCP/ESICM/SCCM policy statement: responding to requests for potentially inappropriate treatments in intensive care units. Am J Respir Crit Care Med. 2015;191(11):1318–30. https://doi.org/10.1164/rccm.201505-0924ST.
35. Robinson EM, Cadge W, Zollfrank AA, Cremens MC, Courtwright AM. After the DNR: surrogates who persist in requesting cardiopulmonary resuscitation. Hast Cent Rep. 2017;47(1):10–9. https://doi.org/10.1002/hast.664.

Chapter 20
The Role of the Pharmacist in Family Engagement in the Intensive Care Unit and During Transitions of Care

Joanna L. Stollings

Introduction

The ABCDEF bundle is an interprofessional, intensive care unit (ICU) bundle:

- Assess, prevent, and manage pain.
- Both spontaneous awakening trials (SATs) and spontaneous breathing trials (SBTs).
- Choice of Analgesia and sedation.
- Delirium-assess, prevent, and manage.
- Early mobility and exercise.
- Family engagement and empowerment.

It integrates the prevention and treatment of pain, agitation, and delirium, resulting in a reduction in duration of mechanical ventilation, a decrease in ICU-acquired delirium and weakness, and optimization of family engagement and empowerment [1]. Utilization of the ABCDEF Bundle promotes interprofessional care [2–7] and improves patient outcomes [2, 3]. A reduction in ICU mortality has been demonstrated with the degree of bundle compliance [8].

Post-intensive care syndrome (PICS) is a term that refers to new or worsening impairment in mental health, physical function, and cognition following critical illness. The development of physiological conditions including posttraumatic stress, depression, complicated grief, and anxiety in family members of critically ill patients has been termed post-intensive care syndrome-family (PICS-F) [9]. Coronavirus Disease 2019 (COVID-19) has resulted in over six million deaths [10]. Survivors of COVID-19 have resulted in long-term effects team Post-Acute

J. L. Stollings (✉)
Department of Pharmaceutical Services, Vanderbilt University Medical Center, Nashville, TN, USA
e-mail: joanna.stollings@vumc.org

© The Author(s), under exclusive license to Springer Nature Switzerland AG 2025

A. J. Vance et al. (eds.), *Families in the Intensive Care Unit*,
https://doi.org/10.1007/978-3-031-83786-9_20

COVID-19 Syndrome (PACS). PACS occurs 4 weeks to 6 months after the acute infection and can affect the neurologic, cardiovascular, respiratory, gastrointestinal, endocrine, renal, dermatologic, and hematologic organ systems [11]. The 2017 Society of Critical Care Medicine (SCCM) Guidelines for Family-Centered Care outline the best evidence available for providing support for family members of critically ill patients in the ICU [12]. The guidelines suggest that routine interprofessional care be used to improve family satisfaction and to reduce conflict between the clinicians and the family [12]. Although numerous studies have demonstrated the role of the pharmacist in enhancing compliance with the different letters of the ABCDEF bundle [13–20] and the utilization of a pharmacist in a PICS clinic has been described [21–23], the role of the pharmacist with family engagement and empowerment or PICS-F has not been defined.

The ABCDEF Bundle

The pharmacist has a unique role engaging the family and assisting with implementation of the ABCDEF Bundle.

A: Assess, prevent, and manage pain, is the first place that the pharmacist can interact with the family to aid in the recognition and treatment of the patient's pain. Numerous complications including nosocomial infections, increased duration of mechanical ventilation, and delirium have been associated with inadequate pain management [24]. Utilization of opiates for treatment of pain in critically ill patients has been associated with a heightened risk of delirium in some studies [25–29] and a lower risk of delirium in others [25, 30]. Pain assessment in critically ill patients is imperative due to the risk for the development of delirium secondary to untreated pain. The pain, agitation/sedation, delirium, immobility, and sleep disruption in adult patients in the ICU (PADIS) guidelines [31] state that all adult critically ill patients be routinely assessed for pain. The reference standard for pain assessment is self-reporting of pain [32]. Additionally, some patients do not wish to have pain treated with opiates due to the fear of development of addiction. Through incorporation of the family into discussions about the importance of accurate pain assessment and treatment when indicated, the pharmacist and family can act together to aid in the patient receiving appropriate pain treatment.

B, C: Both SATs and SBTs, and C, Choice of Analgesia and sedation, are another place where the pharmacist can empower the family in assisting with patient. When turning off the patient's sedation and analgesia, the patient can become agitated. The pharmacist can educate the family to calm the patient first, potentially preventing the use of analgesia/sedation. Additionally, a survey of ICU health care practitioners found that only 44% of respondents practice spontaneous awakening trials on greater than half of ICU days [33].

D: Pharmacists can provide family education on the letter D, Delirium-assess, prevent, and manage, including utilization of both nonpharmacologic, e.g., noise reduction strategies [12] and pharmacologic therapy.

E:The letter E, Early mobility and exercise, can be performed by nurses, physical therapists, occupational therapists, and physicians. With many institutions experiencing a shortage of physical and occupational therapists and the busy schedules of nurses, physicians, and mid-level providers, early mobility is sometimes overlooked as a means to involve the family in patient care. Pharmacists can recommend consulting with physical/occupational therapy during interprofessional rounds.

F: By doing all of the above listed letters and aiding the interprofessional team in inviting the family to participate in interprofessional rounds [12], the pharmacist can promote the letter F, Family engagement and empowerment. By allowing a family member to assist with the patient's care, it improves confidence and competence in the caregiving role in addition to improving psychological health during and after the ICU stay [12]. The 2020 Position Paper on Critical Care Pharmacy Services recommends that pharmacists educate patients and families both during acute illness and at transitions of care [34].

Medication Reconciliation at Transitions of Care

The Centers for Medicare and Medicaid Services started the Readmissions Reduction Program, which decreased payments to hospitals with excess 30-day readmissions in 2012 [35]. A transition of care is defined as when a patient leaves a particular unit or health care facility and moves to a different location (e.g., a different area of a hospital, a different facility, or home) [36]. Over the last decade, transitions of care have been deemed as a significant risk for adverse drug events (ADEs) [37, 38]. ADEs have been shown to increase hospital length of stay, health care costs, and mortality [39, 40]. Medication reconciliation is defined as verifying medication indication, discrepancies, and resolving all medication-related issues at all transitions of care [41]. Pharmacists conducted medication histories when compared to other health care practitioners have been shown to have a lower rate of errors [42–46]. The Joint Commission on Accreditation of Healthcare Organizations declared "sustaining and properly communicating correct medication information" to be a National Patient Safety Goal in 2011 in response to the growing amount of data demonstrating medication errors at transitions of care.

The goal of pharmacists when performing medication reconciliation during each transition of care is to gauge understanding of the medications, ensure adherence, determine any barriers to medication management, and evaluate for support systems. Having the family in addition to the patient present during medication reconciliation is key. When the pharmacist is communicating with the patient and family, the pharmacist should use a structured communication approach such as the **VALUE** pneumonic:

Table 20.1 Benefits of family presence during pharmacist discharge counseling

Ensure patient and family understanding of what medications that he or she will be taking post-discharge
Verify that the patient and family know how to take all of their medications (e.g. what time of day, with food, without food, etc.)
Clarify what side effects to watch out for
Explain what other medications to avoid
Determine what pharmacy will be utilized to obtain medications
Provide any other needed counseling

Value comments made by the family,
Acknowledge family emotions.
Listen.
Understand the patient as a person.
Elicit family questions [12].

The family member can help recall which medications that patient takes, potentially provide a medication list, or direct the pharmacist to which pharmacy to call to obtain a medication list. The additional benefits of having a family member or members present during medication reconciliation at transitions of care are provided in Table 20.1.

A survey of pharmacists that had participated in admission medication reconciliation recommendations for improving care transitions found that sometimes patients were out of the room or undergoing a procedure and could not have counseling. Additionally, patients were often too delirious or sleepy to receive counseling [47]. Given that the incidence of delirium has been reported to be between 20% and 50% among non-ventilated ICU patients and 60% and 80% of ventilated patients, this is not surprising. Additionally, the pharmacist encouraged the family members during the admission medication reconciliation to be present at the discharge medication reconciliation to help the patient better understand their new medication regimen as they transfer to home [47]. With the degree of delirium and sedation in ICU patients, involvement of the family in medication reconciliation at all transitions of care is imperative.

Deprescribing

Elderly patients with cognitive impairment or low health literacy [48] or those with polypharmacy (taking five to nine concomitant medications) are three examples of patient populations at higher risk for ADEs during transitions of care [38]. Additionally, the number of medications a patient is receiving has been shown to be a risk factor for drug–drug interactions [49], increased mortality in the elderly [50], and delirium [51]. “Deprescribing” is defined as tapering or stopping medications to reduce polypharmacy and improve patient outcomes. The following five-step protocol for deprescribing has been recommended:

1. Determine that each medication has an appropriate indication.
2. When determining the number of medications that should be discontinued, the overall potential harm of the medications should be considered.
3. Determine if each individual drug should be discontinued.
4. Prioritize which medications should be discontinued first.
5. Start and monitor a drug discontinuation plan.

In the ICU, deprescribing can be further enhanced in the ICU by determining if medication has a current indication [52]. For example, a patient using nasal steroids for allergies does not need this restarted while in the ICU.

The 2018 PADIS guidelines suggest not routinely using haloperidol or an atypical antipsychotic to treat delirium. The Modifying the Impact of the ICU-Associated Neurological Dysfunction-USA (MIND USA) Study is a multicenter, randomized, placebo-controlled study of 566 patients showing that haloperidol and ziprasidone did not reduce delirium, time on the ventilator, ICU or hospital length of stay, or death compared with placebo. Arrhythmias, parkinsonism (extrapyramidal symptoms), neuroleptic malignant syndrome, study drug discontinuation, and other safety concerns were extremely low across all three groups [53]. Antipsychotics remain viable for the short-term control of agitation (e.g., alcohol or drug withdrawal) or severe anxiety with the need to avoid respiratory suppression (e.g., heart failure, COPD, or asthma).

The AID-ICU trial is a multicenter, randomized, placebo-controlled trial of 963 patients with delirium randomized to haloperidol or placebo. The mean number of days alive and out of the hospital did not differ between the haloperidol and the placebo group [54]. Despite this, numerous surveys have shown that prescribers utilize haloperidol or atypical antipsychotics for the treatment of delirium in the ICU. A single-center, prospective cohort study of 172 ICU survivors found that 42 (24%) of these were prescribed an antipsychotic at discharge [55]. Multiple other studies have demonstrated the continuation of antipsychotics at hospital discharge following ICU admission [56–61]. Risk factors associated with the utilization of antipsychotics include ventricular arrhythmias, excess sedation, akathisia, and hypotension [62]. Additionally, a population-based, retrospective cohort study found that new use of atypical antipsychotics was associated with an increased risk of death compared with nonuse in elderly patients with dementia [63]. These studies demonstrate the importance of discontinuing these medications following ICU admission especially given that clinicians may be reluctant to stop medications that were started in the ICU. The family can serve as resource to clarify home medications and allow clinicians to feel more comfortable with describing medications utilized temporarily.

New and old sedative prescriptions are also commonly prescribed for post-critical illness in adults. A population-based cohort study of 250,428 ICU survivors ≥66 years who had not filled sedative prescriptions ≤6 months pre-hospitalization was conducted. One in 15 sedative-naïve older adult ICU survivors filled a new sedative ≤7 days 50 of discharge, of whom more than half filled persistent prescriptions [64]. This highlights another area for pharmacists to focus on as patients transition care.

Stress ulcer prophylaxis with acid suppressive therapy is commonly continued in patients following an ICU admission. Quality improvement initiatives have been developed to decrease this practice. In one study, in the pre-intervention group, 7% of patients were discharged inappropriately compared to none of the patients in the post-intervention group ($p = 0.22$) [65]. The inappropriate continuation of acid-suppressive therapy at hospital discharge following ICU stay has been documented in other studies [65–68]. Numerous complications have been associated with proton pump inhibitor use including hospital-acquired *Clostridium difficile* infection, pneumonia, hip fracture, and dementia [69–73]. If a current indication such as mechanical ventilation or gastrointestinal bleed does not exist, the family can be a valuable resource to verify if the patient has gastroesophageal reflux disease or another indication that merits continuation.

A qualitative study of focus groups including pharmacists, general practitioners, and specialist physicians was conducted to investigate perspectives of health care providers on deprescribing of anticholinergic and sedative medications. Lack of accountability was the most common reason that anticholinergics and sedatives were not discontinued. Pharmacists were frustrated with general practitioners for not stopping anticholinergic and sedative medications. Irritation was expressed by the general practitioners that the specialist physicians did not take ownership of deprescribing and vice versa [74]. Since family members are quite often present at all physician visits and hospital admissions, they are logical members to assist with deprescribing. Family can serve as a means of communication between multiple physicians.

The frequency of prescribed potentially inappropriate medications, medications potentially harmful to the elderly based on prior research and knowledge of pharmaceutical effect, and actually inappropriate medications, the benefit of the drug was outweighed by the harm after considering clinical circumstances, was described in a single-center study of 120 elderly adult ICU survivors [75]. Using the 2003 Beers criteria and additional medication safety data published after 2003, charts were reviewed and medications were identified as potentially inappropriate medications. At five specific points within the hospital stay, admission, medical/surgical unit admission, ICU admission, ICU discharge, and hospital discharge, medications were evaluated to determine if actually inappropriate medications were started. The following were the most common categories of potentially inappropriate medications identified at hospital discharge: opioids, anticholinergic medications, antidepressants, and drugs causing orthostasis. Of these potentially inappropriate medications, 36% were considered to be actually inappropriate medications by a team consisting of a hospitalist, geriatrician, and a clinical pharmacist. The potentially inappropriate medication categories at hospital discharge with the highest positive predictive values for being actually inappropriate medications were anticholinergics (55%), nonbenzodiazepine hypnotics (67%), benzodiazepines (67%), atypical antipsychotics (71%), and muscle relaxants (100%). In multivariate analysis, the number of discharges and potentially inappropriate medications were independently predicted by the number of preadmission potentially inappropriate medications ($p < 0.001$), discharge to somewhere other than home ($p = 0.03$), and

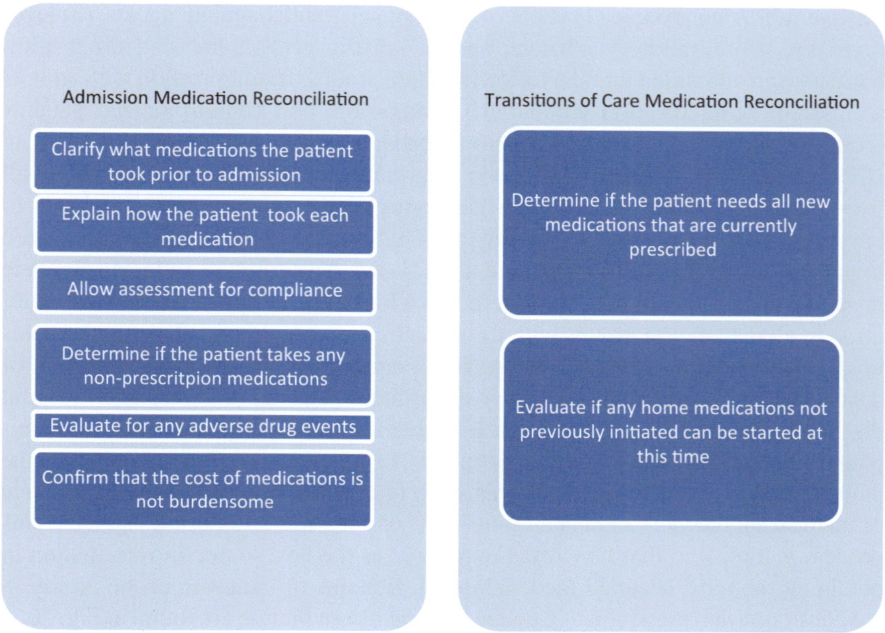

Fig. 20.1 Benefits of family presence during pharmacist admission medication reconciliation and at transitions of care

discharge from a surgical service ($p < 0.001$). Nearly 2/3 of actually inappropriate medications were initiated in the ICU.

Many of these medications initiated in the ICU or at any other time within the hospitalization may have been appropriately initiated for the patient's current clinical situation. However, failure to discontinue these medications once no longer indicated can lead to inappropriate and prolonged use increasing the potential for adverse drug events and drug/drug interactions. The importance of reviewing patients' medication lists daily and during transitions of care is emphasized by this study. The involvement of the family in this process is imperative in determining exactly what medications the patient takes at home to facilitate the deprescribing process. Benefits of inclusion of the family in the transition of medication reconciliation are found in Fig. 20.1.

Reinitiation of Home Medications

In contrast to the inappropriate continuation of medications after hospital discharge, another problem is failure to initiate patients' home maintenance medications upon hospital admission. A large Canadian cohort study of 396,380 elderly patients evaluated records of hospital and outpatient medications prescribed from at least one of the five following groups: (1) statins, (2) antiplatelet/anticoagulant agents, (3) levothyroxine, (4) respiratory inhalers, and (5) gastric acid-suppressing drugs [76]. Patients were classified into the following three groups: hospitalization with an ICU admission, hospitalization without ICU admission, and nonhospitalized patients (controls). Compared to the control group, patients admitted to a hospital without an ICU stay were significantly more likely to have medications discontinued within all five of the medication groups. Likewise, control group patients were less likely to have medications discontinued among all five of the medication groups compared to patients admitted to a hospital with an ICU stay. Compared to patients who were hospitalized without an ICU stay, there was a higher risk of medication discontinuation in all medication groups with the exception of respiratory inhalers in patients hospitalized with an ICU admission. In all study patients, the composite risk of death, hospitalization, and emergency department visits up to 1 year after hospital discharge was found to be significantly higher in patients in which a statin or antiplatelet or anticoagulant was discontinued. To prevent errors of omission in the patient's discharge medication list, this study once again emphasizes the importance of medication reconciliation at all transitions of care. Inclusion of the family in this process is logical in that they often may serve as the best source of information in obtaining the most accurate medication list. Benefits of inclusion of the family in the admission and transition of care medication reconciliation are found in Fig. 20.1.

Discharge Counseling

Following hospital discharge, up to 20% of patients experience an adverse drug event, with approximately 60% being associated with a medication and being deemed preventable [77–79]. These adverse events have been associated with emergency department visits, hospital admissions, and costly health care utilization [80–83].

Readmissions occurred in 20% of Medicare recipients within 30 days of discharge and in 34% within 90 days of discharge in one study [81]. Physicians in the hospital may start new medications and stop the use of other medications, while the patient still has the other medications at home [84]. Once the patient is discharged, it is unclear why medications that the patient should be taking. A survey showed that <60% of patients understood the indications for their new medication at discharge and only 12% conveyed awareness of a known side effect [85].

Discharge counseling is an important patient safety initiative. Pharmacists are the logical individuals to provide discharge counseling given their medication expertise. A survey of pharmacists found that uniformly, all pharmacists found counseling on medications at discharge facilitated understanding among patients about their medication regimens [47]. Pharmacist counseling on medications at discharge is cost-effective [86], improves patient satisfaction, and increases medication adherence [87]. However, the impact of pharmacists' on readmission has not been consistently demonstrated [80, 88–91].

Discharge medication counseling should include the plan for filling medications, troubleshooting anticipated and potential barriers to adherence, utilization of adherence aids such as a pill box, and a teach-back approach to verify understanding. Having the family in addition to the patient present during discharge counseling is imperative and has been reported to be helpful by pharmacists [47]. The additional benefits of having a family member or members present during pharmacist discharge counseling are provided in Table 20.1.

As part of a randomized controlled trial, the frequency and predictors of nonadherence with medications post-discharge in patients that had received discharge medication counseling by a pharmacist were evaluated. Patients who lived alone were less likely to fill their prescriptions than patients who were married or that did not live alone (odds ratio 2.2, 95% confidence interval: 1.01–4.8, p–0.047). Nonadherence was more likely to be demonstrated in patients that were discharged on >10 medications (odds ratio 2.3, 95% confidence interval: 1.05–4.98, $p = 0.036$). Patients who had lower incomes were less likely to have prescriptions filled univariate analysis ($p = 0.04$). However, this was not demonstrated in multivariate analysis [92].

Given the known predictors of nonadherence with medications post-discharge, the pharmacist can engage the family of patients that meet these criteria to enhance compliance. For a patient that lives alone, family can be counseled regarding this known risk factor and given the suggestion of calling or visiting the patient, getting a neighbor to remind the patient about medications, or potentially getting a caregiver involved if needed. For patients who are discharged on >10 medications, the pharmacist could provide a pill box or an adherence aid to assist the patient and family with adherence. Additionally, the pharmacist could provide counseling to the patient and family about incorporating medication administration into activities of daily life such as eating and setting medication timers. For patients with lower incomes, the pharmacist can discuss with the patient and family about medication coupons and programs to assist with obtaining medications in indigent patients.

Several barriers have been identified to medication discharge counseling. Currently, families are not engaged in transitions of care [93]. Patients who were in a hurry to leave the hospital were less receptive to being counseled. Involvement of the family in the discharge counseling process may give the pharmacist a second advocate to the importance of this activity. Due to need for quick turn over of patient beds for the next patient, pharmacists felt hurried to go through the discharge medication process. Pharmacists also were suspicious that patients did not ask as many questions as needed [47]. By including the family in the discharge medication reconciliation process, the pharmacist can ask questions to gauge both the patients' and family members' understanding. Even with these identified barriers, pharmacists still considered discharge counseling an essential part of the patient's health care stay.

Post ICU Clinics

A post-ICU clinic is one means of aiding the transition back to a primary care provider following an ICU stay. Many specific issues are seen in patients following an ICU stay that primary care providers may not be familiar with. Additionally, primary care providers may be familiar with the tools to diagnose and manage these complications. An interprofessional team of providers that staff a post-ICU clinic can assist in the diagnosis and treatment of PICS by using their expertise about specific complications related to critical care. Given that 50% of patients who are readmitted within 30 days of discharge did not visit a primary care provider post-hospitalization, it is not surprising that lack of understanding of medications contributed to readmissions to readmissions [38]. Review of medications, reconciliation, and counseling should all be considered essential parts of a patient's visit to a post-ICU clinic. A pharmacist is the ideal person to perform these tasks [21–23]. There are multiple studies highlighting the important role of pharmacists in post-ICU clinics (Table 20.2). There is no specific data evaluating the pharmacist's role in PACS clinic; however, their role is very similar to those that work in a PICS clinic, it is imperative that the pharmacist involve the family in the complete medication use process [47]. The steps of the complete medication use process are listed in Table 20.3. These steps include not only asking the patient questions but allowing the family to participate as well to obtain the most complete medication information. This process also should alleviate symptoms of PICS-F as the medication review, reconciliation, and counseling from a medication expert can instate confidence in the family member about the patient's quite often complicated medication regimen.

Table 20.2 Summary of pharmacists' interventions in post-ICU clinics

Citation	Population	Design	Outcomes
Stollings et al. *Ann of Pharm* 2018 [94]	56 patients seen in a PICS clinic	Prospective, observational cohort study	• Median of 4 medication interventions per patient • Medication discontinuation in 22 patients (39%) and initiation in 18 (32%) patients • ADE in 9 patients (16%), 2 of which were serious* and 1 was life threatening** • 18 ADE preventative measures were implemented • Influenza vaccine administration in 13 patients (23%) and pneumococcal vaccine administration in 2 patients (4%)
MacTavish et al. *BMJ open Qual.* 2019 [95]	47 patients seen in a PICS clinic intensive care syndrome: Promoting Independence and return to employment (InS:PIRE) 5-week rehabilitation program for ICU survivors assessing medication-related problems (single-center)	Prospective, observational cohort study	• 69 MRP identified in 81% of patients • Drug omissions identified in 29% of patients • Dose adjustments made in 19% of patients • Treatment duration clarification in 17% of patients • 44 of the 69 MRPs were deemed severe • 55% were not aware of any medication changes at discharge • 60% of patients vocalized concerns to the PharmD regarding their medications • Drug classes requiring the most intervention included CV (26%), analgesics (22%), and respiratory (10%)

(continued)

Table 20.2 (continued)

Citation	Population	Design	Outcomes
MacTavish et al. *Ann am Thorac Soc*. 2020 [96]	183 patients seen in InS:PIRE (multi-center)	Prospective, observational cohort study	• 115 patients (62.8%) requiring ≥1 intervention • Treatment duration clarification occurred 44 times • Counseling occurred 33 times • Drug omissions were identified 27 times • 171 clinically significant PharmD interventions were made • 27.4% increase in regular analgesia when comparing before ICU to PICS clinic visit: • 16.3% increase in opioid use when comparing before ICU to PICS clinic visit
Bottom-Tanzer et al. *journal of trauma and acute care surgery*. 2021 [97]	82 surgical and trauma ICU survivors in PICS clinic	Retrospective, single-center study	• PharmD performed medication reconciliations on 96.5% of visits with 94.6% having 1 or more actionable change • 116 interventions were performed by the PharmD with 19 dose adjustments, 23 medication initiation, 27 medication discontinuations, and 47 counseling sessions

(continued)

Table 20.2 (continued)

Citation	Population	Design	Outcomes
MacTavish et al. *BMJ open Respir res.* 2021 [98]	78 COVID-19 survivors in PICS clinic	Prospective, observational study	• Full medication review in 78 patients • 29.5% of patients had previous medications discontinued which were never restarted after discharge • 32 CV medications were new or increased doses (50% anticoagulants, 16% antiarrhythmics 25% statins/ antihypertensives) • 37 CNS medications were new or increased doses (84% analgesics and 16% mental health/ insomnia agents) • 23 (29.5%) patients required analgesics prior to hospitalization, which increased to 39 (50%) after discharge
Mohammad et al. *JACCP: Journal of the American College of clinical pharmacy.* 2022 [99]	52 control vs 52 intervention patients with sepsis, septic shock, and/or respiratory failure survivors in PICS clinic	Retrospective, observational cohort analysis within 6 months of hospital discharge	• 84 MRP in control vs 110 MRP identified in intervention group • Reduction in interventions and MRP from initial visit compared to follow-up in intervention arm: 3.5 vs. 2.4 • Most common drugs with MRP were neurologic and CV

(continued)

Table 20.2 (continued)

Citation	Population	Design	Outcomes
Stollings et al. *J intensive care med*. 2023 [100]	472 patients that received a full medication review in 12 ICU-RCs	Prospective, observational study	• Pharmacy interventions made in 397 (84% of patients) • Median of 2 pharmacy interventions per patient • Medications were stopped in 124 (26%) of patients • Medications were started in 91 (19%) of patients • A dose was decreased in 51 (11%) patients • A dose was increased in 43 (9%) patients • There was no difference in the total number of medications that the patient was prescribed at the start and end of the patient visit • ADE preventive measures were implemented in 115 (24%) patients • ADE events were identified in 69 (15%) patients • Medication interactions were identified in 30 (6%) patients

ADE Adverse drug reaction, *CMM* comprehensive medication management, *CNS* central nervous system, *CV* cardiovascular, *ICU* intensive care unit, *MICU* medical intensive care unit, *MRP* medication related problem, *PharmD* doctor of pharmacy, *QI* quality improvement, *SAT* spontaneous awakening trial, *SBT* spontaneous breathing trial

Table 20.3 Medication-related questions asked at a post-intensive care syndrome clinic

Questions for the patient	Questions for the family member
1. Why do you take each of these medications?	1. Do you know what reason the patient takes each of these medications?
2. What dose and how often do you take each of these medications?	2. Do you know what dose and how often the patient takes each of these medications?
3. How do you take each medication (i.e., what time of day and with eals)?	3. How does the patient take each of these medications?
4. How often do you miss a dose? What do you do if you miss a dose?	4. How often does the patient miss a dose? What does he or she do if he or she misses a dose?
5. Does you use a pill box?	5. Does the patient use a pill box?
6. What side effects have you experienced with these medications?	6. What side effects has the patient experienced from these medications?
7. How much and how often do you use your pain medications?	7. How much and often does the patient use their pain medications?
8. Does you use any over the counter medications?	8. Does the patient use any over the counter medications?
9. Does you take any herbal medications?	9. Does the patient take any herbal medications
10. Do you visit one pharmacy?	10. Does the patient visit one pharmacy?
11. Do you ask your physician or pharmacist prior to taking any over-the-counter or herbal medications?	11. Does the patient ask their physician or pharmacist prior to taking any over-the-counter or herbal medications?
12 is the cost of medications problematic?	12. Is the cost of the patient's medications problematic?
13. Do you smoke?	13. Does the patient smoke?
14. Do you drink alcohol?	14. Does the patient drink alcohol?
15. Do you use illicit drugs?	15. Does the patient use illicit drugs?
16. Do you take your blood pressure at home?	16. Does the patient take their blood pressure at home?
17. Do you have regular bowel movements?	17. Does the patient have regular bowel movements?
18. Have you had an influenza vaccine?	18. Has the patient had an influenza vaccine?
19. Have you had a pneumococcal vaccine?	19. Has the patient had a pneumococcal vaccine?
20. Do you need refills of any medications?	20. Does the patient need any refills of any medications?

Conclusion

A pharmacist is a key member in family engagement both in the ICU and during transitions of care. Empowering the family to assist with the conduction of the ABCDEF bundle, performing medication reconciliation at all transitions of care, promoting deprescribing, performing discharge counseling, and serving as an integral member of an interprofessional post-ICU clinic team are all roles of the pharmacist in facilitating family engagement and empowerment.

Financial Support None.

Conflicts of Interest and Sources of Funding Joanna L. Stollings has no conflicts of interest to disclose.

References

1. Marra A, Ely EW, Pandharipande PP, Patel MB. The ABCDEF bundle in critical care. Crit Care Clin. 2017;33(2):225–43.
2. Balas MC, Vasilevskis EE, Olsen KM, Schmid KK, Shostrom V, Cohen MZ, Peitz G, Gannon DE, Sisson J, Sullivan J, et al. Effectiveness and safety of the awakening and breathing coordination, delirium monitoring/management, and early exercise/mobility bundle. Crit Care Med. 2014;42:1024.
3. Pandharipande P, Banerjee A, McGrane S, Ely EW. Liberation and animation for ventilated ICU patients: the ABCDE bundle for the back-end of critical care. Crit Care. 2010;14(3):157.
4. Carrothers KM, Barr J, Spurlock B, Ridgely MS, Damberg CL, Ely EW. Contextual issues influencing implementation and outcomes associated with an integrated approach to managing pain, agitation, and delirium in adult ICUs. Crit Care Med. 2013;41(9 Suppl. 1):S128–35.
5. Balas MC, Vasilevskis EE, Burke WJ, Boehm L, Pun BT, Olsen KM, Peitz GJ, Ely EW. Critical care nurses' role in implementing the "ABCDE bundle" into practice. Crit Care Nurse. 2012;32(2):35–47.
6. Morandi A, Brummel NE, Ely EW. Sedation, delirium and mechanical ventilation: the 'ABCDE' approach. Curr Opin Crit Care. 2011;17(1):43–9.
7. Vasilevskis EE, Ely EW, Speroff T, Pun BT, Boehm L, Dittus RS. Reducing iatrogenic risks: ICU-acquired delirium and weakness—crossing the quality chasm. Chest. 2010;138(5):1224–33.
8. Barnes-Daly MA, Phillips G, Ely EW. Improving hospital survival and reducing brain dysfunction at seven California community hospitals: implementing PAD guidelines via the ABCDEF bundle in 6,064 patients. Crit Care Med. 2017;45(2):171–8.
9. Needham DM, Davidson J, Cohen H, Hopkins RO, Weinert C, Wunsch H, Zawistowski C, Bemis-Dougherty A, Berney SC, Bienvenu OJ, et al. Improving long-term outcomes after discharge from intensive care unit: report from a stakeholders' conference*. Crit Care Med. 2012;40(2):502–9.
10. Guideline Clinical Management of COVID-19 Patients: Living Guideline [http://apps.who.int/bookorders.]
11. Excellence NIfHaC. COVID-19 Rapid Guidelines: Managing the Longterm-effects of COVID-19.
12. Davidson JE, Aslakson RA, Long AC, Puntillo KA, Kross EK, Hart J, Cox CE, Wunsch H, Wickline MA, Nunnally ME, et al. Guidelines for family-centered care in the neonatal, pediatric, and adult ICU. Crit Care Med. 2017;45(1):103–28.
13. Marshall J, Finn CA, Theodore AC. Impact of a clinical pharmacist-enforced intensive care unit sedation protocol on duration of mechanical ventilation and hospital stay. Crit Care Med. 2008;36(2):427–33.
14. Stollings JL, Foss JJ, Ely EW, Ambrose AM, Rice TW, Girard TD, Wheeler AP. Pharmacist leadership in ICU quality improvement: coordinating spontaneous awakening and breathing trials. Ann Pharmacother. 2015;49(8):883–91.
15. MacLaren R, Plamondon JM, Ramsay KB, Rocker GM, Patrick WD, Hall RI. A prospective evaluation of empiric versus protocol-based sedation and analgesia. Pharmacotherapy. 2000;20(6):662–72.

16. Devlin JW, Marquis F, Riker RR, Robbins T, Garpestad E, Fong JJ, Didomenico D, Skrobik Y. Combined didactic and scenario-based education improves the ability of intensive care unit staff to recognize delirium at the bedside. Crit Care. 2008;12(1):R19.
17. Gesin G, Russell BB, Lin AP, Norton HJ, Evans SL, Devlin JW. Impact of a delirium screening tool and multifaceted education on nurses' knowledge of delirium and ability to evaluate it correctly. Am J Crit Care. 2012;21(1):e1–11.
18. Swan JT. Decreasing inappropriate unable-to-assess ratings for the confusion assessment method for the intensive care unit. Am J Crit Care. 2014;23(1):60–9.
19. Louzon P, Jennings H, Ali M, Kraisinger M. Impact of pharmacist management of pain, agitation, and delirium in the intensive care unit through participation in multidisciplinary bundle rounds. American journal of health-system pharmacy : AJHP. 2017;74(4):253–62.
20. Marino J, Bucher D, Beach M, Yegneswaran B, Cooper B. Implementation of an intensive care unit delirium protocol: an interdisciplinary quality improvement project. Dimens Crit Care Nurs. 2015;34(5):273–84.
21. Stollings JL, Bloom SL, Huggins EL, Grayson SL, Jackson JC, Sevin CM. Medication management to ameliorate post-intensive care syndrome. AACN Adv Crit Care. 2016;27(2):133–40.
22. Stollings JL, Caylor MM. Postintensive care syndrome and the role of a follow-up clinic. Am J Health-Syst Pharmacy. 2015;72(15):1315–23.
23. Huggins EL, Bloom SL, Stollings JL, Camp M, Sevin CM, Jackson JC. A clinic model: post-intensive care syndrome and post-intensive care syndrome-family. AACN Adv Crit Care. 2016;27(2):204–11.
24. Chanques G, Jaber S, Barbotte E, Violet S, Sebbane M, Perrigault PF, Mann C, Lefrant JY, Eledjam JJ. Impact of systematic evaluation of pain and agitation in an intensive care unit. Crit Care Med. 2006;34(6):1691–9.
25. Pandharipande P, Cotton BA, Shintani A, Thompson J, Pun BT, Morris JA Jr, Dittus R, Ely EW. Prevalence and risk factors for development of delirium in surgical and trauma intensive care unit patients. J Trauma. 2008;65(1):34–41.
26. Dubois MJ, Bergeron N, Dumont M, Dial S, Skrobik Y. Delirium in an intensive care unit: a study of risk factors. Intensive Care Med. 2001;27(8):1297–304.
27. Ouimet S, Kavanagh BP, Gottfried SB, Skrobik Y. Incidence, risk factors and consequences of ICU delirium. Intensive Care Med. 2007;33(1):66–73.
28. Van Rompaey B, Elseviers MM, Schuurmans MJ, Shortridge-Baggett LM, Truijen S, Bossaert L. Risk factors for delirium in intensive care patients: a prospective cohort study. Crit Care. 2009;13(3):R77.
29. Pisani MA, Murphy TE, Araujo KL, Slattum P, Van Ness PH, Inouye SK. Benzodiazepine and opioid use and the duration of intensive care unit delirium in an older population. Crit Care Med. 2009;37(1):177–83.
30. Agarwal V, O'Neill PJ, Cotton BA, Pun BT, Haney S, Thompson J, Kassebaum N, Shintani A, Guy J, Ely EW, et al. Prevalence and risk factors for development of delirium in burn intensive care unit patients. J Burn Care Res. 2010;31(5):706–15.
31. Devlin JW, Skrobik Y, Gelinas C, Needham DM, Slooter AJC, Pandharipande PP, Watson PL, Weinhouse GL, Nunnally ME, Rochwerg B, et al. Clinical practice guidelines for the prevention and management of pain, agitation/sedation, delirium, immobility, and sleep disruption in adult patients in the ICU. Crit Care Med. 2018;46(9):e825–73.
32. Peacock S, Patel S. Cultural influences on pain. Rev Pain. 2008;1(2):6–9.
33. Patel RP, Gambrell M, Speroff T, Scott TA, Pun BT, Okahashi J, Strength C, Pandharipande P, Girard TD, Burgess H, et al. Delirium and sedation in the intensive care unit: survey of behaviors and attitudes of 1384 healthcare professionals. Crit Care Med. 2009;37(3):825–32.
34. Lat I, Paciullo C, Daley MJ, MacLaren R, Bolesta S, McCann J, Stollings JL, Gross K, Foos SA, Roberts RJ, et al. Position paper on critical care pharmacy services: 2020 update. Crit Care Med. 2020;48(9):e813–34.

35. Rodrigues CR, Harrington AR, Murdock N, Holmes JT, Borzadek EZ, Calabro K, Martin J, Slack MK. Effect of pharmacy-supported transition-of-care interventions on 30-day readmissions: a systematic review and meta-analysis. Ann Pharmacother. 2017;51(10):866–89.
36. College A, of Clinical P, Kirwin J, Canales AE, Bentley ML, Bungay K, Chan T, Dobson E, Holder RM, Johnson D, Lilliston A, et al. Process indicators of quality clinical pharmacy services during transitions of care. Pharmacotherapy. 2012;32(11):e338–47.
37. Leendertse AJ, Egberts AC, Stoker LJ, van den Bemt PM, Group HS. Frequency of and risk factors for preventable medication-related hospital admissions in The Netherlands. Arch Intern Med. 2008;168(17):1890–6.
38. College A, of Clinical P, Hume AL, Kirwin J, Bieber HL, Couchenour RL, Hall DL, Kennedy AK, LaPointe NM, Burkhardt CD, Schilli K, et al. Improving care transitions: current practice and future opportunities for pharmacists. Pharmacotherapy. 2012;32(11):e326–37.
39. Bates DW, Spell N, Cullen DJ, Burdick E, Laird N, Petersen LA, Small SD, Sweitzer BJ, Leape LL. The costs of adverse drug events in hospitalized patients. Adverse drug events prevention study group. JAMA. 1997;277(4):307–11.
40. Hug BL, Keohane C, Seger DL, Yoon C, Bates DW. The costs of adverse drug events in community hospitals. Joint Commission J Qual Patient Safety/Joint Commission Resour. 2012;38(3):120–6.
41. Agrawal A, Wu WY. Reducing medication errors and improving systems reliability using an electronic medication reconciliation system. Joint Commiss J Qual Patient safety/Joint Commiss Resour. 2009;35(2):106–14.
42. Reeder TA, Mutnick A. Pharmacist- versus physician-obtained medication histories. Am J Health-Syst Pharmacy. 2008;65(9):857–60.
43. Pippins JR, Gandhi TK, Hamann C, Ndumele CD, Labonville SA, Diedrichsen EK, Carty MG, Karson AS, Bhan I, Coley CM, et al. Classifying and predicting errors of inpatient medication reconciliation. J Gen Intern Med. 2008;23(9):1414–22.
44. Patel E, Pevnick JM, Kennelty KA. Pharmacists and medication reconciliation: a review of recent literature. Integr Pharm Res Pract. 2019;8:39–45.
45. Bajeux E, Alix L, Cornee L, Barbazan C, Mercerolle M, Howlett J, Cruveilhier V, Line-Iehl C, Cador B, Jego P, et al. Pharmacist-led medication reconciliation at patient discharge: a tool to reduce healthcare utilization? An observational study in patients 65 years or older. BMC Geriatr. 2022;22(1):576.
46. Studer H, Imfeld-Isenegger TL, Beeler PE, Ceppi MG, Rosen C, Bodmer M, Boeni F, Hersberger KE, Lampert ML. The impact of pharmacist-led medication reconciliation and interprofessional ward rounds on drug-related problems at hospital discharge. Int J Clin Pharm. 2023;45(1):117–25.
47. Haynes KT, Oberne A, Cawthon C, Kripalani S. Pharmacists' recommendations to improve care transitions. Ann Pharmacother. 2012;46(9):1152–9.
48. Davis TC, Wolf MS, Bass PF 3rd, Thompson JA, Tilson HH, Neuberger M, Parker RM. Literacy and misunderstanding prescription drug labels. Ann Intern Med. 2006;145(12):887–94.
49. Qato DM, Alexander GC, Conti RM, Johnson M, Schumm P, Lindau ST. Use of prescription and over-the-counter medications and dietary supplements among older adults in the United States. JAMA. 2008;300(24):2867–78.
50. Jyrkka J, Enlund H, Korhonen MJ, Sulkava R, Hartikainen S. Polypharmacy status as an indicator of mortality in an elderly population. Drugs Aging. 2009;26(12):1039–48.
51. Inouye SK, Charpentier PA. Precipitating factors for delirium in hospitalized elderly persons. Predictive model and interrelationship with baseline vulnerability. JAMA. 1996;275(11):852–7.
52. Scott IA, Hilmer SN, Reeve E, Potter K, Le Couteur D, Rigby D, Gnjidic D, Del Mar CB, Roughead EE, Page A, et al. Reducing inappropriate polypharmacy: the process of deprescribing. JAMA Intern Med. 2015;175(5):827–34.

53. Girard TD, Exline MC, Carson SS, Hough CL, Rock P, Gong MN, Douglas IS, Malhotra A, Owens RL, Feinstein DJ, et al. Haloperidol and ziprasidone for treatment of delirium in critical illness. N Engl J Med. 2018;379(26):2506–16.
54. Andersen-Ranberg NC, Poulsen LM, Perner A, Wetterslev J, Estrup S, Hastbacka J, Morgan M, Citerio G, Caballero J, Lange T, et al. Haloperidol for the treatment of delirium in ICU patients. N Engl J Med. 2022;387(26):2425–35.
55. Tomichek JE, Stollings JL, Pandharipande PP, Chandrasekhar R, Ely EW, Girard TD. Antipsychotic prescribing patterns during and after critical illness: a prospective cohort study. Crit Care. 2016;20(1):378.
56. Kram BL, Kram SJ, Brooks KR. Implications of atypical antipsychotic prescribing in the intensive care unit. J Crit Care. 2015;30(4):814–8.
57. Jasiak KD, Middleton EA, Camamo JM, Erstad BL, Snyder LS, Huckleberry YC. Evaluation of discontinuation of atypical antipsychotics prescribed for ICU delirium. J Pharm Pract. 2013;26(3):253–6.
58. Flurie RW, Gonzales JP, Tata AL, Millstein LS, Gulati M. Hospital delirium treatment: continuation of antipsychotic therapy from the intensive care unit to discharge. Am J Health Syst Pharm. 2015;72(23 Suppl. 3):S133–9.
59. Rowe AS, Hamilton LA, Curtis RA, Davis CR, Smith LN, Peek GK, Reynolds VW. Risk factors for discharge on a new antipsychotic medication after admission to an intensive care unit. J Crit Care. 2015;30(6):1283–6.
60. D'Angelo RG, Rincavage M, Tata AL, Millstein LS, Gulati MS, Flurie RW, Gonzales JP. Impact of an antipsychotic discontinuation bundle during transitions of care in critically ill patients. J Intensive Care Med. 2019;34(1):40–7.
61. Zhang Y, Wilkins JM, Bessette LG, York C, Wong V, Lin KJ. Antipsychotic medication use among older adults following infection-related hospitalization. JAMA Netw Open. 2023;6(2):e230063.
62. Glassman AH, Bigger JT. Antipsychotic drugs: prolonged QTc interval, torsade de pointes, and sudded death. Am J Psychiatry. 2001;158:1774–84.
63. Gill SS, Bronskill SE, Normand SLT, Anderson GM, Sykora K, Lam K, Bell CM, Lee PE, Fischer HD, Herrmann N, et al. Antipsychotic drug use and mortality in older adults with dementia. Ann Intern Med. 2007;146(11):775–86.
64. Burry LD, Bell CM, Hill A, Pinto R, Scales DC, Bronskill SE, Williamson D, Rose L, Fu L, Fowler R, et al. New and persistent sedative prescriptions among older adults following a critical illness: a population-based cohort study. Chest. 2023;163(6):1425–36.
65. Tasaka CL, Burg C, VanOsdol SJ, Bekeart L, Anglemyer A, Tsourounis C, Rennke S. An interprofessional approach to reducing the overutilization of stress ulcer prophylaxis in adult medical and surgical intensive care units. Ann Pharmacother. 2014;48(4):462–9.
66. Murphy CE, Stevens AM, Ferrentino N, Crookes BA, Hebert JC, Freiburg CB, Rebuck JA. Frequency of inappropriate continuation of acid suppressive therapy after discharge in patients who began therapy in the surgical intensive care unit. Pharmacotherapy. 2008;28(8):968–76.
67. Pavlov A, Muravyev R, Amoateng-Adjepong Y, Manthous CA. Inappropriate discharge on bronchodilators and acid-blocking medications after ICU admission: importance of medication reconciliation. Respir Care. 2014;59(10):1524–9.
68. Shin S. Evaluation of costs accrued through inadvertent continuation of hospital-initiated proton pump inhibitor therapy for stress ulcer prophylaxis beyond hospital discharge: a retrospective chart review. Ther Clin Risk Manag. 2015;11:649–57.
69. Gomm W, von Holt K, Thome F, Broich K, Maier W, Fink A, Doblhammer G, Haenisch B. Association of proton pump inhibitors with risk of dementia: a pharmacoepidemiological claims data analysis. JAMA Neurol. 2016;73(4):410–6.
70. Lazarus B, Chen Y, Wilson FP, Sang Y, Chang AR, Coresh J, Grams ME. Proton pump inhibitor use and the risk of chronic kidney disease. JAMA Intern Med. 2016;176(2):238–46.

71. Miano TA, Reichert MG, Houle TT, MacGregor DA, Kincaid EH, Bowton DL. Nosocomial pneumonia risk and stress ulcer prophylaxis: a comparison of pantoprazole vs ranitidine in cardiothoracic surgery patients. Chest. 2009;136(2):440–7.
72. Khalili H, Huang ES, Jacobson BC, Camargo CA Jr, Feskanich D, Chan AT. Use of proton pump inhibitors and risk of hip fracture in relation to dietary and lifestyle factors: a prospective cohort study. Br Med J. 2012;344:e372.
73. Barletta JF, Sclar DA. Proton pump inhibitors increase the risk for hospital-acquired Clostridium difficile infection in critically ill patients. Crit Care. 2014;18(6):714.
74. Kouladjian L, Gnjidic D, Reeve E, Chen TF, Hilmer SN. Health care practitioners' perspectives on deprescribing anticholinergic and sedative medications in older adults. Ann Pharmacother. 2016;50(8):625–36.
75. Morandi A, Vasilevskis EE, Pandharipand PP, Girard TD, Solberg LM, Neal EB, Koestner T, Torres RE, Thompson JL, Shintani AK, et al. Inappropriate medications in elderly ICU survivors: where to intervene? Arch Intern Med. 2011., In press;171:1032.
76. Bell CM, Brener SS, Gunraj N, Huo C, Bierman AS, Scales DC, Bajcar J, Zwarenstein M, Urbach DR. Association of ICU or hospital admission with unintentional discontinuation of medications for chronic diseases. JAMA. 2011;306(8):840–7.
77. Forster AJ, Clark HD, Menard A, Dupuis N, Chernish R, Chandok N. Adverse events among medical patients after discharge from hospital (vol 170, p. 345, 2004). Can Med Assoc J. 2004;70(5):771.
78. Forster AJ, Murff HJ, Peterson JF, Gandhi TK, Bates DW. The incidence and severity of adverse events affecting patients after discharge from the hospital. Ann Intern Med. 2003;138(3):161–7.
79. Pirmohamed M, James S, Meakin S, Green C. Adverse drug reactions as cause of admission to hospital—admissions to ear, nose, and throat departments were not mentioned-Reply. Br Med J. 2004;329(7463):460.
80. Jack BW, Chetty VK, Anthony D, Greenwald JL, Sanchez GM, Johnson AE, Forsythe SR, O'Donnell JK, Paasche-Orlow MK, Manasseh C, et al. A reengineered hospital discharge program to decrease rehospitalization: a randomized trial. Ann Intern Med. 2009;150(3):178–87.
81. Jencks SF, Williams MV, Coleman EA. Rehospitalizations among patients in the medicare fee-for-service program REPLY. N Engl J Med. 2009;361(3):312.
82. Friedman B, Basu J. The rate and cost of hospital readmissions for preventable conditions. Med Care Res Rev. 2004;61(2):225–40.
83. Raschetti R, Morgutti M, Menniti-Ippolito F, Belisari A, Rossignoli A, Longhini P, La Guidara C. Suspected adverse drug events requiring emergency department visits or hospital admissions. Eur J Clin Pharmacol. 1999;54(12):959–63.
84. Kripalani S, Jackson AT, Schnipper JL, Coleman EA. Promoting effective transitions of care at hospital discharge: a review of key issues for hospitalists. J Hosp Med. 2007;2(5):314–23.
85. Kerzman H, Baron-Epel O, Toren O. What do discharged patients know about their medication? Patient Educ Couns. 2005;56(3):276–82.
86. Chinthammit C, Armstrong EP, Warholak TL. A cost-effectiveness evaluation of hospital discharge counseling by pharmacists. J Pharmacy Pract. 2012;25(2):201–8.
87. Sarangarm P, London MS, Snowden SS, Dilworth TJ, Koselke LR, Sanchez CO, D'Angio R, Ray G. Impact of pharmacist discharge medication therapy counseling and disease state education: pharmacist assisting at routine medical discharge (project PhARMD). Am J Med Qual. 2013;28(4):292–300.
88. Al-Rashed SA, Wright DJ, Roebuck N, Sunter W, Chrystyn H. The value of inpatient pharmaceutical counselling to elderly patients prior to discharge. Br J Clin Pharmacol. 2002;54(6):657–64.
89. Kilcup M, Schultz D, Carlson J, Wilson B. Postdischarge pharmacist medication reconciliation: impact on readmission rates and financial savings. J Am Pharm Assoc. 2013;53(1):78–84.

90. Walker PC, Bernstein SJ, Jones JN, Piersma J, Kim HW, Regal RE, Kuhn L, Flanders SA. Impact of a pharmacist-facilitated hospital discharge program: a quasi-experimental study. Arch Intern Med. 2009;169(21):2003–10.
91. Holland R, Desborough J, Goodyer L, Hall S, Wright D, Loke YK. Does pharmacist-led medication review help to reduce hospital admissions and deaths in older people? A systematic review and meta-analysis. Br J Clin Pharmacol. 2008;65(3):303–16.
92. Wooldridge K, Schnipper JL, Goggins K, Dittus RS, Kripalani S. Refractory primary medication nonadherence: prevalence and predictors after pharmacist counseling at hospital discharge. J Hosp Med. 2016;11(1):48–51.
93. Manias E, Bucknall T, Hughes C, Jorm C, Woodward-Kron R. Family involvement in managing medications of older patients across transitions of care: a systematic review. BMC Geriatr. 2019;19(1):95.
94. Stollings JL, Bloom SL, Wang L, Ely EW, Jackson JC, Sevin CM. Critical care pharmacists and medication management in an ICU recovery center. Ann Pharmacother. 2018;52(8):713–23.
95. MacTavish P, Quasim T, Shaw M, Devine H, Daniel M, Kinsella J, Fenelon C, Kishore R, Iwashyna TJ, McPeake J. Impact of a pharmacist intervention at an intensive care rehabilitation clinic. BMJ Open Qual. 2019;8(3):e000580.
96. MacTavish P, Quasim T, Purdie C, Ball M, Barker L, Connelly S, Devine H, Henderson P, Hogg LA, Kishore R, et al. Medication-related problems in intensive care unit survivors. Learning from a multicenter program. Ann Am Thorac Soc. 2020;17(10):1326–9.
97. Bottom-Tanzer SF, Poyant JO, Louzada MT, Ahmed SE, Boudouvas A, Poon E, Hojman HM, Bugaev N, Johnson BP, Van Kirk AL, et al. High occurrence of postintensive care syndrome identified in surgical ICU survivors after implementation of a multidisciplinary clinic. J Trauma Acute Care Surg. 2021;91(2):406–12.
98. MacTavish P, McPeake J, Breslin A, Forrest R, Kishore R, MacGregor F, Oprey A, Quasim T, Shaw M. Evaluation of medication changes following severe COVID-19 infection: a multicentre evaluation. BMJ Open Respir Res. 2021;8(1)
99. Mohammad RA, Eze C, Marshall VD, Coe AB, Costa DK, Thompson A, Pitcher M, Haezebrouck E, McSparron JI. The impact of a clinical pharmacist in an interprofessional intensive care unit recovery clinic providing care to intensive care unit survivors. J Am Coll Clin Pharm. 2022;5(10):1027–38.
100. Stollings JL, Poyant JO, Groth CM, Rappaport SH, Kruer RM, Miller E, Whitten JA, McIntire AM, McDaniel CM, Betthauser KD, et al. An international, multicenter evaluation of comprehensive medication management by pharmacists in ICU recovery centers. J Intensive Care Med. 2023;8850666231176194:957.

Chapter 21
Engaging Families in Rehabilitation for The Critically Ill

Kimberley Haines, Lauren Phillips, and Andrea Marshall

Introduction—Toward More Compassionate Care

Family members are increasingly recognized as valued members of the healthcare team [1–4]. This can help to ensure the delivery of person-centered care that values, respects, and incorporates family participation and presence to benefit the patient. The benefit to the patient is quality individualized care through the maintenance of the important psychological and advocacy roles that families provide. This spectrum of participation should be guided by the patients' preferences and ability of staff to provide the necessary support to the family, as well as consideration of pre-existing relationships of the patient with different family members.

This principle of engaging families can be applied to rehabilitation across transitions of care from the intensive care unit (ICU) to home, under the premise of—"*invite, educate and support*" [5]. Approaches to engaging families in rehabilitation of the critically ill can be informed by a conceptual framework describing the tenets of family-centered care [6]: "Families are considered experts in what helps and hurts them, are indispensable, invaluable partners for policy-makers, professionals and advocates, are not called or treated as dependent but should be considered as equals with whom to collaborate and empower. Family-centred policies and

K. Haines (✉)
Department of Critical Care, Melbourne Medical School, The University of Melbourne, Melbourne, VIC, Australia
e-mail: Kimberley.Haines@wh.org.au

L. Phillips
Physiotherapy Department, Western Health, Melbourne, VIC, Australia

A. Marshall
Menzies Health Institute and School of Nursing and Midwifery, Griffith University, Gold Coast Campus, Southport, QLD, Australia

Intensive Care Unit, Gold Coast University Hospital, Southport, QLD, Australia

© The Author(s), under exclusive license to Springer Nature Switzerland AG 2025
A. J. Vance et al. (eds.), *Families in the Intensive Care Unit*,
https://doi.org/10.1007/978-3-031-83786-9_21

practices promote peer and community-based systems of care and mutual support, democratization and gender equity."

Previously, critical care rehabilitation trials were designed from the perspective of health professionals; interventions were applied *to* the patient [7–9]. Patients and families were overlooked in design and implementation; however, families are an under-utilized resource. Increasingly, we recognize the need to design interventions *with* ICU patients and their families—at much higher levels of engagement than before [10]. Our hypothesis is that greater partnership will result in improved outcomes for both patients and families, although this requires testing. As we begin this process, research is needed to better understand and refine the following concepts of family engagement in rehabilitation, specifically in the following areas:

1. What types of rehabilitative activities do patients want for their families to support them, and what activities do families want to participate in—within the acute (ICU, general hospital wards) and subacute (rehabilitation wards, community care) settings and how can we best support them?
2. Are family and patient outcomes improved following critical illness, with the addition of family engagement in rehabilitation?
3. What are the potential barriers and facilitators to implementing family involvement in rehabilitation in clinical care and in research?

Implementing engagement strategies via a blanket approach should not be the goal but, rather, creating a culture where patients and families can have control and decisional input to individualize their own care [4]. Orchestrating opportunities where families are, with patient consent, invited to be involved in an active role, may address shared emotional needs between family and patient, and invest in the long-term outcomes and recovery trajectories for both. These complexities and challenges may be made worse during times of illness and stress (and the converse may be true). It should be highlighted that there are practical challenges to obtaining consent of the patient whilst critically ill, and the risk of coercion which needs to be managed carefully. Consent from the patient to have their families involved in their care should be sought at the earliest and most appropriate time in the patient's recovery. Attention should also be paid to cultural and religious considerations, family dynamics, and which family member(s) might be most appropriate to engage. Ascertaining this information is likely to be best sought via the next of kin and/or decision-maker, nursing, and medical staff.

Few studies engaging families in rehabilitation for patients exist within and/or beyond the ICU to describe the "what, why, when and how" this could be effective. As a result, this chapter draws on existing research and theories describing family participation, and how this might be applied and integrated within rehabilitation of the critically ill. As in all clinical care, suggestions made within this chapter should be considered in the context of whether they are likely to benefit any specific patient's recovery.

Transitions of Care and Rehabilitation

The ICU is only one point on the patient and family journey, in which the burden of critical illness extends from pre-ICU through to the post-hospital phase [11]. Across this spectrum of care, the question has been rightly posed—*"who is visiting whom?"* recognizing that we as healthcare providers may simply be visitors in the lives of patients and families, and not the other way around [4]. Given that families are often the primary caregivers to the patient (or the patient may be the caregiver/decision-maker) prior to and following hospitalization, effort should be made to ensure this role is not made redundant within the ICU setting. It is also important to be inclusive of families who may not have been in a primary caregiver role to the patient if the patient did not require caregiving support pre-morbidly. Where possible, families should be empowered to maintain their role across the transitions of care (Fig. 21.1). While this may be the aspirational goal of engagement, barriers exist such as the power differential in the clinician and family relationship, and routines are often designed to suit clinicians and not families. Furthermore, early on in critical illness, families may be unable to engage due to the cognitive and emotional load and stressors of having a critically ill family member. As the patient recovers (as the risk of dying potentially decreases), families may be in attendance less at the bedside, as they begin to resume other aspects of their family role such as caring for children and returning to employment. While the nature of the tasks in which families can engage families will change as the patient acuity changes (Fig. 21.1), regular opportunities should be given to facilitate participation as the patient and family wish.

Rehabilitation has been defined by the World Health Organization as an enablement process to attain "*optimal physical, sensory, intellectual, psychological and social functional levels*" [12]. The fundamental goal of rehabilitation is to achieve participation meaningful to the individual. Family is integral in this process. Families can serve as patient advocates and an important conduit with the clinical team to provide information on the patient's premorbid health status as well as their

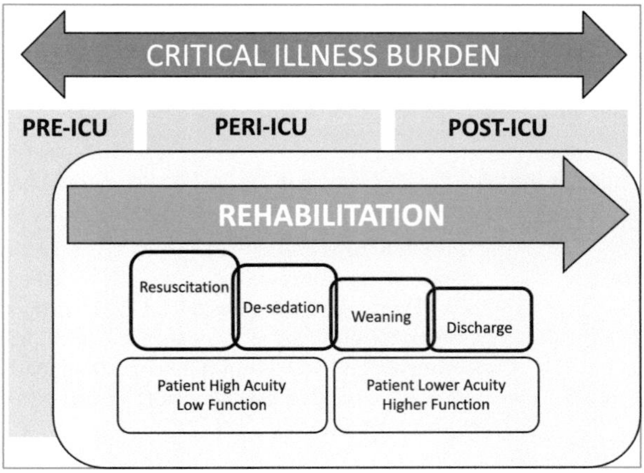

Fig. 21.1 Transitions of care and rehabilitation In ICU

hobbies and interests. Families can also be involved in activities at the bedside to provide physical assistance and encourage and motivation to participate in rehabilitation. These concepts are captured within the International Classification of Functioning, Disability and Health (ICF) [13, 14]. Used extensively in rehabilitation settings, this model of disability categorizes the disability of acute illness into categories: damage to body structures, limitations in activity, restriction in social roles, and health-related quality of life [13]. The ICF illustrates interrelating steps culminating in varying levels of disablement and considers the effect other modifiers may have on patient recovery such as social environment and caregiver support [15]. The functional limitations patients experience following critical illness can become restrictions dependent on their social infrastructure [13]. It is therefore crucial that families are integrated early within the rehabilitation process—if this is what the patient and family want (recognizing that there may be many families who do not want to engage in this way). There are three overarching concepts for integrating families within the rehabilitation process:

1. Benefit to the family—channeling psychological distress into a purposeful active role.
2. Benefit to the patient—humanizing the illness and recovery experience through provision of emotional support, maintenance of patient identity, social structures, and connectedness to the outside world.
3. Benefit to staff and health system—partnering with families as a supporting resource to deliver therapeutic interventions outside of constrained therapy time.

The provision of rehabilitation within and beyond the ICU is often led and largely underpinned by the allied health professions. Allied health represents the third pillar of healthcare that complements medicine and nursing [16]. Allied health professionals have diagnostic and therapeutic skills with a particular focus on provision of therapy to restore function, participation, and community reintegration. Table 21.1 depicts various allied health therapeutic roles and potential for engagement of families in rehabilitative activities particular to their profession.

Table 21.1 Allied health professions, therapeutic roles, and rehabilitation

Allied health profession	Therapeutic role	Types of rehabilitative activities families could be engaged in related to each professional group
Physical therapy	Multi-system assessment of respiratory, cardiovascular, neurological, and musculoskeletal systems to formulate individualized treatment plans and use of functional activities to rehabilitate and restore physical condition [17, 18]	Assistance with activities of daily living, in bed exercises/activities (e.g., bridging, rolling), out-of-bed exercises (e.g., sit to stand, walking), other physically therapeutic activities such as stretching and massage

(continued)

Table 21.1 (continued)

Allied health profession	Therapeutic role	Types of rehabilitative activities families could be engaged in related to each professional group
Occupational therapy	Facilitation of task performance by improving relevant performing skills or developing and teaching compensatory strategies to overcome lost performance skills [19, 20]	A recent systematic review has described the future role of the ICU occupational therapy role to include: Participation in self-care activities, cognitive interventions, psychologic interventions to reduce depression and anxiety, modifying physical and social environment [20]. This might include assisting with activities of daily living and self-care, cognitive stimulation, and use of adaptive devices (e.g., helping patients assistance with activities of daily living, helping the patient to use adaptive utensils at meal times, using wheelchairs, assisting with appropriate levels of cognitive stimulation and engagement such as reading newspaper, playing cards) [20]
Speech-language therapy	Assessment and management of communication, swallowing difficulties, and tracheostomy weaning [21] through rehabilitation, goals, programs, equipment, and advice to optimize and maintain function [22–24]	Assistance with communication devices to facilitate/augment communication [22, 24] (e.g., helping patient to use a communication board or app). Being aware of swallowing difficulties and preparation of suitable food and fluid consistencies following discharge from hospital
Dietetics	Assessment of nutritional status and provision of nutrition support and counseling to optimize nutrition and support health-promoting behaviors [25–27]. Dieticians may also provide advice to the multi-professional team on the optimal way to manage the nutritional needs of all critically ill patients	Physically assisting the patient at meal times to help them eat and encouraging them to consume oral nutrition supplements to meet their nutritional requirements [28] or bringing preferred food from home to do this
Psychology	Diagnosis and treatment of mental and behavioral health problems to enhance health-promoting behaviors, treatment adherence and functional ability [29]	Assisting patient to use a mindfulness app or helping them practice other psychological support techniques such as resilience and coping. Advocating for patients to be able to participate in activities that support their psychological Well-being such as going outside, listening to music, bringing their pet in to visit or engaging in animal-assisted therapy [30]
Social work	Psychosocial support and counseling as well as crisis intervention, psychosocial assessment, facilitation of communication, end-of-life care, and practical assistance [31]	Assisting and maintaining patient engagement with outside world and their social networks (e.g., bringing in photos and news or correspondences from family and friends)

[a]Also known as physiotherapy in Australia, UK, South Africa, Europe, New Zealand, and other countries [32]

Engaging Families at the Bedside in ICU

As critical care clinicians, we must recognize that families are potentially in crisis. We have a significant opportunity to lessen that distress. We need to focus our efforts of care not only on the patient in the bed but those at the bedside, as the two are inextricably linked. Treating one without consideration of the other may be ineffective and in some cases detrimental.

The theoretical context underpinning the engagement of families in rehabilitation in the ICU is supported by the theory of facilitated sense-making. This theory recognizes the value of an active role for family members where clinicians help them make sense of what they are experiencing through an iterative process as the patient condition changes [17]. This process of practically engaging families in rehabilitation can help them make sense of what is happening and gives meaning to their new and changing role [17]. All health professionals play an important part in supporting and facilitating family engagement in the ICU—it is no single profession's responsibility and the team must work together to support this practice. Allied health professionals are well positioned to support family engagement in rehabilitation. Nurses have the greatest contact time with families and will be able to assess family readiness for engagement and support engagement across a range of different activities. Intensive care physicians and other medical professionals can support and encourage families to partner with health professionals in supporting rehabilitation activities.

With this in mind, there may be many practical low-cost, high-value rehabilitative activities in which to engage families. If a patient is acutely unwell, this should not preclude family engagement in rehabilitative activities but, rather, an adaptive approach can be taken. Some examples of rehabilitative activities families may want to participate are provided in Fig. 21.2, focused on assisting patients with activities of daily living. By encouraging and supporting families to help the patient carry out these tasks they are engaging in rehabilitation and restoration of function and participation. For example, physical therapists might be responsible for supporting families to do exercises, speech-language therapists might set up a communication board, and occupational therapists might devise cognitive engagement exercises and teach families how to engage the patient to use these strategies (Fig. 21.2). However, these activities are not exclusive to a particular professional group and should be shared amongst the team.

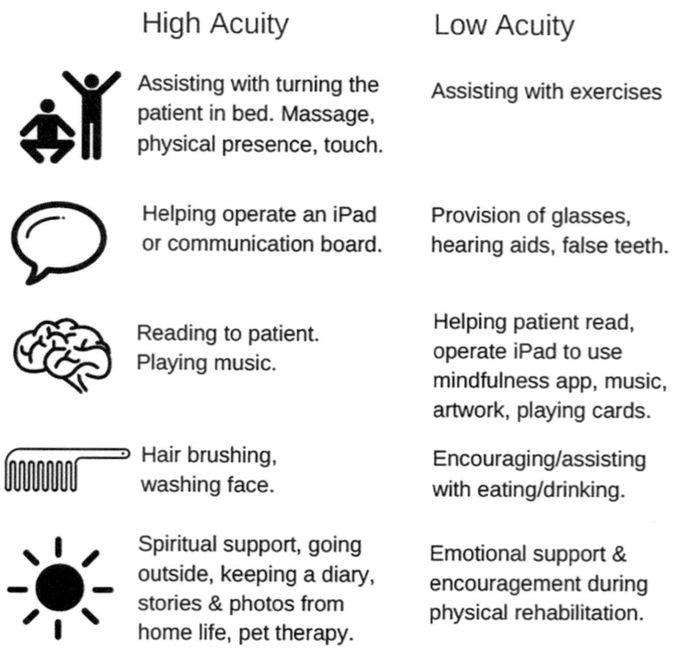

Fig. 21.2 Types of rehabilitative activities to invite family participation

A Spectrum of Participation

A spectrum of engagement by families in rehabilitation and care tasks may be influenced by gender, social, cultural, and religious factors. At one end of the spectrum, families may feel more comfortable to simply maintain their role as a family member where participation at the bedside may be defined by companionship, emotional support, and reassurance, with therapeutic benefit to both. At the other end of the spectrum, some families may wish to be consistently and very involved in care and rehabilitation.

This spectrum is particularly important to consider within the context of diversity within families. For example, differences in caregiver roles (spouse, sibling, parent), trans-generational, single-parent, and "blended" families [18], "families of origin" and "families of choice" which may be relevant to people who identify as LGBTQI [19], cultural differences where the entire family unit expect to be involved in care, those from migrant or asylum family roles where they may be under additional duress external to ICU as well as other possible circumstances. It is essential to consider the healthcare needs of caregivers from all backgrounds. To achieve equity and not just equality, we must ensure that we better understand the unique needs of families in order to achieve optimal outcomes as a result of our care. Some suggested strategies are listed in Box 21.1.

Box 21.1 Strategies for Supporting and Engaging Families

1. Spend time getting to know the caregiver to establish their needs and preferences. Some potential questions to do this might include:
   What's important to you as a caregiver?
   Who's important to you as a caregiver?
   What are your preferences for how we communicate with you?
   What aspects of care do you expect to be involved in or would like to be involved in?
   How do you think you can best support your loved one's rehabilitation?
   What do you need from us to help you during this time? Is there anything you would like us to do differently?
2. With consent of caregiver, communicate a summary of these preferences to rest of team (via medical records or whiteboard in bed space) to avoid duplication so knowledge can be built upon.
3. Be aware of own subconscious biases. Avoid assumptions based on appearance.

Importantly, wherever families (and patients) are on this participation spectrum, their involvement should be supported by an environment and systems. This allows the individuals, in partnership with staff, to tailor their participation and integration with patient care.

What Is the Evidence?

There are very few studies currently describing family engagement in rehabilitation of the critically ill, instead much of the literature describes involvement in bedside care (which may incorporate aspects of rehabilitation). Table 21.2 outlines key findings where families have been engaged or participated in rehabilitation or other aspects of care. These are presented from the perspective of clinicians, families, and patients.

Overall, Table 21.2 shows the majority of staff, families, and patients were supportive of family participation in a range of care activities, many of which could be classified as rehabilitative. However, in practice, very few families actually participated in the care of the patient. This suggests that while beliefs and attitudes may be positive toward participation, implementation strategies may be required to facilitate the engagement of families in care and rehabilitative activities.

Table 21.2 Engagement of families in bedside care

Study	Sample size	Design	Key findings
Felten-Barentsz et al. (2021) [20]	10 family members	Qualitative	**Families:** Believed that physical activity in the ICU improves recovery. Participating in this activity decreased feelings of powerlessness and uselessness
Van Delft et al. (2021) [21]	18 articles	Review	**Patients:** 77% of patients favored participation of their family in care **Families:** 85–97% of family members were willing to participate **Staff:** 96% of staff agreed with the concept of involving families in physical care
Willigen et al. (2020) [22]	5 former ICU patients and 5 family members	Qualitative	There was agreement across participants that physical rehabilitation should be started as soon as possible after admission to ICU and exhaustion was highlighted as the biggest challenge to participation. In addition to aiding physical recovery, physical rehabilitation in the ICU may also provide psychological support for both patients and relatives
Sottile et al. (2015) [23]	55 former ICU patients and 49 family members	RCT	**Patients:** Reported that PT was both extremely necessary and beneficial. Patients reported moderate degrees of difficulty and exertion associated with PT sessions. Overall, patients were extremely satisfied with their PT experience **Families:** Reported that PT was both extremely necessary and beneficial. Family members perceived PT as being moderately difficult and causing moderate discomfort to the patient. Overall, family members were extremely satisfied with the PT experience
Blom et al. (2013) [24]	7 family members	Qualitative	**Families**: Being allowed to participate in patient care was important with four components: 1. Participation in care and being close to the patient—"being there" as well as "doing." 2. Confidence in the care the patient receives 3. Support needed for involvement in caregiving 4. Vulnerability—An atmosphere needs to be created that supports and invites families to participate
Rukstele et al. (2013) [5]	N/A	Review	Adoption of a philosophical approach and establishing a foundation for patient and family-centered care (steering committee created, staff education, open visiting, addressing myths/fears). Engaging families in mobilization through—*invite* (welcome pack), *educate* (brochure on implications of immobility, demonstrate task, provision of written instructions, determine what role meets patient and family needs), *support* (encourage families to bring items from home, engage patient in outside world)

(continued)

Table 21.2 (continued)

Study	Sample size	Design	Key findings
Garrouste-Orgeas et al. 2010 [25]	101 patient-family pairs	Observational	**Staff**: The majority of physicians and nurses were favorable to family participation in a range of care tasks (washing/cleaning, transfers, massage to prevent pressure injuries)
			Families: 97% were willing to participate and were favorable to a range of 13 care tasks. Only 14% participated in care spontaneously. 58% and 26% had symptoms of anxiety and depression, respectively. There was a nonsignificant relationship between symptoms and willingness to participate
			Patients: Of the 44/101 who were able to complete the retrospective phone interview, 77% were favorable to their families participating in care. Of the remaining proportion who did not want care from their families, reasons included: Desire to preserve image, unwillingness to be assisted, embarrassment, nurses better-skilled, physical modesty
Azoulay et al. (2003) [26]	2754 staff 544 families	Observational	**Staff**: 88% felt participation in care (e.g., feeding, bathing, tracheal suctioning) should be offered to families. Only 60% of these had involved family in care. Of the staff who felt families should not participate, 66% believed that it might contribute to family suffering
			Families: 33% wanted to participate. Predictors of desire were related to patient severity of illness on admission, ICU LOS, family factors (age, not of European descent, previous experience of ICU in the family, emotional burden and effectiveness of information, more time wanted for information). Most common reason for not wanting to participate was staff did their job perfectly (85%). Families may not have understood what participation in care meant and potential benefits
Hammond et al. (1995) [27]	27 nurses 20 families	Mixed methods	**Staff**: 96% agreed with concept of involving families in physical care. Major theme: There were problems of role adaptation for nurses and families involved and building relationships **Families**: 85% wanted to be involved in physical care of the patient, 15% did not. Major theme: Adapting to the demanding ICU environment and identifying boundaries of their new role as caregiver

How Might We Practically Do This?

Adopting an approach to family engagement in rehabilitation requires a philosophical and paradigmatic shift toward embracing true family-centered care that is facilitated by leadership, teamwork, patience and compassion. In the ICU, we need to borrow more from models of rehabilitative care where families are viewed as integral to the recovery process. In stroke rehabilitation, for example, families would be regularly involved in interprofessional team meetings to set goals, understand more about patient needs/preferences and plan for return home. The concept of a 24-h model of rehabilitation in subacute settings is one idea to actively promote rehabilitation around the clock to engage all members of the team to approach care in this way and reduce inactivity common on hospital wards. Families are viewed as an essential part of this philosophy of care where they may be able to continue the patient's exercises with them and help them with eating or cognitive tasks outside of the relatively short periods of therapy time.

To adopt such an approach in the ICU may require a cultural shift in practice away from what is easiest for the clinicians, to what is best for the patient and their family and how we can create opportunities throughout the 24-hour period that are based on patient goals (The difficulty of this cultural shift should neither be understated, nor overstated, as it is already underway in many ICUs). For example, it may be easiest and take less time to turn a patient in bed where staff do most of the activity compared to setting up the environment, using verbal and physical prompts to facilitate the patient to complete the task. Prompting and supporting the patient may take more time, but will have greater rehabilitative benefit. To then go a step further to engage the families in this sort of care may require even more time and skill from the staff, but again may have rehabilitative benefit to the family. Over time, attitudes from staff toward families may change from that of hindrance to help.

Other strategies might include the early adoption of joint goal setting between the patient, family, and interprofessional team. This might take the form of an interprofessional team ward round (medical, nursing, and allied health) for complex, long-stay ICU patients, where families are welcomed in this process. Allied health professionals often receive training in how to set rehabilitative goals with patients and families and can serve as an important resource in the healthcare team by actively leading and role modeling these discussions. A key question often asked by allied health professionals when establishing therapeutic alliance is: "what matters to you?" [20] These can help define short-, medium-, and long-term rehabilitation goals which can be captured as a daily care plan and made visible on whiteboards at the bedside to help remind all those caring for the patient and avoid daily reinvention when staff members change. Example headings that could be used on a whiteboard at a patient's bedside to display their care plan might include:

1. My goals are….
2. People important to me are….
3. I communicate by….
4. I would like to know….

Table 21.3 Practical strategies and considerations to support family engagement

Target group	Strategy
Staff	A systems-based approach may help support the partnership between staff and families. Strategies might include prompts in electronic medical records or nursing care plans reminding staff to invite families to participate, structuring of ward rounds to engage with families, operationalizing family-centered care in guidelines and policies, education for staff about how to engage and coach families as partners and better understanding regarding the role of family as advocate [30]
Patient	Preferences and goals are clear, accessible to the patient, and documented goal-driven care plan. Being aware of those patients who are more likely to be alone without family support and considering other ways their rehabilitation could be supported such as engaging therapy assistants and volunteers
Family	Written or verbal information provided in the waiting room and at the bedside about participating in patient care that gives direction about the types of tasks families can do to help the patient's recovery, education about standard steps and milestones of recovery, how to participate as well as facilitate (e.g., some tasks may appear difficult for the patient to undertake but there may will be therapeutic benefit to them completing rather than family doing it for them), understanding the partnership with staff, facilitating accessibility to the patient (e.g., open visiting hours)

5. From home I need….
6. My expected date of discharge is….
7. My planned discharge destination is….

Families can also be easily involved in clinician handover at the bedside as they can provide the nuances of care that may not otherwise be handed over about the patients' preferences. Families remain the constant advocate for the patient and if we engage them in this way we recognize them as expert members of the team, which may help us, be more effective and efficient as clinicians through the creation of therapeutic alliance. Furthermore, it may help therapists provide more patient-centered care, as families know what is most important to patients. Table 21.3 displays some practical strategies to support the implementation of family engagement. In addition, many useful "work tools" to support the implementation of the Society of Critical Care Medicine's Family-Centered Care Guidelines are available [21].

Thinking Beyond ICU

It is important we consider how to prepare families in their ongoing journey beyond the ICU. Many families and patients report challenges when transitioning from the high monitored environment of the ICU to the general wards [22] and from the wards to home. Strategies to improve these transitions of care could be achieved through:

- Meeting informational needs –written or verbal communication about what to expect when leaving ICU or hospital that addresses patient factors, family factors, health system factors, and how to access ongoing support.
- In some cases, introducing the patient and family to the ward environment and staff prior to discharge from ICU (e.g., long-ICU stay, highly complex). This might also include allied health clinician handover between the ICU and ward with involvement of the patient and family. This may help to alleviate anxiety and carry forward important aspects of clinical care to ensure rehabilitative gains are not lost and goals reaffirmed. While this may not always be practical (even though we can transport the sickest of ICU patients for procedures), it requires a shift in thinking about what is important and when and re-arranging resources to be more patient and family-centered wherever possible.

Beyond hospital discharge, families often go on to support patients in their struggle to achieve functional independence by assisting them physically, psychologically, and socially [23]. This can impact the psychosocial outcomes of families [24]. This role-shift for spouses has been described as a "*dynamic process initially triggered by the critical illness incident and later influenced by the patient's gradual recovery*," involving four elements [23]: committing to caregiving, acquiring caregiving skills, negotiating level of caregiver, and gradually leaving the caregiving role. This study is particularly useful as it provides insights to the challenges faced by families in the post-ICU phase of recovery. The authors suggest the findings can inform clinicians' efforts in preparing families of what to expect following hospitalization and the development of targeted supportive interventions delivered by either the primary or secondary healthcare sector.

Allied health professionals and other rehabilitation specialists play an important role in facilitating this transition from hospital to home. To empower families and support the transition out of hospital, common strategies include:

- Regular involvement of families in patient goal setting on admission and throughout the subacute stay.
- Regular family meetings with the healthcare team to discuss questions or concerns. Families are provided with updates on patient progress from the various professional and discussion of the estimated discharge date and destination occurs.
- Involvement in caregiver training sessions and education with allied health professionals about how to use specialist equipment, how to assist the patient with activities of daily living or ongoing physical rehabilitation tasks, how to meet dietary and communication or swallowing requirements. This ensures families are safely and confidently able to meet the patient care needs post-discharge.
- Involvement in trial of care sessions for more complex discharges. Families are invited and encouraged to stay with the patient for a 24-hour period on the ward to receive additional education and exposure to the patient's care requirements while remaining in a supported and safe environment. This often serves the purpose of informing the team and ongoing decision-making about whether the patient and family are likely to cope post-discharge.

- Meeting informational needs about Post-Intensive Care Syndrome (showing them the Society of Critical Care Medicine's Thrive resources), what to expect following discharge and where to go for support and help such as in-person or online peer support groups [25].
- Ensuring appropriate referrals to community providers are made so the patient and family are linked in with ongoing support.

Conclusion

There is little evidence to guide our practice in engaging families in rehabilitation of the critically ill. These data are important to generate to help us better understand how family involvement in rehabilitation might modify patient disability and whether families benefit from engagement. In the absence of data, we need to consider how we, as ICU clinicians, can promote a more family-centered environment in the ICU, extending to inclusion of family in rehabilitative activities where appropriate. To empower families in the rehabilitation arc, we need to be open and willing to learn *from* and *with* patients and their families, which may lead to better outcomes.

Acknowledgments We would like to thank Fenella Gill, Marc Nickels, and Laurie Grealish for their review of this second edition.

References

1. Davidson JE, Powers K, Hedayat KM, Tieszen M, Kon AA, Shepard E, et al. Clinical practice guidelines for support of the family in the patient-centered intensive care unit: American College of Critical Care Medicine Task Force 2004–2005. Crit Care Med. 2007;35(2):605–22. https://doi.org/10.1097/01.CCM.0000254067.14607.EB.
2. Beesley SJ, Hopkins RO, Francis L, Chapman D, Johnson J, Johnson N, et al. Let them in: family presence during intensive care unit procedures. Ann Am Thorac Soc. 2016;13(7):1155–9. https://doi.org/10.1513/AnnalsATS.201511-754OI.
3. Cypress BS. Family presence on rounds: a systematic review of literature. Dimens Crit Care Nurs. 2012;31(1):53–64. https://doi.org/10.1097/DCC.0b013e31824246dd.
4. Berwick DM, Kotagal M. Restricted visiting hours in ICUs: time to change. JAMA. 2004;292(6):736–7. https://doi.org/10.1001/jama.292.6.736.
5. Rukstele CD, Gagnon MM. Making strides in preventing ICU-acquired weakness: involving family in early progressive mobility. Crit Care Nurs Q. 2013;36(1):141–7. https://doi.org/10.1097/CNQ.0b013e31827539cc.
6. Briar Lawson K, Lawson H, Hennon C, Jones A. Family-centered policies and practices: international implications. New York: Columbia University Press; 2001.
7. Denehy L, Skinner EH, Edbrooke L, Haines K, Warrillow S, Hawthorne G, et al. Exercise rehabilitation for patients with critical illness: a randomized controlled trial with 12 months of follow-up. Crit Care. 2013;17(4):R156. https://doi.org/10.1186/cc12835.

8. Morris PE, Berry MJ, Files DC, Thompson JC, Hauser J, Flores L, et al. Standardized rehabilitation and hospital length of stay among patients with acute respiratory failure: a randomized clinical trial. JAMA. 2016;315(24):2694–702. https://doi.org/10.1001/jama.2016.7201.
9. Schweickert WD, Pohlman MC, Pohlman AS, Nigos C, Pawlik AJ, Esbrook CL, et al. Early physical and occupational therapy in mechanically ventilated, critically ill patients: a randomised controlled trial. Lancet. 2009;373(9678):1874–82. https://doi.org/10.1016/S0140-6736(09)60658-9.
10. Haines KJ, Kelly P, Fitzgerald P, Skinner EH, Iwashyna TJ. The untapped potential of patient and family engagement in the organization of critical care. Crit Care Med. 2017;45(5):899–906. https://doi.org/10.1097/CCM.0000000000002282.
11. Angus DC, Carlet J, Brussels RP. Surviving intensive care: a report from the 2002 Brussels roundtable. Intensive Care Med. 2003;29(3):368–77. https://doi.org/10.1007/s00134-002-1624-8.
12. World Health Organization: Rehabilitation; 2017. http://www.who.int/topics/rehabilitation/en/. Accessed 11 May, 2017.
13. Iwashyna TJ, Netzer G. The burdens of survivorship: an approach to thinking about long-term outcomes after critical illness. Semin Respir Crit Care Med. 2012;33(4):327–38. https://doi.org/10.1055/s-0032-1321982.
14. World Health Organization. International classification of functioning, disability and health. Geneva, Switzerland: World Health Organization; 2001.
15. Herridge MS, Cameron J. Models of rehabilitative care after critical illness. In: Stevens RD, Hart N, Herridge MS, editors. Textbook of post-ICU medicine. Oxford, UK: Oxford University Press; 2014.
16. Philip K. Allied health: untapped potential in the Australian health system. Aust Health Rev. 2015;39(3):244–7.
17. Davidson JE. Facilitated sensemaking: a strategy and new middle-range theory to support families of intensive care unit patients. Crit Care Nurse. 2010;30(6):28–39. https://doi.org/10.4037/ccn2010410.
18. Shudy M, de Almeida ML, Ly S, Landon C, Groft S, Jenkins TL, et al. Impact of pediatric critical illness and injury on families: a systematic literature review. Pediatrics. 2006;118(Suppl. 3):S203–18. https://doi.org/10.1542/peds.2006-0951B.
19. Hash KAMM. Caregiving in the LGBT community. In: Springer, editor. Annual review of gerontology and geriatrics, vol. 37; 2017. p. 77.
20. Barry MJ, Edgman-Levitan S. Shared decision making--pinnacle of patient-centered care. N Engl J Med. 2012;366(9):780–1. https://doi.org/10.1056/NEJMp1109283.
21. Davidson JE, Aslakson RA, Long AC, Puntillo KA, Kross EK, Hart J, et al. Guidelines for family-centered care in the neonatal, pediatric, and adult ICU. Crit Care Med. 2017;45(1):103–28. https://doi.org/10.1097/CCM.0000000000002169.
22. Bench SD, Day T, Griffiths P. Involving users in the development of effective critical care discharge information: a focus group study. Am J Crit Care. 2011;20(6):443–52. https://doi.org/10.4037/ajcc2011829.
23. Agard AS, Egerod I, Tonnesen E, Lomborg K. From spouse to caregiver and back: a grounded theory study of post-intensive care unit spousal caregiving. J Adv Nurs. 2015;71(8):1892–903. https://doi.org/10.1111/jan.12657.
24. Haines KJ, Denehy L, Skinner EH, Warrillow S, Berney S. Psychosocial outcomes in informal caregivers of the critically ill: a systematic review. Crit Care Med. 2015;43:1112. https://doi.org/10.1097/CCM.0000000000000865.
25. Mikkelsen ME, Jackson JC, Hopkins RO, Thompson C, Andrews A, Netzer G, et al. Peer support as a novel strategy to mitigate post-intensive care syndrome. AACN Adv Crit Care. 2016;27(2):221–9. https://doi.org/10.4037/aacnacc2016667.

Chapter 22
Animal-Assisted Interactions in the ICU

Breanna Hetland and Christina Bach

Introduction

Treatment advancements and improvements in the quality of ICU care have led to a sustained decrease in ICU mortality. However, for more than half of ICU survivors, physical, psychological, and cognitive deficits resulting from an ICU hospitalization persist after the critical illness has resolved [1]. These deficits are known as post-intensive care syndrome (PICS) and include modifiable risk factors such as delirium, decreased mobility, sedation, and an overall negative ICU experience [2]. Unrelieved and distressing symptoms throughout the hospitalization can increase the incidence of PICS and are traumatic for patients and their families. Common symptoms reported by patients in the ICU include fatigue, sleeplessness, anxiety, restlessness, pain, sadness, fear, and confusion [3–5]. Sedative and analgesic medications have historically been given as first-line treatment to lessen the patient's symptom burden, but these medications can lead to poor outcomes. Therefore, critical care clinicians and researchers have increased their focus on nonpharmacological symptom management strategies to reduce the modifiable risk factors associated with PICS and promote a more humanized, patient-centered care environment [6]. Animal-assisted interactions (AAIs) are a means to facilitate the holistic management of patient symptoms, promote overall wellness in the ICU, and improve the ICU experience for patients, families, and staff [6, 7].

The bond between people and animals is a mutually beneficial and dynamic relationship influenced by behaviors essential to health and well-being [8]. The long-term health benefits of animals to the human mind, body, and spirit have been

B. Hetland
University of Nebraska Medical Center College of Nursing, Omaha, NE, USA
e-mail: breanna.hetland@unmc.edu

C. Bach
Baptist Health, Jacksonville, USA

© The Author(s), under exclusive license to Springer Nature Switzerland AG 2025
A. J. Vance et al. (eds.), *Families in the Intensive Care Unit*,
https://doi.org/10.1007/978-3-031-83786-9_22

well-documented for centuries [9]. Specific to healthcare, animal companionship can help mitigate stress, improve wellness, and promote recovery from illness [6, 9]. AAIs have been used in various acute and subacute settings to reduce anxiety, stress, and pain and promote overall engagement in care. However, they have not been widely adopted in the ICU because of heightened concerns regarding patients' severity of illness, technical equipment, and infection risk. Research continues to evolve, but early evidence suggests that the use of AAIs in the ICU is both safe and effective and should be considered for regular use during critical illness to positively benefit patients, family members, and staff [6, 10, 11].

Types of Animal-Assisted Interactions

AAIs describe interventions that intentionally incorporate animals in health, education, and human service for therapeutic purposes to improve health and wellness. Many terms for AAIs are used in the literature, with the two most common being animal-assisted therapies (AATs) and animal-assisted activities (AAAs) [11]. AATs are goal-oriented, structured interventions designed to improve physical, social, emotional, and/or cognitive function [12, 13]. Trained providers work with the animal and its handler to meet specific therapeutic criteria, which are then evaluated as part of the treatment process and documented in the electronic medical record [13, 14]. Alternatively, AAAs are more informal interactions used to promote motivation, education, or recreation and enhance recovery and quality of life [14]. AAAs can be as simple as a visit with a patient and their family members or more prescriptive and goal oriented. Skilled human–animal teams undergo introductory training, preparation, and assessment to be allowed to deliver AAAs in specific healthcare environments. In both AATs and AAAs, animals must meet temperament, behavioral, and suitability criteria individualized for the environment in which they are to work [15, 16]. Additionally, the animal handler must have adequate knowledge about the animal's behavior, needs, health, and indicators of stress [15]. Typically, both the animal and the handler are evaluated by a multidisciplinary team consisting of professionals with expertise in animal behavior, therapy, and related fields. It is common for hospitals to collaborate with established therapy animal registration and certification organizations to facilitate the training, evaluation, and registration process for therapy animals and their handlers. These organizations set forth specific requirements and guidelines for both animals and handlers seeking registration. Criteria may include passing temperament tests, completing training programs, and meeting health and vaccination standards [15, 16].

Animals Used in AAI

It is important to note the difference between service animals, emotional support animals, therapy animals, resident animals, and personal pets. Service animals are individually trained to perform specific tasks to assist their owner with a disability as defined by the Americans with Disabilities Act. The use of service animals does not constitute AAI. Emotional support animals require no specific training or licensing but are supported in writing by a qualified physician or mental health professional [14].

Most animals who participate in AAIs are volunteer therapy animals. Along with their handlers, volunteer therapy animals undergo training, certification, and registration with an AAI organization to safely visit patients and staff in the healthcare setting. A variety of therapy animals are used to deliver AAI. While therapy dogs are commonly used in the inpatient environment, cases using other species, such as cats, rabbits, birds, miniature pigs, alpacas, guinea pigs, and horses, are documented. Resident animals are a subset of therapy animals owned by a healthcare facility where they live full-time. Professionals employed by the facility are responsible for training, handling, and caring for the resident animal. They may be used for both AAT and AAA with patients, families, and staff in the facility [14]. Personal pets are often considered integral members of the family. With an increased focus on patient and family-centered care, more hospitals are allowing personal pets to visit patients. It is important to note that personal pet visitation policies differ from those regarding trained service or therapy animals [17, 18].

Emerging technologies offer creative opportunities for AAI in the ICU. With increasing sophistication, robot animals (Fig. 22.1) can be an alternative for AAI in patient populations that are considered too high risk for live animal interactions, such as those undergoing bone marrow transplants or extracorporeal membrane oxygenation [19]. Research indicates that using robot animals in these settings has similar effects to that of live animals [20–22]. Additionally, the COVID-19 pandemic prompted new audiovisual and virtual technology applications that allow for alternative AAI visits in situations where visitation is restricted [23]. Virtual AAIs can be delivered using video chat, prerecorded videos, live on-demand videos, or through slideshows of therapy animal photos. This alternative form of delivery benefits various patient populations, and professional nursing organizations support it as a therapeutic intervention to reduce stress in ICU staff members. Virtual AAI visits can be especially beneficial to boost staff morale and reduce stress and anxiety because they allow for quick access during the workday without taking time away from patient care or requiring staff to be present outside work hours [23].

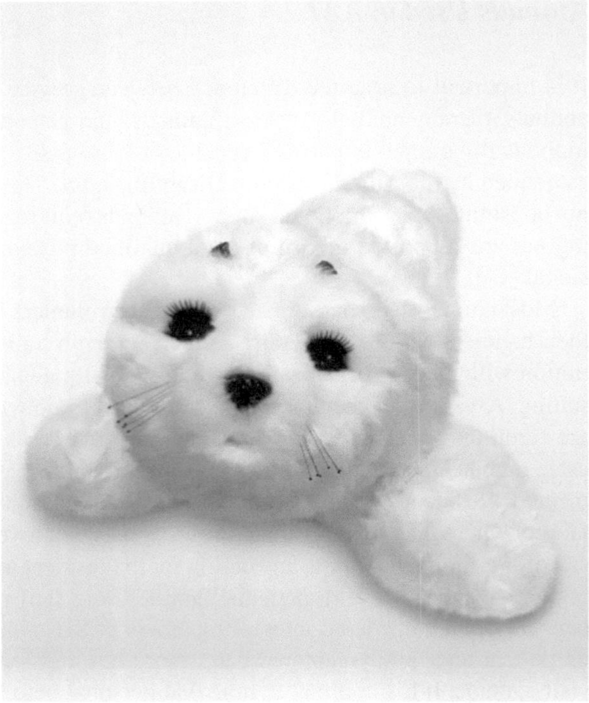

Fig. 22.1 PARO seal: a robotic animal

AAI in the ICU

AAIs have been successfully implemented in acute and subacute care settings with patients, their family members, and staff. AAIs are a way to reduce suffering, improve reality orientation, increase engagement, and lessen the physiological burden for the ICU patient [6]. In addition, they may enhance mood, reduce stress and anxiety, and improve job satisfaction and engagement among healthcare professionals [11, 24, 25]. AAIs can be tailored to meet the needs of diverse situations, making this intervention desirable to many patients, especially those in the ICU who may have additional constraints due to their illness [7, 22].

In ICU-specific studies, patients, families, and clinicians report strong satisfaction with and support for AAIs. The evidence supporting AAIs in critical care is still in its early stages, mainly consisting of positive but anecdotal reports [11]. A 2022 scoping review identified only six primary research studies evaluating AAIs in the ICU, five of which were published within the last 3 years [11]. Several case studies have shown patients exhibiting positive responses such as getting out of bed or speaking for the first time during an animal visit [7, 26]. Other evidence results from observational studies, quality improvement projects, or pilot studies with relatively small sample sizes. Still, current research shows promise that AAIs have the potential to enhance the emotional, psychological, social, and physical well-being of the entire critical care community. Additional studies need to be done to refute assumed safety concerns and guide the development of evidence-based practice recommendations for the use of AAIs in the ICU [11].

Therapeutic Activities During AAI in the ICU

Animals in the ICU can offer various therapeutic activities depending on the needs and abilities of the patient, family, or clinical staff. In some cases, passive activities such as observation and visitation are more than sufficient to achieve the goals of the AAI. For example, patients may benefit simply from the distraction of watching a dog perform learned skills. End-of-life care may also be a good time to bring in therapeutic animals to support grieving family members. In other cases, with appropriate infection prevention measures, animals can sit with patients at the head of the bed during uncomfortable procedures such as spinal taps. Other, more dynamic activities can target therapeutic goals related to speech, memory, balance and endurance, memory, self-esteem, fine motor, and sensory stimulation [27]. Patients can work on their gate or stamina by walking with the dog. If their mobility is limited, they can practice fine motor skills and upper extremity strength by doing things such as brushing, petting, feeding, or dressing the animal with accessories like a bandana [27].

Supporting Evidence for the Use of AAI in the ICU

Psychological and Emotional Well-being of Patients

Patients and families describe the ICU experience as isolating, overwhelming, and powerless [28–30]. AAI is a useful tool that can promote psychological and emotional well-being by decreasing anxiety and stress, reducing loneliness, and improving mood [11, 27, 31–34]. In one study, 86% of patients reported improved anxiety levels after working with dogs during therapy sessions [27]. Testimonials from patients and families who experienced AAIs during an inpatient stay reported that the animal sessions induced relaxation, resulting in a positive change in attitude and encouraging sleepiness [27]. In a recent systematic review of qualitative evidence to support AAIs in various inpatient and outpatient settings, the authors reported that AAIs fostered feelings of normalcy, enhanced self-esteem and companionship, and offered a distraction from pain and distress [24]. Anecdotal stories from patients and families who interacted with therapy dogs in a burn ICU illustrated the ability of AAIs to improve patient mood and self-esteem [27, 35]. Because the animals do not see the scars of burn patients, they allow patients in these units to feel accepted and distract them from physical changes they may have associated with their injuries. The distraction provided by animal visits lessens the patient's focus on their illness, facilitating their overall engagement in recovery [24]. As insurance reimbursement agencies put greater emphasis on patient experience as a quality indicator of healthcare facility performance, the use of animals to improve patient well-being warrants further investigation [36].

Family and Provider ICU Experience

The potential benefits of AAIs extend beyond the patient, positively impacting family members and healthcare staff. In a systematic review of AAI in the ICU, interactions with animals were well received by clinicians and families, with an overall satisfaction ranging from 93% to 100% across all studies [11]. In a study with pediatric patients, family and staff were surveyed on the use of AAI in the acute care setting. The survey included items on the parents' and staff's perceptions of AAI and its effect on the child during hospitalization. Eighty-four percent ($n = 42$) of parents perceived a great benefit of their child's interaction with the therapy dog, and 100% ($n = 118$) of parents and staff viewed them as very worthwhile to include in the acute care hospital setting. Parents were grateful for the relief from anxiety and distraction the therapy dogs provided for their children [37]. Anecdotal stories from using a therapy dog in a pediatric burn ICU highlight many situations where patients were withdrawn, refusing to speak or interact with parents and staff. Once the dog was brought into the room, the children began to talk and laugh with their parents and interact with providers [38].

Animals are often welcome visitors in high-stress environments. With increased concern for moral distress and burnout in healthcare, interventions to support the well-being of staff are critical to the quality of healthcare delivered. AAIs may reduce burnout by improving unit morale. An AAI staff wellness program evaluated the effectiveness of therapy dog walkabout visits in the emergency department and ICU [39]. After 9 months, 91% of staff agreed or strongly agreed that the program seemed to be inversely related to staff stress. Staff also reported an increase in morale, with an overall 94% satisfaction rate and 97% supporting the continuation of the program. Key themes from qualitative feedback included feelings of being cared for by the organization, improved unit environment, and increased staff wellness [39]. In a recent exploratory study, investigators gathered feedback on the experiences and perceptions of hospital staff in acute settings who participated in an inpatient AAI program [36]. Staff felt AAI decreased staff stress, promoted social interactions and interactions with patients, and provided comfort and company to patients [36].

Meaningful Communication and Connection

Interactions with animals in the ICU environment can prompt more genuine connection and break down communication barriers between providers, patients, and family members. A recent study evaluating personal pet visitations in the ICU found that the presence of a pet resulted in storied conversations, fostered empathy, and offered a greater understanding of the patient's psychosocial condition [18]. AAIs improved rapport by allowing patients and families to see the more personal sides of their providers and by offering opportunities to share stories about their personal pet experiences. Providers said that pets promoted a connection between them and their patients and acted as a "social lubricant" by encouraging easy interactions and safer conversations in such a high-stress environment. Patients, families, and clinicians alike have commented about the joy, support, and pain relief that AAIs provide [40]. This improved camaraderie extends beyond the patient-provider connection. In one AAI program, the animal helped clinicians engage in peer-to-peer conversations and bolstered unit morale during visits to the unit [39].

AAIs elicit communicative responses from patients that can contribute to therapeutic outcomes. Many anecdotal stories can be found in the literature that detail a nonresponsive patient smiling for the first time or attempting to reach out toward the animal. These types of responses, albeit subtle, are incredibly encouraging to providers and families alike [18]. Additionally, providers described instances when they could better determine a patient's cognitive status and orientation level because of a visit from a pet. In one visit, a patient who was thought to be comatose attempted to communicate and indicated comprehension after a visit from her personal pet [18]. In another case, a patient who was reported to have had no purposeful movement began stroking the dog's fur after having her hand placed on its head. After a few minutes, she was petting the dog along his entire back and regained full consciousness the following day [35].

Mobility

Mobility is essential to physical and mental recovery in the ICU, shown to benefit patients throughout hospitalization and improve outcomes at hospital discharge. Patients who engage in higher levels of activity during their ICU stay have a lower incidence of pressure injuries, a more positive ICU experience, and reduced anxiety levels [41–43]. Active mobility during hospitalization can improve physical function, preserve muscle strength, and increase the number of delirium-free days at hospital discharge when compared to individuals who remain immobile. While the benefits of increased mobilization are documented in various settings and populations, patients in the ICU have profoundly low levels of activity and spend most of their time sedentary or immobile. Common barriers to mobility include patient anxiety, fear, sedation, fatigue, symptoms of pain, and lack of motivation, all issues that AAI can help address [44, 45].

AAIs are an innovative strategy to encourage and promote mobility in the ICU and improve motivation to engage in critical care rehabilitation. In a study evaluating canine-assisted ambulation, heart failure patients were more willing to ambulate when offered a chance to walk with a dog and were less likely to refuse therapy [46]. Interestingly, 19% of patients approached by study staff initially refused to ambulate but changed their minds when offered a chance to participate in the canine-assisted ambulation intervention. Patients who participated in the intervention walked nearly twice as far as those who did not [46]. These results are similar to another study with adult heart transplant patients who walked a further distance and for a longer duration with a dog compared to those who walked without a dog [47].

Working closely with animals during physical and occupational therapy can improve reality orientation, provide cognitive stimulation, and increase attention span—all of which can help reduce the risk of developing delirium in the ICU [25]. AAIs can also improve behavioral activation by providing the extra energy a patient needs to feel motivated enough to move [24, 48]. Qualitative feedback from one study includes the following patient quotes: "Knowing the dog was there helped me and motivated me to get out of bed" and "Having the therapy dog brightens my day and gives me more motivation" [27].

Physiologic Burden, Sedation, and Pain Medication

Various studies demonstrate the effectiveness of AAIs in reducing physiological burden for both adult and pediatric hospitalized patients. Additionally, AAIs may be an effective tool to reduce the amount of sedative and pain medications commonly used in the ICU to reduce agitation, anxiety, and pain [7]. Unfortunately, these medications have a dose-dependent relationship with multiple adverse outcomes such as mortality, delirium, prolonged mechanical ventilation, and long-term physical, psychological, and cognitive impairments after discharge [2, 49]. Reducing the amount of medication given to maintain the lowest sedation level possible while maintaining safety is imperative to improve outcomes for critically ill individuals.

Although ICU-specific studies to date that focus on measuring stress biomarkers before and after AAIs have shown no particular response to stress [31], it is well known that interactions with animals can reduce levels of stress hormones such as cortisol, norepinephrine, and epinephrine [25]. One study of patients hospitalized for advanced heart failure did find that patients had lower neurohormonal levels and cardiopulmonary pressures after a visit from a therapy dog [34]. Another study found that 20-minute sessions with a therapy dog after surgery led to favorable neurological and cardiovascular responses for pediatric patients in the immediate postoperative period. AATs could facilitate rapid recovery of alertness and activity after anesthesia, modify pain perception, and induce an emotional prefrontal response [50]. After interacting with a dog, patients reported less pain, increased feelings of comfort, and had reduced heart and respiratory rates [32, 33].

Safety Considerations When Implementing AAIs in the ICU

Safety is a primary concern for all ICU patients, regardless of the intervention. AAIs require additional safety considerations for all involved—patient, family, staff, animal, and animal handler. Presumed risks of AAIs in critical care populations include allergic reactions, physical trauma (scratches and skin tears), and risk of transmission of zoonotic diseases between the animal and the patient [7]. While published guidelines recommend that animals be restricted from visiting patients who are in critical care or isolation, these recommendations are not supported by strong clinical evidence and are based mostly on epidemiologic lab studies [15, 16]. In a systematic review of AAIs in the ICU, no adverse events were reported related to AAIs in any of the studies [11]. In fact, the CDC has never documented a case of infection from pet visitation, and anecdotal evidence is plentiful from programs across the country that have never experienced zoonotic infection [26]. Further research would help safely expand AAI programs to more ICUs, but the following sections highlight best practices from current programs.

Patient and Family

It is important to assess the patient's background, clinical condition, and physical and psychological needs for their suitability to interact with an animal prior to each AAI session [7, 11]. This assessment should be conducted in collaboration with the patient (if able), their family, and clinical staff. The patient's diagnosis and medical background may exclude them from participating in AAIs. For example, those with severe allergies, reactive airway disease, significant immunosuppression, or large open wounds may not be safe to interact with an animal. Additionally, in the case where a patient is in isolation precautions that cannot be safely accommodated, they may still benefit from watching an animal outside their door doing tricks and interacting with others [38]. The patient's overall desire for an animal interaction should be considered. Tools such as the Pet Attitude Scale may be used to assess whether they like animals, have a pet at home, or have had any previous negative experiences with animals [31, 51]. Decisions regarding the appropriate level of physical engagement a patient can tolerate should be based on the patient's range of motion, eyesight, hearing, and presence of any lines or tubes. Ideally, the patient is alert, interactive, and cooperative. However, if they are sedated, patients and their family members may still benefit from physically touching the animal, having the animal lay next to them, or overhearing conversations about the animal among family, clinical staff, and animal handlers.

Clinical Staff and Animal Handlers

Depending on the type of AAI being administered, the clinical staff and animal handler may be one and the same. Anyone responsible for delivering AAIs in the ICU should receive education and training specific to critical care, such as information about technical equipment, frequently used terminology, and the roles of healthcare team members. They require a baseline understanding of the severity of illness seen in the ICU, including clinical signs of decompensation and potential psychological stressors, such as fatigue, pain, and anxiety. They must be able to modify sessions based on the patient's level of consciousness and mobility to accommodate individual patient needs and responses to animal interactions. It is imperative that they be briefed on the best ways to respond to difficult situations in the ICU, such as a decompensating patient, distressed family member, combative patient, and medical emergencies in adjoining rooms. Shadowing experiences in the ICU without the animal will help volunteer handlers understand the environment prior to AAI sessions [7]. Additionally, all should follow hospital policy regarding attire, wear a visible badge, and undergo education on confidentiality and privacy rules in the healthcare setting [38].

Animal

Clinicians and researchers implementing AAIs should consider the size of the animal. Smaller animals may be more appropriate for ventilated patients or those with multiple pieces of attached equipment. Hypoallergenic animal breeds may be preferred since many critically ill patients suffer from significant respiratory compromise [7]. Animals should be clean, well-groomed, in good health, and up-to-date on their immunizations with regular health and behavioral status evaluations [52]. A clean sheet should be placed under the animal before the animal gets on the bed or chair with a patient and discarded after the interaction [38]. Animals used in AAIs have a calm temperament, are people-oriented, and remain unphased by hospital smells, sounds, and surfaces [7, 38]. Therapy or resident animals should be limited to 2 h of working time per day or shorter depending on the animal [27].

Environment

Families, healthcare staff, and animal handlers must work together to prepare and maintain a safe environment for sessions involving AAIs. This includes reviewing all lines and tubes to prevent dislodgement, covering areas of open skin, and providing adequate lighting. All participants should wash their hands before and after each interaction. The patient should be offered glasses or hearing aids if applicable and sitting upright in bed if medically appropriate. The room temperature should be adjusted as needed with consideration for both the patient's and the animal's comfort. The handler should be aware of the best way to safely exit the room and the unit with the animal in the case of a medical emergency or crisis [7].

Recommendations for Building and Sustaining AAI Programs in the ICU

As the evidence supporting the use of AAIs continues to evolve, experts in the field have begun publishing best practices related to AAI programs in the ICU [6, 9]. Regardless of the type of AAI, policies, and procedures should be in place to ensure proper infection control and promote safety [7]. Medical facilities are responsible for providing sufficient training for AAI teams and frequent evaluations of the AAI staff, volunteer animal handlers, and the animal's behavior. Patients, families, and staff need education regarding AAI policies, the benefits of AAIs, and the use of AAI services at the facility [7]. Also, staff should be frequently queried for their perception of how AAI programs are going in their units [7].

Establishing a program champion who is consistently in the ICU and has credibility with staff and leadership is important to create the system change needed to build AAI programs. Champions must establish clear program goals with milestones and measurable outcomes. While patient outcomes are paramount, assessing the impact of AAIs on family and staff well-being should also be considered. Program champions should collaborate with key stakeholders such as medical directors, infection control clinicians, and volunteer coordinators (if using volunteer AAI teams) who can help identify potential barriers prior to implementation efforts. There should be multidisciplinary efforts to create clear policies and procedures that include program goals and evaluation plans, describe roles and responsibilities, and outline the logistics of animal visits, including what to do when there is an issue such as an accident or concern with temperament. Hospitals can partner with reputable AAI organizations that have credibility registering teams specifically for the hospital environment. These organizations can help identify animal teams most appropriate for the ICU. Lastly, carefully construct inclusion and exclusion criteria prior to launching the program to start with a cohort of patients most likely to have successful animal interactions [6, 9].

Future Considerations

While AAI continues to be a valuable tool to support patients, families, and clinical staff in acute and subacute settings, more research is needed to understand the specific psychophysiological responses that lead to improved outcomes. Current evidence is subjective, largely relying on self-report and qualitative feedback. Most ICU-specific studies use quasi-experimental, observational designs with small sample sizes. Additionally, few studies have implemented a control group for comparison making it difficult to generalize findings across critical care populations. Future studies should consider more rigorous designs with creative controls, such as visits with just human interaction alone or with plush, robotic, or virtual animals [53]. The exact amount of time required with an animal remains unclear, and studies are needed to determine the ideal quality, frequency, and length of animal visits, as well as the physiological mechanisms that elicit positive responses in the ICU [32].

Further discussion among experts about measurable outcomes and input from stakeholders regarding the most valuable outcomes to patients, families, and providers is warranted. For example, researchers may consider whether there is a correlation between the presence of a pet and decreased amounts of sedative and analgesic medications, increased treatment compliance, improved immune function, ventilator weaning, greater family satisfaction scores, or reduced provider burnout and turnover [38]. ICU patients may be ideal candidates for researchers to measure plasma or serum biomarkers because many ICU patients have indwelling-catheter vascular access [31].

Advances in animal robotics, virtual reality, and audiovisual technologies offer alternative opportunities to deliver AAI in the ICU [20–22, 54]. These technologies may be just as clinically effective while providing greater flexibility and using fewer resources. In addition, the infection control barriers encountered with live animal programs can be mitigated [22]. Regarding infection risk, current rules surrounding best practice for animal visitation in the ICU are not necessarily evidence-based but instead grounded in worry of what "could happen." [55] Broad sweeping, one-size-fits-all policies for AAIs in the ICU are not in the best interest of patients or their families [17]. ICU animal visitation should be considered case-by-case, guided by clear policies and procedures, rather than categorically prohibiting it [17].

References

1. Geense WW, Zegers M, Peters MA, et al. New physical, mental, and cognitive problems 1 year after ICU admission: a prospective multicenter study. Am J Resp Crit Care Med. 2021;203(12):1215–521. https://doi.org/10.1164/rccm.202009-3381OC.
2. Lee M, Kang J, Jeong YJ. Risk factors for post–intensive care syndrome: a systematic review and meta-analysis. Aust Crit Care. 2020;33(3):287–94. https://doi.org/10.1016/j.aucc.2019.10.004.
3. Puntillo KA, Neuhaus J, Arai S, et al. Challenge of assessing symptoms in seriously ill intensive care unit patients: can proxy reporters help? Crit Care Med. 2012;40(10):2760–7. https://doi.org/10.1097/CCM.0b013e31825b94d8.
4. Barr J, Fraser GL, Puntillo K, et al. Clinical practice guidelines for the management of pain, agitation, and delirium in adult patients in the intensive care unit. Crit Care Med. 2013;41(1):263–306. https://doi.org/10.1097/CCM.0b013e3182783b72.
5. Ka P, Arai S, Cohen NH, et al. Symptoms experienced by intensive care unit patients at high risk of dying. Crit Care Med. 2010;38(11):2155–60. https://doi.org/10.1097/CCM.0b013e3181f267ee.

6. Hosey MM, Jaskulski J, Wegener ST, Chlan LL, Needham DM. Animal-assisted intervention in the ICU: a tool for humanization. Crit Care. 2018;22(1):22. Published 2018 Feb 12. https://doi.org/10.1186/s13054-018-1946-8.
7. Hetland B, Bailey T, Prince-Paul M. Animal assisted interactions to alleviate psychological symptoms in patients on mechanical ventilation. Am J Hosp Palliat Care. 2017;19(6):516–23.
8. American Veterinary Medical Association (AVMA). Human-animal bond. https://www.avma.org/one-health/human-animal-bond. Updated 2023. Accessed January 26, 2023.
9. Halm MA. The healing power of the human-animal connection. Am J Crit Care. 2008;17(4):373–6.
10. Hetland B, Hickman R, McAndrew N, Daly B. Factors that influence active family engagement in care among critical care nurses. AACN Adv Crit Care. 2017;28(2):160–70. https://doi.org/10.4037/aacnacc2017118.
11. Lovell T, Ranse K. Animal-assisted activities in the intensive care unit: a scoping review. Intensive Crit Care Nurs. 2022;73(103304):103304. https://doi.org/10.1016/j.iccn.2022.103304.
12. International Association of Human-Animal Interaction Organizations. Definitions for animal assisted intervention and guidelines for wellness of animals involved; 2018. https://iahaio.org/best-practice/white-paper-on-animal-assisted-interventions/
13. Mills JT 3rd, Yeager AF. Definitions of animals used in healthcare settings. US Army Med Dep J. 2012:12–7.
14. American Veterinary Medical Association (AVMA). Animal-assisted interventions: definitions. https://www.avma.org/resources-tools/avma-policies/animal-assisted-interventions-definitions. Updated 2023. Accessed January 26, 2023.
15. Lefebvre SL, Golab GC, Christensen E, et al. Guidelines for animal-assisted interventions in health care facilities. Am J Infect Control. 2008;36(2):78–85. https://doi.org/10.1016/j.ajic.2007.09.005.
16. Murthy R, Bearman G, Brown S, et al. Animals in healthcare facilities: recommendations to minimize potential risks. Infect Control Hosp Epidemiol. 2015;36(5):495–516. https://doi.org/10.1017/ice.2015.15.
17. Barchas D, Melaragni M, Abrahim H, Barchas E. The best medicine: personal pets and therapy animals in the hospital setting. Crit Care Nurs Clin North Am. 2020;32:167–90. https://doi.org/10.1016/j.cnc.2020.01.002.
18. Yamasaki J. The communicative role of companion pets in patient-centered critical care. Patient Educ Couns. 2018;101(5):830–5. https://doi.org/10.1016/j.pec.2017.12.014.
19. Steffani Nolte. Therapy seal helps ICU patients at Nebraska medicine. 3 News Now; 2019. Accessed January 31, 2023. https://www.3newsnow.com/news/local-news/therapy-seal-helps-icu-patients-at-nebraska-medicineb.
20. Hetland B. Robot rehab: AAI with robot during inpatient pediatric rehab. ClinicalTrials.gov identifier: NCT05275543. Updated January 9, 2023. Accessed January 31, 2023. https://clinicaltrials.gov/ct2/show/NCT05275543.
21. Hetland B. Animal assisted interactions with animal robot during PT/OT in the ICU (PARO). ClinicalTrials.gov identifier: NCT05075395. Updated November 2, 2023. Accessed January 31, 2023. https://clinicaltrials.gov/ct2/show/NCT05075395.
22. Lindquist R, Tracy MF, Snyder M. Complementary therapies in nursing. 9th ed. New York, NY: Springer Publishing; 2023. p. 264.
23. Mabe KS. Implementing a virtual animal assisted therapy intervention to improve stress in trauma intensive care unit nurses during COVID-19. [Doctoral dissertation]. Chapel Hill, NC: University of North Carolina Chapel Hill; 2021.
24. Shen RZZ, Xiong P, Chou UI, Hall BJ. "We need them as much as they need us": a systematic review of the qualitative evidence for possible mechanisms of effectiveness of animal-assisted intervention (AAI). Complement Ther Med. 2018;41:203–7. https://doi.org/10.1016/j.ctim.2018.10.001.
25. Malik J. Animal-assisted interventions in intensive care delirium: a literature review. AACN Adv Crit Care. 2021;32(4):391–7. https://doi.org/10.4037/aacnacc2021708.

26. Cullen L, Titler L, Drahozal R. Family and pet visitation in the critical care unit. Crit Care Nurs. 1999;19(3):84–7.
27. Pruskowski KA, Gurney JM, Cancio LC. Impact of the implementation of a therapy dog program on burn center patients and staff. Burns. 2020;46(2):293–7. https://doi.org/10.1016/j.burns.2019.11.024.
28. Imanipour M, Kiwanuka F, Akhavan R, Masaba S, Alemayehu YH. Family members' experiences in adult intensive care units: a systematic review. Scand J Caring Sci. 2019;33(3):569–81. https://doi.org/10.1111/scs.12675.
29. Rotondi AJ, Chelluri L, Sirio C, et al. Patients' recollections of stressful experiences while receiving prolonged mechanical ventilation in an intensive care unit. Crit Care Med. 2002;30(4):746–52. https://doi.org/10.1097/00003246-200204000-00004.
30. Baumgarten M, Poulsen I. Patients' experiences of being mechanically ventilated in an ICU: a qualitative metasynthesis. Scand J Caring Sci. 2015;29(2):205–14. https://doi.org/10.1111/scs.12177.
31. Branson S, Boss L, Hamlin S, Padhye NS. Animal-assisted activity in critically ill older adults: a randomized pilot and feasibility trial. Biol Res Nurs. 2020;22(3):412–7. https://doi.org/10.1177/1099800420920719.
32. Coakley AB, Mahoney EK. Creating a therapeutic and healing environment with a pet therapy program. Complement Ther Clin Pract. 2009;15(3):141–6. https://doi.org/10.1016/j.ctcp.2009.05.004.
33. Phung A, Joyce C, Ambutas S, et al. Animal-assisted therapy for inpatient adults. Nursing. 2017;47(1):63–6. https://doi.org/10.1097/01.NURSE.0000504675.26722.d8.
34. Cole KM, Gawlinski A, Steers N, Kotlerman J. Animal-assisted therapy in patients hospitalized with heart failure. Am J Crit Care. 2007;16(6):575–8.
35. Miller J. Animal-assisted therapy: the bond that heals. World Crit Care Nurs. 1999;3(1):12–5.
36. Abrahamson K, Cai Y, Richards E, Cline K, O'Haire ME. Perceptions of a hospital-based animal assisted intervention program: an exploratory study. Complement Ther Clin Pract. 2016;25:150–4. https://doi.org/10.1016/j.ctcp.2016.10.003.
37. Uglow LS. The benefits of an animal-assisted intervention service to patients and staff at a children's hospital. Br J Nurs. 2019;28(8):509–15. https://doi.org/10.12968/bjon.2019.28.8.509.
38. Hastings T, Burris A, Hunt J, Purdue G, Arnoldo B. Pet therapy: a healing solution. J Burn Care Res. 2008;29(6):874–6. https://doi.org/10.1097/BCR.0b013e31818b9df8.
39. Caton N, Campbell K, Brumwell T, et al. Pups assisting wellness for staff (P.A.W.S.): evaluating the impact of canine-assisted interventions on critical care staff wellness. Healthc Manage Forum. 2021;34(2):119–22. https://doi.org/10.1177/0840470420960162.
40. Horowitz S. Animal-assisted therapy for inpatients: tapping the unique healing power of the human–animal bond. Altern Complement Therapies. 2011;16(6):339–43. https://doi.org/10.1089/act.2010.16603.
41. Corner EJ, Murray EJ, Brett SJ. Qualitative, grounded theory exploration of patients' experience of early mobilisation, rehabilitation and recovery after critical illness. BMJ Open. 2019;9(2):e026348. https://doi.org/10.1136/bmjopen-2018-026348.
42. Klein K, Mulkey M, Bena JF, Albert NM. Clinical and psychological effects of early mobilization in patients treated in a neurologic ICU: a comparative study. Crit Care Med. 2015;63(4):865–73. https://doi.org/10.1097/CCM.0000000000000787.
43. Azuh O, Gammon H, Burmeister C, et al. Benefits of early active mobility in the medical intensive care unit: a pilot study. Am J Med. 2016;129(8):866–71. https://doi.org/10.1016/j.amjmed.2016.03.032.
44. Wang J, Ren D, Liu Y, Wang Y, Zhang B, Xiao Q. Effects of early mobilization on the prognosis of critically ill patients: a systematic review and meta-analysis. Int J Nurs Stud. 2020;110:103708. https://doi.org/10.1016/j.ijnurstu.2020.103708.
45. Zhang L, Hu W, Cai Z, et al. Early mobilization of critically ill patients in the intensive care unit: a systematic review and meta-analysis. PLoS One. 2019;14(10):11–21. https://doi.org/10.1371/journal.pone.0223185.

46. Abate SV, Zucconi M, Boxer BA. Impact of canine-assisted ambulation on hospitalized chronic heart failure patients' ambulation outcomes and satisfaction: a pilot study. J Cardiovasc Nurs. 2011;26(3):224–30.
47. Walden M, Lovenstein A, Randag A, et al. Methodological challenges encountered in a study of the impact of animal-assisted intervention in pediatric heart transplant patients. J Pediatr Nurs. 2020;53:67–73. https://doi.org/10.1016/j.pedn.2020.04.017.
48. Snipelisky D, Burton MC. Canine-assisted therapy in the inpatient setting. South Med J. 2014;107(4):265–73. https://doi.org/10.1097/SMJ.0000000000000090.
49. Shehabi Y, Bellomo R, Kadiman S, et al. Sedation intensity in the first 48 hours of mechanical ventilation and 180-day mortality: a multinational prospective longitudinal cohort study. Crit Care Med. 2018;46(6):850–9. https://doi.org/10.1097/CCM.0000000000003071.
50. Calcaterra V, Veggiotti P, Palestrini C, et al. Post-operative benefits of animal-assisted therapy in pediatric surgery: a randomised study. PLoS One. 2015;10(6):e0125813. https://doi.org/10.1371/journal.pone.0125813.
51. Munsell L, Canfield M, Templer DI, Tangan K, Arikawa H. Modification of the pet attitude scale. Soc Anim. 2004;12(2):137–42. https://doi.org/10.1016/j.jpsychores.2008.02.002.
52. Centers for Disease Control and Prevention. Guidelines for environmental infection control in health-care facilities: recommendations of CDC and the healthcare infection control practices advisory committee (HICPAC). MMWR Morb Mortal Wkly Rep. 2003:154–6. https://www.cdc.gov/infectioncontrol/pdf/guidelines/environmental-guidelines-P.pdf
53. Kowalski MO, Smith C, Cole DA, et al. A multicenter study of animal-assisted activity and anxiety among older adults hospitalized in acute care settings. Appl Nurs Res. 2021;60:151447. https://doi.org/10.1016/j.apnr.2021.151447.
54. Chubak J, Pocobelli G, Ziebell RA, et al. Effects of the COVID-19 pandemic on animal-assisted activities in pediatric hospitals. [published online ahead of print, 2022 Sep 30]. J Pediatr Health Care. 2022; https://doi.org/10.1016/j.pedhc.2022.09.011. S0891–5245(22)00281–4
55. Davidson JE, Hudson CA. Family-centered care: a reflection. Crit Care Nurs Clin North Am. 2020;32(2):xv–x. https://doi.org/10.1016/j.cnc.2020.04.001.

Chapter 23
How to Study the Family ICU Syndrome: A Basic Approach to Research Methodology

Christiane S. Hartog and Anna-Henrikje Seidlein

> …not everything that can be counted counts, and not everything that counts can be counted.—William Bruce Cameron (1963)

Introduction: Why Perform Clinical Research?

While we all agree that we need to provide high-quality care, we cannot be sure of what we are doing unless we measure what we do. Measuring processes and outcomes gives us a sense of knowing where we are compared to where we want to be. The preceding chapters in this book have defined the scope and different angles of understanding, engaging, and supporting families in the ICU. If we want to improve understanding and management of the Family Intensive Care Unit Syndrome (FICUS), we must know how to develop and answer *meaningful* research questions. In this chapter, we will look at some general aspects of successful clinical research and how these might reflect on the study of FICUS.

C. S. Hartog (✉)
Department of Anaesthesiology and Intensive Care, Charité Universitätsmedizin Berlin, Berlin, Germany

A.-H. Seidlein
Institute of Ethics and History of Medicine, University Medicine Greifswald, Greifswald, Germany

Interdisciplinary Surgical Intensive Care Unit, University Medicine Greifswald, Greifswald, Germany

Institute for Nursing Science and Interprofessional Learning, University Medicine Greifswald, Greifswald, Germany
e-mail: Anna-Henrikje.Seidlein@med.uni-greifswald.de

© The Author(s), under exclusive license to Springer Nature Switzerland AG 2025

A. J. Vance et al. (eds.), *Families in the Intensive Care Unit*,
https://doi.org/10.1007/978-3-031-83786-9_23

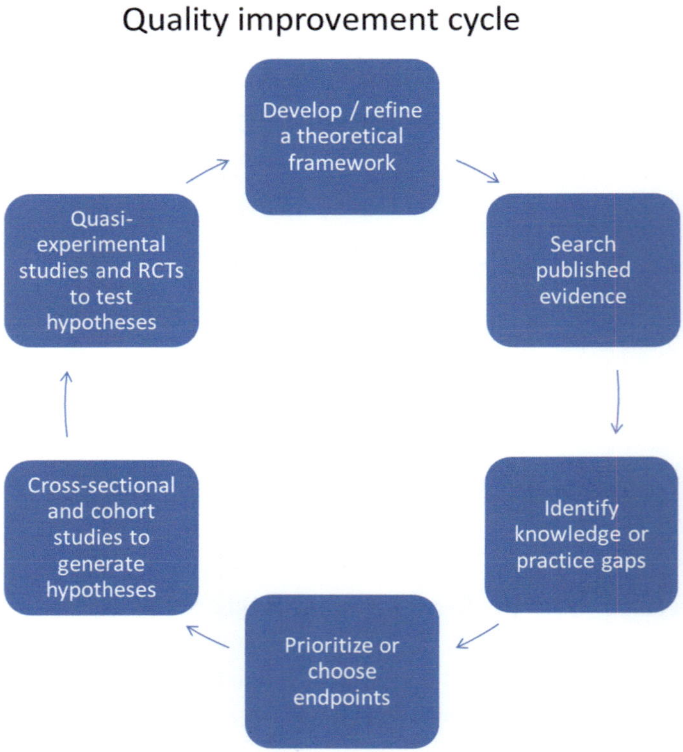

Fig. 23.1 The continuous cycle of quality improvement

While this chapter cannot extensively cover the subject of devising and carrying out clinical research, it will deal more specifically with the question how to study FICUS in a continuing cycle of quality improvement projects (Fig. 23.1). The important aspects that will be covered are: (1) theoretical framework and the research question; (2) choosing and measuring study endpoints; (3) appropriate study designs; and (4) considering complex clinical interventions.

Theoretical Framework and the Research Question

As Polit & Beck [1] state, "High quality studies achieve a high level of *conceptual integration"* (p. 126). Thus, the first step should be to conceptualize FICUS considering existing research, theories, and models to develop a conceptual rationale. It becomes rapidly obvious that FICUS is a multifaceted syndrome incorporating a large variety of domains that may interact with one another in many ways. FICUS is an emerging concept, and there is no universally accepted framework. Rather, different ways exist to conceptualize the problem [2]. Future research will probably modify or converge the heterogeneous concepts. It is therefore all the more important to keep an open mind and, if necessary and appropriate, to consider qualitative research designs, which enable a deeper understanding and the uncovering of previously unrecognized and thus unconsidered aspects [3, 4]. In addition, the Covid 19 pandemic has shown that circumstances of care and support, and thus also the experience of the families, can change very quickly [5]. As a result, conceptual adjustments might be necessary due to shifts in circumstances.

It is critical to remember that the kind of concept you favor will strongly determine the kind of research you will build on it. Developing a valid framework can be a research project in itself.

A potential framework which might be useful in future studies of FICUS can be found in Fig. 23.2. It is our own preliminary attempt to bring together different potential conceptualizations, which are described in more detail below. It is likely not complete or accurate; future research may substantially change it as our understanding of the syndrome FICUS evolves over time.

One potential conceptualization might be based on the work by Netzer et al. [6]

FICUS

(1) Syndrome and risk factors (maladaptive reasoning, personal and family conflicts, stressful emotions, sleeplessness, anticipatory grief, and cognitive bias).

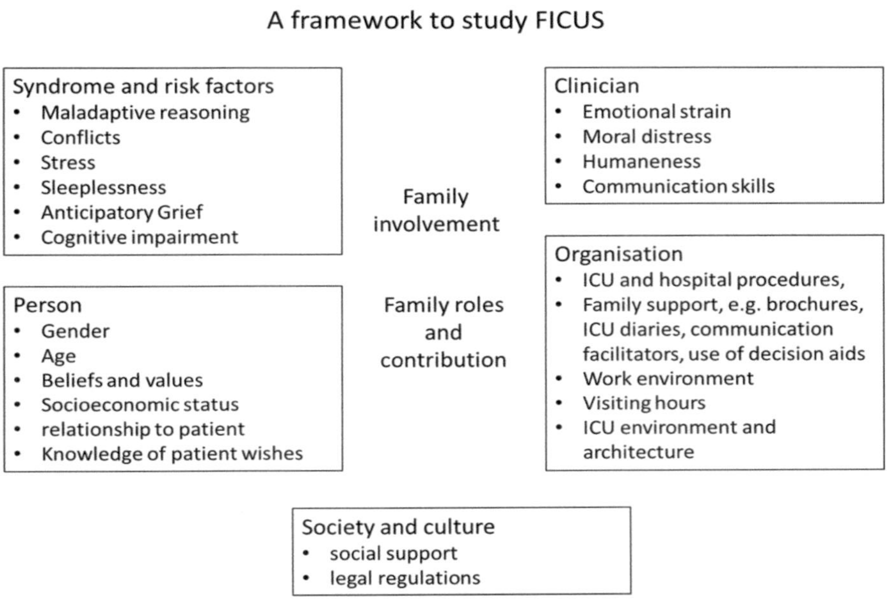

Fig. 23.2 A potential framework for the study of FICUS

(2) Person (gender, age, beliefs, values, socioeconomic status, relationship to patient, and knowledge of patient wishes).
(3) Clinicians (emotional strain, moral distress, humaneness, communication skills).
(4) Organization (ICU and hospital procedures, measures of family support, e.g., brochures, ICU diaries, communication facilitators, and use of decision aids, quality of the work environment, visiting hours, ICU environment and architecture), and.
(5) Sociocultural context (social support, legal regulations).

Some examples of potential research questions which are based on this framework are as follows:

- Do certain personal traits of the family member increase the risk for FICUS, for instance, gender, age, degree of relationship to the patient, level of education, and psychological morbidity?
- Can different organizational models reduce FICUS, for instance, open visiting hours, presence of communication facilitators, and use of decision aids or information brochures?
- Can interventions that reduce clinician stress mitigate FICUS?

Another way to conceptualize FICUS is to build on family involvement (based on Olding et al. [7]).

Involvement of Family Members in the ICU

(1) Involvement as presence.
(2) Involvement as receiving care and having needs met (specifically support, comfort, information, proximity, and reassurance).
(3) Involvement as communicating and receiving information.
(4) Involvement as decision-making.
(5) Involvement as contributing to care.

Potential research questions that are based on this framework might address whether FICUS correlates positively or negatively with involvement or which type of involvement is preferable in terms of environmental impact.

A third way to conceptualize FICUS might be from the viewpoint of the roles that families play in the ICU. McAdam et al. derived these roles from qualitative research [8]:

Family Roles and Contributions

(1) Active presence.

(2) Patient protector.
(3) Facilitator.
(4) Historian.
(5) Coach.
(6) Voluntary caregiver.

Potential research questions based on this framework might address which roles correlate specifically with FICUS, and whether empowerment of the family to fulfil these roles will have a beneficial effect.

Choosing and Measuring Study Endpoints

After you have developed a research question ("why"), you need to choose the variables which can describe exposure, intervention, and outcome (PICO-scheme). In general, quality improvement in the ICU should use quality measures which, apart from being valid, should also be reliable, responsive, interpretable, and feasible [9] (Table 23.1). Reliable means that the measure has good re-test properties and is not influenced by the person who measures it. A reliable measure yields the same results even when assessed by a different rater (inter-rater reliability) or at different times provided the variable has not changed (intra-rater reliability). A measure should also be responsive, i.e., respond to effective interventions or changes. For instance, the health-related quality of life (HRQL) measure SF-36 may not be responsive to changes due to different management of ICU survivors, because SF-36 is not specific for ICU survivors and lacks important domains [10]. An interpretable measure is one that should be easily understood by stakeholders including clinicians, ICU, and hospital leadership. A feasible measure is one that can be easily collected with available resources.

Table 23.1 Some examples of process and outcomes measures (modified after Curtis et al. [9])

	Process measure	Outcome measure
Do patients and families care about this?	May not be important	Yes, important
Do clinicians care about this?	Yes, monitors delivery of healthcare	Yes, shows the results of healthcare
Obtain from routine data?	Sometimes	Sometimes
Useful for feedback and quality improvement?	Yes, shows what clinicians are actually doing	Yes, but indirectly because outcomes are affected by a variety of processes
Directly measures prevention?	Yes	No
Need for risk adjustment?	No	Yes
Time needed for measurement?	Less	More (long-term outcomes)
Sample size requirements?	Smaller	Larger

However, studying FICUS requires endpoints that are family-centered. Such endpoints are novel, and their psychometric properties are likely not well established. Therefore, establishing quality measures in FICUS will necessarily entail some methodological research about the properties of measures. It may be helpful to consider a timeline that starts before ICU admission and continues beyond the ICU (Fig. 23.3).

First, there is the challenge to develop a concise but comprehensive measure of the syndrome itself, essential to determine (1) who has it and who has not (sensitivity, specificity, cut-off score) and (2) if someone has it, to what extent does he/she have it. The latter is important if you want to measure changes (responsiveness to change). For instance, when measuring burnout, self-rating questionnaires are used consisting of several scales or domains with defined psychometric properties such as the Maslach Burnout Inventory. A cut-off can be used to determine who has burnout and who has not. A frequently used outcome in family-centered care is the mental well-being of family members. Grief, depression, anxiety, stress, or helplessness can be measured by specific, validated instruments. However, it is yet unknown whether all of these typically make up the FICUS syndrome, to what extent and how to define a cut-off.

Further outcomes to measure are variables that are expected to have an effect on FICUS. Prior to the ICU, particularly for patients with a scheduled ICU stay, family members should be appropriately informed and prepared for their potential future role and involvement in the ICU. Advance care planning, i.e., the facilitated development of a written document that contains patient's treatment preferences, has the potential to increase compliance with end-of-life preferences and reduce family stress [11]. Goal-concordant care is one interesting new outcome that can be assessed during and after treatment in the ICU [12, 13]. Family members want the

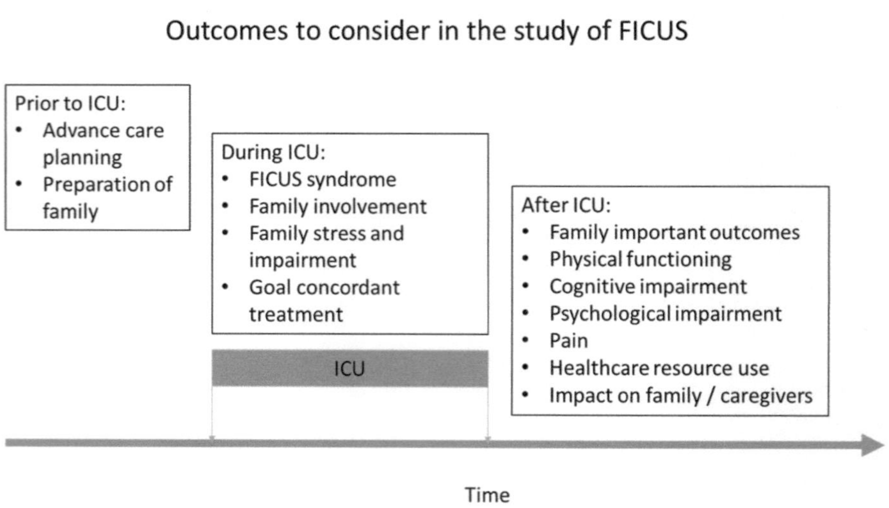

Fig. 23.3 Timeline of outcomes to consider in the study of FICUS

care their loved ones receive to be concordant with patient-identified goals, respecting any treatment limitation the patient has placed on clinical care. Patient-identified goals could be to return to work, be comfortable in one's own home, or stay alive even if this entails living in a nursing home. The incidence of goal-discordant care requires measurement of (1) patient goals, (2)treatment limitations if any, (3)treatments received, and (4) judgments regarding concordance; all of these provide multiple challenges which need to be overcome [13]. Another way to approach goal concordance is to evaluate preference-sensitive decisions as opportunities for shared decision-making with families. These are treatment decisions that should trigger clinicians to clarify patient goals for instance a permanent feeding tube, a suprapubic urinary catheter, or a tracheotomy [14]. Within this context, time-limited trials are increasingly discussed as a way to promote goal-concordant care [15]. Future research should address ways to operationalize goal concordance and establish correlation with other FICUS-related measures such as learned helplessness, acute stress, or moral distress of staff (just to name a few).

Several research groups have started to develop core outcome measures for intensive care which involve the patient and family perspective. Health-related quality of life (HRQL) is often used as a patient-important outcome, but generic measures like Short Form 36 Health Survey (SF-36) or EuroQol-5D (EQ-5D) have significant gaps in their coverage, for instance, cognitive functioning, relationships and family support and healthcare use [10]. Moreover, patients and families differ from researchers in their rating of the importance of outcomes after survivorship. They confer less importance to survival and more importance to pain, physical functioning and symptoms, fatigue, healthcare resource utilization, and impact on family or caregivers [16]. The FS-ICU provides a summary assessment of experienced care and communication in the ICU from the perspective of families but has been found to be unresponsive in interventional studies. Other domains that are important to patients and family members are facilitated continuity of care following ICU discharge, family participation in bedside care, and decision aids for end-of-life decision-making [17].

An important decision is the choice of the *primary endpoint*, as this will determine the sample calculation. The primary endpoint is obviously the most important, it is chosen to answer the research question and test the hypothesis. It also determines sample size calculation. Secondary endpoints are interesting because they provide background information. However, it must be kept in mind that the findings from secondary endpoints are only hypothesis-generating.

Given the multidimensionality of the syndrome and the many confounders that have an impact, the challenge of selecting a single primary endpoint as well as the time point to measure it is a great one. For instance, Curtis et al. conducted a randomized controlled two-center trial to test an intervention that used facilitators who supported communication between clinicians and families, adapted communication to family needs, and mediated conflict. The primary outcome was a measure of family members' symptoms of depression, but the intervention was associated with decreased depressive symptoms at 6 months ($p = 0.017$), not at 3 months as expected; moreover, symptoms of anxiety or post-traumatic stress did not change. Thus, the result leaves open questions about the effect of the intervention on the families' emotional burden; however, secondary outcomes showed a reduction in ICU and hospital length of stay in the intervention group with considerable financial savings [18]. Another challenge is the low response rates that are encountered in follow-up studies [19]. Recruiting families after the ICU can be subject to recruiting bias, with data suggesting that respondents are more satisfied with care than nonrespondents. In addition, answers may be subject to recall bias which may be particularly true when recalling specific stressors [20] or degree of compliance with patient preferences.

Appropriate Study Designs

Basically, a distinction must be drawn between qualitative and quantitative study designs, which both are relevant in the context of FICUS (Fig. 23.4). The latter can be further differentiated into nonexperimental (observational), quasi-experimental, and experimental (interventional) studies. The hierarchy of evidence places multi-centre randomized controlled trials (RCT) above observational and cross-sectional studies; they have the strongest explanatory power regarding causal relationships. However, the restrictions and challenges which are inherent in the study of FICUS, as described above, will limit the range of feasible study designs. As FICUS is an emerging concept, the study of FICUS will evolve in parallel. Initially, well-designed explorative studies are needed before a high-evidence RCT can be successfully designed and conducted.

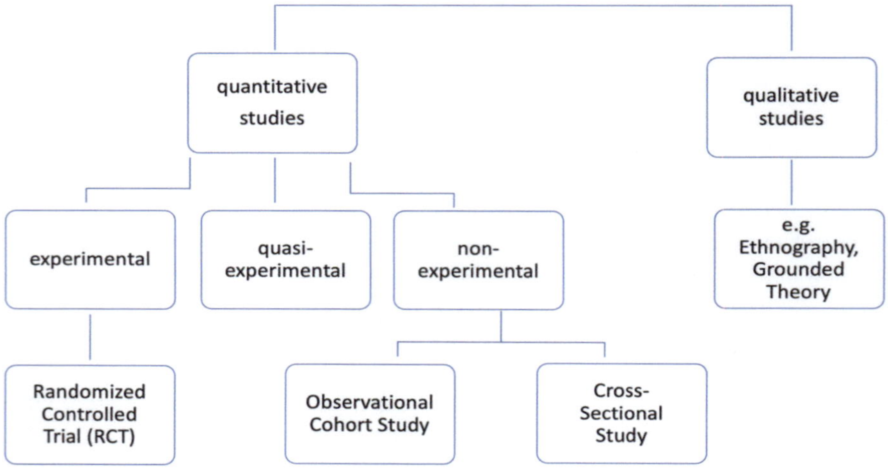

Fig. 23.4 Study designs to consider when studying FICUS

Qualitative Studies

Qualitative research is rooted within the interpretative paradigm (i.e., hermeneutics, phenomenology, and symbolic interactionism). Qualitative research aims to reconstruct and understand meaning in the social world [21]. Therefore, it focuses on individuals' beliefs, experiences, and motivations. Consequently, the methods of data collection are, for example different forms of field observation, interviews, or video analysis. Accordingly, the types of data collected are narrative, comprising "thick descriptions" in observation protocols and interview transcripts. Statistical representativeness is not the primary objective of qualitative research; however, achieving data "saturation" [22] is a common goal and generalizability is reached using other procedures such as typification or theory building (e.g., Grounded Theory Methodology). The quality criteria for conducting and reporting qualitative research differ substantially from those of quantitative research [23].

Qualitative and quantitative designs are not only mutually exclusive but can complement each other meaningfully. Qualitative research often does the groundwork without which it would not be possible to examine the phenomena and concepts quantitatively. It unfolds its great value especially in areas where little is known about the subject, the phenomenon to be studied, and the specific problem. The openness that comes with qualitative research allows for the discovery of new aspects or previously unknown phenomena. It enables us to learn more about the experiences of the individuals concerned from their own perspective (from the inside) and to give them a voice.

Quantitative Studies

1. Cross-sectional studies

   This type of study measures the prevalence of certain outcomes, perceptions, or states of being at a given time point or short period of time. It takes a "snapshot" in a general sample. In contrast to cohort studies, the sample consists of unselected participants who are not followed up over several time points. Population-based cross-sectional studies are valuable to assess the prevalence of a condition or disease. They allow the development of hypotheses about risk factors and causal relationships. Limitations include lack of knowledge about preexisting risk factors, length of exposure, and antecedent-consequent bias, i.e., it is unknown whether the outcome is a result or a preexisting condition.
2. Observational cohort study

   An observational study examines a cohort, which is defined as a group of people who share a common characteristic. Researchers often define inclusion and exclusion criteria to select participants. Cohorts can be studied retrospectively by looking back in time after the outcome has occurred or prospectively by following a cohort into the future. Observational cohort studies are useful to study risk and outcome rates and temporal relationships between outcome and exposure. Their quality is determined by how well participants represent the condition to be studied (generalisability), how complete the cohort is at baseline (participation rate) as well as by the attrition rate during follow-up (loss-to-follow-up). Limitations include expense and time, given that individuals must be followed up for longer periods of time.

3. Quasi-experimental design for improvement initiatives

   These research designs test causal hypotheses but lack the random allocation of participants to intervention and control groups. Usually, the intervention is tested against no intervention or standard of care. Participants either choose the treatment or control intervention or are assigned by administrators, or the intervention is implemented as the new standard of care. This design can be used retrospectively, i.e., after the intervention was put in place or prospectively, i.e., before an intervention is instituted. These studies are often used in quality improvement initiatives. To account for the limitation—lack of randomization—additional statistical methods are sometimes used to create comparison groups that are as similar as possible at baseline, i.e., before the intervention, for instance, propensity score matching. While the quasi-experimental design is often used in quality improvement projects, observed differences between groups can be due to an imperfect match or environmental changes over time rather than the intervention.

4. Randomized controlled trial

   The RCT directly compares different treatment groups. Participants are randomly assigned to either group. In addition, validity can be increased by double- or triple-blinding (participants, statisticians, and investigators). Treatment crossovers can also add to the validity but also infer the problem of carry-over effects. The stepped wedge cluster design ensures that all included trial sites will eventually benefit from the intervention [24]. The RCT is considered to provide the most direct evidence for the causal effect of an intervention and provides evidence of the highest level. However, some drawbacks exist as well. Because of stringent in- and exclusion criteria, the study population may not be generalizable to the "normal" patients in the unit. Selective analysis (including analysis of intent-to-treat rather than per-protocol) or loss-to-follow-up can diminish the validity. Subgroup analysis is often performed, but even when preplanned, results are merely hypothesis-generating. Lastly, RCTs are costly and time-consuming. As Niven and colleagues point out "RCTs and quality improvement efforts are not mutually exclusive. In an ideal world, they should be complementary" [25]—especially for FICUS, the two must be considered together because the goal is always to improve the situation of the patients' relatives from their point of view.

Complex Interventions

The ultimate aim of studying FICUS is to develop, implement, and evaluate interventions that will mitigate or prevent it. Such interventions will typically be complex interventions. For instance, one intervention that alleviated relatives' psychological stress after 90 days consisted of a brochure and a communication strategy, which was taught to clinicians and practiced in family conferences; the control group received usual care [26]. Another intervention employed communication facilitators who supported communication between clinicians and families adapted communication to family needs, and mediated conflicts versus usual care versus usual care; this intervention was delivered in the context of a multicentre RCT [18].

Complex interventions are complex because they contain a number of interactive components both in the experimental as well as in the control group, a number of difficult behaviors required by those delivering or receiving the intervention, a number of groups or organizational levels targeted by the intervention, a number and variability of outcomes and they allow for a degree of flexibility or tailoring the intervention during the implementation [27]. It is therefore recommended to develop interventions systematically, using the best available evidence and appropriate theory, a step-wise approach which tests each component and target to understand and control uncertainties, and develop it along a line from exploratory on to pilot and then more definitive studies.

Skivington et al. [27] divide complex interventions into four phases: (1) development or identification of the intervention; (2) feasibility; (3) evaluation; and (4) implementation. Each phase comprises the same set of six common core elements, which are "considering context," "developing and refining programme theory," "engaging stakeholders," "identifying key uncertainties," "refining the intervention," and "economic considerations." In addition, you might perform a gap analysis in your unit or in several units. For instance, the Gap Analysis Tool for Family-Centered Care measures areas with need for improvement [28, 29]. Moreover, patients and family members are increasingly being engaged during the planning and conduct of clinical research. This is especially fruitful when addressing healthcare delivery where patients and family-led research has been shown to be feasible and can identify opportunities for improving care [19].

Lastly, evaluating the results of complex interventions may be difficult. As described above, the difficulties include choosing relevant endpoints and times when to measure them. To quote: "If the result is negative, we are left wondering whether the intervention is inherently ineffective (either because the intervention was inadequately developed or because all similar interventions are ineffective), whether it was inadequately applied or applied in an inappropriate context, or whether the trial used an inappropriate design, comparison groups or outcomes. If there is a positive effect, it can be hard to judge how the results of the trial might be applied to a different context" [30].

Concluding Remarks

FICUS is an umbrella concept that helps to consider a variety of relevant symptoms and outcomes perceived by those affected. This allows us to take a much-needed holistic view but at the same time results in particular challenges in terms of research methodology. Furthermore, the theoretical framework and conceptualization of FICUS is still in a state of "work in progress"—this dynamic must be adequately taken into account when conceptualizing research projects. Particular elements of the FICUS symptom complex, but also the overall concept in the interplay of the different elements, still need to be investigated further, but face various challenges not only in terms of research design but also research ethics [31]. Future research will also increasingly face the challenge of considering the transitions between FICUS (as a phenomenon during the stay at the ICU) and PICS-F (as a post-ICU syndrome), which again raises considerable research methodological difficulties. To understand and critically appraise published study results (on FICUS), one must have a basic understanding of research methodology. However, developing and conducting empirical studies oneself requires a very robust knowledge of at least epistemology, methodologies, methods, and research ethics. In a nutshell, It requires an interprofessional and interdisciplinary team with different knowledge, skills, and expertise.

References

1. Polit DF, Beck CT. Nursing research. Generating and assessing evidence for nursing practice. 11th ed. Wolters Kluwer; 2020.
2. Saeid Y, et al. Family intensive care unit syndrome: an integrative review. Iran J Nurs Midwifery Res. 2020;25(5):361–8.
3. Saeid Y, et al. The family intensive care unit syndrome: a qualitative content analysis. Nurs Crit Care. 2022;27(3):401–9.
4. Aghaie B, et al. A Whirlpool of stress in families of intensive care unit patients: a qualitative multicenter study. Crit Care Nurse. 2021;41(3):55–64.
5. Bartoli D, et al. The lived experiences of family members of Covid-19 patients admitted to intensive care unit: a phenomenological study. Heart Lung. 2021;50(6):926–32.
6. Netzer G, Sullivan DR. Recognizing, naming, and measuring a family intensive care unit syndrome. Ann Am Thorac Soc. 2014;11(3):435–41.
7. Olding M, et al. Patient and family involvement in adult critical and intensive care settings: a scoping review. Health Expect. 2016;19(6):1183–202.
8. McAdam JL, Arai S, Puntillo KA. Unrecognized contributions of families in the intensive care unit. Intensive Care Med. 2008;34(6):1097–101.
9. Curtis JR, et al. Intensive care unit quality improvement: a "how-to" guide for the interdisciplinary team. Crit Care Med. 2006;34(1):211–8.
10. Lim WC, et al. Conceptualizing and measuring health-related quality of life in critical care. J Crit Care. 2016;31(1):183–93.
11. Detering KM, et al. The impact of advance care planning on end of life care in elderly patients: randomised controlled trial. Br Med J. 2010;340:c1345.

12. Rutz Voumard R, et al. Goal-concordant care after severe acute brain injury. Front Neurol. 2021;12:710783.
13. Turnbull A, Hartog C. Goal-concordant care in the ICU: a conceptual framework for future research. Intensive Care Med. 2017;
14. Turnbull A, Sahetya S, Needham D. Aligning critical care interventions with patient goals: a modified Delphi study. Hear Lung. 2016;45:517–24.
15. VanKerkhoff TD, et al. Time-limited trials in the intensive care unit to promote goal-concordant patient care. Clin Pulm Med. 2019;26(5):141–5.
16. Dinglas VD, et al. Perspectives of survivors, families and researchers on key outcomes for research in acute respiratory failure. Thorax. 2018;73(1):7–12.
17. Oczkowski SJW, et al. A modified Delphi process to identify clinical and research priorities in patient and family centred critical care. J Crit Care. 2017;42:243–7.
18. Curtis JR, et al. Randomized trial of communication facilitators to reduce family distress and intensity of end-of-life care. Am J Respir Crit Care Med. 2016;193(2):154–62.
19. Curtis JR, et al. Effect of a quality-improvement intervention on end-of-life care in the intensive care unit: a randomized trial. Am J Respir Crit Care Med. 2011;183(3):348–55.
20. Matt B, et al. Relatives' perception of stressors and psychological outcomes—results from a survey study. J Crit Care. 2017;39:172–7.
21. Thompson S, Schick-Makaroff K. Qualitative research in clinical epidemiology. In: Parfrey PS, Barrett BJ, editors. Clinical epidemiology: practice and methods. New York, NY: Springer US; 2021. p. 369–88.
22. Hennink M, Kaiser BN. Sample sizes for saturation in qualitative research: a systematic review of empirical tests. Soc Sci Med. 2022;292:114523.
23. Carter SM, Little M. Justifying knowledge, justifying method, taking action: epistemologies, methodologies, and methods in qualitative research. Qual Health Res. 2007;17(10):1316–28.
24. Hemming K, et al. The stepped wedge cluster randomised trial: rationale, design, analysis, and reporting. Br Med J. 2015;350:h391.
25. Niven AS, et al. The future of critical care lies in quality improvement and education. Ann Am Thorac Soc. 2019;16(6):649–56.
26. Lautrette A, et al. Respective impact of no escalation of treatment, withholding and withdrawal of life-sustaining treatment on ICU patients' prognosis: a multicenter study of the Outcomerea Research Group. Intensive Care Med. 2015;41(10):1763–72.
27. Skivington K, et al. A new framework for developing and evaluating complex interventions: update of Medical Research Council guidance. Br Med J. 2021;374:n2061.
28. Davidson JE, et al. Guidelines for family-centered care in the neonatal, pediatric, and adult ICU. Crit Care Med. 2017;45(1):103–28.
29. Hwang DY, El-Kareh R, Davidson JE. Implementing intensive care unit family-centered care: resources to identify and address gaps. AACN Adv Crit Care. 2017;28(2):148–54.
30. Campbell NC, et al. Designing and evaluating complex interventions to improve health care. Br Med J. 2007;334(7591):455–9.
31. Silverman HJ, Lemaire F. Ethics and research in critical care. Intensive Care Med. 2006;32(11):1697–705.

Index

© The Editor(s) (if applicable) and The Author(s), under exclusive license to Springer Nature Switzerland AG 2025
A. J. Vance et al. (eds.), *Families in the Intensive Care Unit*,
https://doi.org/10.1007/978-3-031-83786-9

MIX
Papier aus verantwortungsvollen Quellen
Paper from responsible sources
FSC® C105338

If you have any concerns about our products,
you can contact us on
ProductSafety@springernature.com

In case Publisher is established outside the EU,
the EU authorized representative is:
Springer Nature Customer Service Center GmbH
Europaplatz 3, 69115 Heidelberg, Germany

Printed by Libri Plureos GmbH
in Hamburg, Germany